Urban Mortality Change
in England and Germany, 1870–1913

Liverpool Studies in European Population
General Editor DAVID SIDDLE

Urban Mortality Change
in England and Germany, 1870–1913

JÖRG VÖGELE

LIVERPOOL UNIVERSITY PRESS

First published 1998 by
LIVERPOOL UNIVERSITY PRESS
Senate House, Abercromby Square
Liverpool, L69 3BX

British Library Cataloguing-in-Publication Data
A British Library CIP record is available

ISBN 0–85323–842–1 *cased*
0–85323–852–9 *paper*

Set in Times New Roman by
Northern Phototypesetting Co. Ltd, Bolton
Printed and bound in the European Union by
Bell and Bain Ltd, Glasgow

To all my friends in Liverpool

DIVINA NATURA DEDIT AGROS,
ARS HUMANA AEDIFICAVIT URBES

M. T. Varro, *De re rustica*

CONTENTS

PLATES

FIGURES

TABLES

ACKNOWLEDGEMENTS

The following analysis represents the results of the research project 'Urban Mortality Change in Britain and Germany, 1870–1910', funded by The Wellcome Trust, London and by the Alexander von Humboldt-Stiftung, Bonn-Bad Godesberg. The project was carried out at the Department of Economic and Social History, University of Liverpool, at the Department of History, University of Konstanz, and at the Institute for the History of Medicine, University of Düsseldorf.

My special thanks go to Robert Lee, University of Liverpool, who accompanied the project from its initial phases to its present conclusion. I would also like to thank Reinhard Spree, formerly University of Konstanz and now at the University of Munich. Our cooperation in Konstanz formed the original basis of my current research. Alfons Labisch, University of Düsseldorf, supported the project in its later stages. His suggestions and ideas were nevertheless substantial for the present work. Crucial support came from Gerry Kearns, University of Cambridge, Naomi Williams and especially from Fiona Lewis, University of Liverpool. Many thanks go to the members of the Institute for European Population Studies, University of Liverpool, and to contributors at the Annual Conference of the Society for the Social History of Medicine, Liverpool, July 1990; 10th International Economic History Conference, Leuven, August 1990; and the History of Public Health and Prevention, Conference at Lovik, Lidingö, Stockholm, 6–8 September 1991. Parts of the analysis were presented at the Wellcome Unit for the History of Medicine, University of Oxford, within the seminar series 'Aspects of North-West European Demographic Regimes', Hilary Term 1993; in the 'Kolloquium zur Landesgeschichte', Historisches Seminar of the Heinrich-Heine-Universität Düsseldorf, 2 June 1993; and at the third meeting of the 'Arbeitskreis für Sozialgeschichte der Medizin der Robert-Bosch-Stiftung', Stuttgart, September 1994.

Further thanks go to Julie Holbrooke, Liverpool; Ulrich Kohler, Mannheim; Ingrid Kreitmeier, Konstanz; Evelyne Schulz, Konstanz; and to Janine Illian, Düsseldorf; Sabine Nimtz, Düsseldorf; Achim Raiser, Düsseldorf.

ABBREVIATIONS

CDR	Crude death rate
IMR	Infant mortality rate
M	Marks
RD	Registration district
SMR	Standardized mortality rate
TB	Tuberculosis
Typhoid	Typhoid fever
Varco	Coefficient of variation

I INTRODUCTION

Chapter 1

INTRODUCTORY REMARKS

In his famous report on the English working class Frederick Engels provides a detailed description of the atrocious living conditions in large English cities and towns in the 1840s (Engels, 1892). This image serves as an archetype for the inhumane characteristics of the early phase of industrialization, under which Britain as the frontrunner in this development suffered the most. Yet, if we take health as an indicator of living conditions, quite a different picture emerges. Manchester, with a mortality rate of 32 (per 1,000 inhabitants) in the 1840s, together with Liverpool, one of the unhealthiest English cities, does not show an exorbitantly high crude mortality rate when compared with German towns and cities in that period. Indeed, Munich registered similar mortality rates to these English cities, and Engels could have found even more unhealthy towns in less industrialized Germany—Breslau,[1] for example, experienced a mortality rate of 33. In fact, German towns and cities had to suffer greater deprivation in the 1860s and 1870s, when a far higher mortality rate was recorded than in the English towns. In both countries, however, urban death rates significantly exceeded those of rural areas and national aggregate figures. In 1861, for example, the life expectancy of a male baby in Liverpool was 26 years, while in Okehampton in Devon, a boy born in the same year could expect to live for about 57 years (Woods, 1984b, p. 40). Referring to these unhealthy conditions in nineteenth-century cities and towns one might speak of an 'urban graveyard effect' or an 'urban penalty' (Kearns, 1988a). Towards the end of the nineteenth century, however, urban mortality improved substantially in relative as well as in absolute terms, the gap between urban and rural mortality narrowed as a consequence, and the 'urban penalty', which had been generally evident throughout Europe in earlier decades, became attenuated or even disappeared entirely. The towns as the bearers of industrialization suffered most as a result of changing living conditions, but they obviously also had the innovative potential to overcome the threats of disease or death, and became the frontrunners in improved health conditions in modern industrialized societies.

The following analysis discusses the prevailing health conditions in the second half of the nineteenth and early part of the twentieth century in terms of changes in urban mortality and the disease panorama. This historical epidemiology serves as an essential prerequisite in evaluating urban advance, as well as scrutinizing the strategies and measures which were adopted as a response to specific health conditions in the major urban centres in order to combat disease. A comparative analysis of the largest towns and cities in England and Germany will provide the framework to delineate more general processes as well as ascertaining the truly distinctive features of each country within the context of the European mortality decline.

---

1 Today Wroclaw, in what is now Poland.

During the last 200 years life expectancy in Europe has risen from between 20 and 40 years to 70 to 80 or even higher. The reason for this decline in mortality remains, as the Nobel Prize winner Robert Fogel puts it, a big puzzle. Traditionally ascribed to advances in medical technology, in recent decades the decline has been attributed only in part to curative medicine. Instead, major determinants under discussion are improved quality and quantity in diet via a rise in standards of living, environmental improvements and preventive medical and hygienic measures. These determinants will be discussed and evaluated in the context of the following analysis of the largest towns both in England and Wales, and in Germany. The health conditions and the mechanisms of mortality change in an urban environment during industrialization in the late nineteenth and early twentieth centuries can be used as a paradigm for conditions in highly urbanized industrial societies. In this respect, the project will further contribute to an evaluation of current international public health strategies, encompassing such issues as the discussion of appropriate strategies in the fight against AIDS, the containment of cholera in South America, the resurgence of tuberculosis and plague, as well as reviewing the implications for the 'Healthy Cities Project' of the World Health Organization.

Chapter 2

APPROACH, METHODS AND AIMS

The nineteenth and early twentieth centuries formed the transition period between the traditional mortality pattern, characterized by high mortality rates, low life expectancy at birth, as well as great epidemics and hunger crises, and the modern mortality pattern, characterized by low mortality rates, high life expectancy, and the predominance of degenerative and man-made diseases.

These changes in mortality trends have been described with the help of the concept of the so-called 'epidemiologic transition' (Omran, 1971; 1977). Focusing on interrelations between patterns of health and socio-economic change, three major successive patterns of mortality have been distinguished:

> (1) *The Age of Pestilence and Famine* when mortality is high and fluctuating, thus impeding sustained population growth. The average life expectancy at birth is low, varying between 20 and 40 years.

> (2) *The Age of Receding Pandemics* when mortality declines progressively; the rate of decline accelerates as severe epidemics become less frequent and later on disappear completely. The average life expectancy at birth increases to about 50 years; population growth is sustained and begins to take off exponentially.

> (3) *The Age of Degenerative and Man-Made Diseases* when mortality continues to decline and eventually reaches stability at a relatively low level. The average life expectancy rises gradually until it exceeds 70 years.

The classic Western model of the 'epidemiologic transition' describes the transition from high (above 30 per 1,000 inhabitants) to low mortality (less than 10 per 1,000) that accompanied the process of modernization in most Western European societies. After a stage of pestilence and famine during the pre-modern and early modern periods, a slow and intermittent rate of declining mortality gradually gave way to a more precipitous decline around the turn of the twentieth century.

The reasons for this remarkable decline in the mortality rate in Western Europe during the 'epidemiologic transition' still remain a puzzle. Until the 1950s declining mortality was widely attributed to improvements in medical therapy and technology. More recently, however, the debate has been vigorously influenced by the work of T. McKeown. McKeown could show that numerous causes of death were in decline long before specific medical therapies were available (McKeown and Record, 1962; McKeown et al., 1972; McKeown, 1976). Using this as a starting point, McKeown discussed various factors and attributed most of the credit for the mortality decline to the improved quantity and quality of diet—to which he particularly attributed the retreat of tuberculosis, a disease which contributed one-half of the total fall in mortality in the second half of the nineteenth century. In second place, he emphasized the role of sanitary reforms, which, he claimed, accounted for the decline in mortality from fevers and diseases of the digestive system, so that McKeown believed it could be held responsible for one-quarter of the secular mortality decline as a whole. One-fifth of the decline he traced back to changes in the virulence of certain disease organisms, as in the case of scarlet fever. Finally, medical intervention is said to have been effective solely in the cases of smallpox and diphtheria serum-therapy and contributed only marginally to the total mortality decline. McKeown's approach to the analysis of the causes behind the mortality decline during this period is essentially reductionist. As the major contributions cannot be ascribed to medical intervention, sanitary reforms or changes in micro-organisms, it is an improvement in the standard of living accompanied by an enhanced nutritional status which remains the major force behind this development.

McKeown's approach to explaining the European mortality decline is a deductive one. As the bulk of the decline in the nineteenth century was registered in the infectious disease group he relates the mechanisms of the downward trend to two primary causes: changes in the exposure to disease and the ability to resist disease. As environmental reform most likely influenced mortality from water-borne and food-borne diseases (diarrhoeal diseases, typhoid fever), the reduction in this disease group provides a yardstick by which to evaluate the impact of sanitary reform on the overall decline. The main killer of that period, tuberculosis, is linked to the standard of living, and as a corollary, the decline in tuberculosis mortality is related directly to improved nutrition, implied by rising living standards.

The impact of McKeown's work cannot be overestimated. His conclusions still form the platform of present-day health campaigns launched by the World Health Organization (WHO).[1] With respect to historical research, there has been an intensive discussion, especially in Britain, of McKeown's methods and conclusions (e.g. Woods and Woodward, 1984; Kearns, 1988a; Szreter, 1988; 1994; Mercer, 1990). Reservations are many.[2] Criticism focuses on the neglect of age-specific mortality rates—changes in the age-composition of the population at risk might have a substantial impact on mortality—and especially on his deductive approach. To what degree can tuberculosis be linked to diet? Or is it rather dependent on housing and working conditions? Furthermore, the effects of specific measures on the diseases might be complex and cumulative in their impact. This, however, cannot be controlled without information about morbidity conditions in a specific population.

---

1 See, for example, Ashton (1992).

2 For a recent survey of the discussion in a broader geographical context, see Schofield et al. (1991). Various contributions of varying quality consider the demographic change and potential variables involved for several Western European states. The state of research in Germany is reflected in the facts that no German author contributed to this volume and national demographic development is not explicitly dealt with. Essential reading for Germany is still Lee (1980). For England J. M. Winter (1982) gives a basic introduction.

Assuming that sanitary reforms had a crucial impact on the control of digestive diseases, predominant in the younger age-groups, this may well have had ramifications in terms of resistance against other diseases, which previously would not have been associated with sanitary reform. For example, Preston and van de Walle (1978) argue that reductions in childhood illness (in particular gastro-intestinal disorders) did not only reduce childhood mortality, but, via an improved physical growth, also increased lifelong resistance to many infectious and non-infectious diseases. Similarly, R. Fogel (1986) emphasizes that individuals at a given living standard will have less resistance to other diseases if they suffer from diarrhoeal disorders, as such illnesses reduce absorption from food intake.

Another major problem with McKeown's analysis is that he used cause-of-death data aggregated on a national level. It has been argued that this led him to ignore the immense differences between urban and rural mortality. However, a substantially higher urban mortality can be found in a number of countries in the nineteenth century.[3] In this context we may speak of an 'urban graveyard effect' or an 'urban penalty'—which affected even small towns, from 2,500 inhabitants upwards. Furthermore, national data obscure the fact that urban mortality began to decline drastically towards the end of the nineteenth century and the 'urban penalty', which had been generally evident throughout Europe in earlier decades, became attenuated or disappeared entirely—despite the increasing population in towns and cities during the urbanization period. Recent research has focused on urban mortality change, emphasizing in particular the interrelationship between urbanization and population development during the demographic and epidemiologic transitions (Woods, 1984a; Kearns, 1988a; 1989; Kearns et al., 1989; Kearns, 1991). It has been suggested that the effect of public health provision on the secular decline in urban mortality has been underestimated (Kearns, 1988a; 1989; Kearns et al., 1989),[4] with the general consensus that there exists a need to re-examine the overall contribution of various public health strategies when attempting to explain mortality changes during the 'epidemiologic transition' (Szreter, 1988). A number of valuable case studies do exist (e.g. Luckin [1984; 1986] and Hardy [1993], on London; Pooley and Pooley [1984] on Manchester; Woods [1984a] on Birmingham). They focus either, more traditionally, on the epidemiology of specific diseases in individual towns, or on the impact of sanitary measures on the health conditions in a specific town. In general they mainly support this view. The problem with the classic approach, however, is that specific contemporary public health strategies may have had an impact on various diseases which lie outside the scope of the specific analysis. Similarly, those studies are unable to evaluate the impact the eradication of a particular disease might have left on the complete disease panorama and on the level and trend of overall mortality.

3 In general see Weber (1899). For England, see Glass (1964); Kearns (1988a); Woods and Woodward (1984). For Germany, see Knodel (1977); Vögele (1991). For France, see Preston and van de Walle (1978). For the USA, see Condran and Crimmins (1980).
4 Similar conclusions were reached for France. See Preston and van de Walle (1978).

In the case of Germany a modern historical epidemiology of the major diseases in the late nineteenth and early twentieth centuries is still in its initial stages.[5] R. Spree (1981b; 1986; 1988) has provided the framework of a historical epidemiology for Imperial Germany. Little concrete research has been undertaken on German urban mortality in general (Vögele, 1991).[6] In those cases in which cities have been included in individual studies, the choice of city often appears haphazard, and there seem to be no coherent criteria for determining their selection (Gottstein, 1927; Bleker, 1983) or diachronic aspects were neglected (Geissler, 1883; Laux, 1985). Even fewer studies exist which concentrate at a micro-level on an individual city (Evans, 1987). Recent medical or social historical research concerning health and mortality issues during the 'epidemiologic transition' have only marginally dealt with urban mortality change (Lee, 1979; 1980; Imhof, 1981a; 1985; Spree, 1981a; 1986; Rothenbacher, 1982).

Rather more limited research has been undertaken on German urban mortality of that period using a coherent sample of towns (Spree, 1981a; Laux, 1985; Vögele, 1991). This has provided a preliminary description of the amount and course of urban mortality in large towns and cities during the nineteenth century in terms of overall mortality development and the changing disease panorama (Vögele, 1991), whereas H.-D. Laux (1985) deals primarily with regional variations in the urban mortality of Prussia in 1905. He stresses the fact that regional location and socio-cultural determinants had the strongest impact on variations in overall mortality, and, in particular, on the incidence of suicide and diseases of the digestive system; whereas the other causes of death were mainly determined by inter-urban variation in environmental conditions. Diseases of the respiratory system were strongly influenced by specific living and working conditions and the degenerative disease complex by the quality of the medical infrastructure. As he does not take into account diachronic aspects of urban mortality, this picture remains rudimentary. Reinhard Spree concentrates on social inequality with reference to the development of people's health during the late nineteenth and early twentieth centuries (Spree, 1981a; 1986). The evidence of increasing social differentials during the last decades of the nineteenth century in the case of infant mortality rates (IMR) which were not identical with class formation, indicates that economic growth was not the sole driving force behind the mortality decline. Although the focus of his work is not exclusively on urban mortality, on a more disaggregated level and referring to single case studies, Spree also stresses the relevance of infrastructural measures in influencing the mortality decline.

A reliable and methodologically robust epidemiological analysis of the important diseases in England and Germany is clearly an essential prerequisite in order to

---

5 For an overview see Otto et al. (1990).
6 For a short summary of the current state of research see Vögele (1991); Kearns et al. (1989).

evaluate the findings of different case studies.[7] However, such an analysis, using a sufficiently large data base to permit effective generalization, is still lacking, despite its paramount importance for examining both the context of changes in the mortality pattern and the various measures designed to control the major diseases.

Furthermore, still less research has been undertaken using a cross-national comparative approach, although such an approach might help to outline more general processes as well as the truly distinctive features of each country. In this context, the selection of England and Germany seems to be an ideal platform. On the one hand, a comparative analysis including England as the frontrunner where industrialization and urbanization were concerned is of special importance. As the first country to be exposed to the specific new health risks of industrialization and urbanization, England had to develop original stategies and measures to combat disease. The specific developments in England will be compared with those in Germany, which, as a central power in continental Europe, followed England with a delay of some decades in an accelerated process of industrialization and urbanization. On the other hand, from a European perspective, the developmental paths of both countries towards industrial society have sufficient features in common to make such a comparison feasible whilst, at the same time, having enough differences to justify such an approach.[8] A preliminary investigation in this direction focused on differences in the development of health services in both states, as well as in Sweden (Kearns et al., 1989). Using mortality change as a framework within which to analyse the interaction of political and economic factors in the management of urban public health, the three cases can be characterized as follows. Rich, liberal England applied environmentalist policies and left the medical profession much to itself. On the other hand, Sweden—the poor mercantilistic power—followed individual-coercion policies and incorporated the medical profession into the state. Germany is characterized as an intermediary in terms of wealth, state ideology and incorporation of the medical profession, and adopted the state insurance model.

A growing number of British-German comparative studies in the history of medicine, mainly PhD theses, are currently being prepared and focus on single diseases, for example on tuberculosis and sexually transmitted diseases, following Paul Weindling's pioneering work on the different strategies in the fight against diphtheria in England, France and Germany (Weindling, 1992a; 1992b). Historians have been particularly interested in comparing social policy and the emergence of the welfare state in Britain and Germany (Mommsen, 1981; Ritter, 1983; 1989; Hennock, 1987). In this context the classic work of Ludwig Teleky should also be mentioned. At the centre of his later work were administrative and public health

---

7 Inexhaustible sources are still the classic nineteenth and early twentieth century epidemiologies. See, for example, Oesterlen (1874); Hirsch (1886); Creighton (1894 and 1965); Grotjahn and Kaup (1912); Grotjahn (1915 and 1923); Gottstein et al. (1925, 1926 and 1927). For a modern attempt to follow this tradition, see Kiple (1993).
8 For an excellent sketch of the political and socio-economic developments see Mommsen (1986).

structures in Germany, England and the United States (Teleky, 1950). Another focus of comparative work, relevant in this context, is on housing policy and town planning (Sutcliffe, 1981; Daunton, 1990; Pooley, 1992).

Almost complementary to these studies, the current project focuses more on actual urban health conditions and their determinants in England and Germany. Despite rapid in-migration to towns during the phase of urbanization in both countries and insanitary conditions, urban mortality rates improved substantially during the period under investigation. This may have been the result of special urban efforts to fight disease. As the towns and cities were especially exposed to major epidemic diseases, they may have developed their own strategies and measures to control them. So, first, the focus of attention will be on mortality change in English and German cities during the late nineteenth and early twentieth centuries, when urban mortality substantially improved and the gap between urban and rural mortality began to close. This will involve an analysis of changes in age-, sex- and cause-specific mortality, as well as the nature, importance, and the geographical and social distribution of the major diseases within an urban context. Different conditions may, on the one hand, have led to the development of different public health strategies, or, on the other hand, have been a consequence of these various policies. In addition, similar strategies to fight disease might even have had different results if they had been applied in the context of different disease panoramas. If increasing urban size was associated with a more rapid transmission of disease, public health and medical strategies in the period under consideration may also have been determined selectively by the differing constitutional power of urban authorities in England and Germany, and by broader geographical and economic factors. Therefore, the role of different public health strategies and types of medical intervention which were introduced during this time in individual cities in both European countries will be analysed—with special emphasis on water supply and sanitation, housing conditions, and overall medical provision. With industrialization and urbanization, living conditions changed significantly. How did this affect the health conditions of urban populations, and what kind of health-related infrastructural measures were planned and undertaken in order to control disease within the framework of contemporary epidemiological, medical, socio-economic and political conditions? In the context of McKeown's debate, the role of developments in the standard of living in both countries will also be discussed. In short, the aims of this investigation are to describe the extent, character and development of the 'urban penalty' as well as to contribute to the debate on the reasons for its diminution or disappearance. Within this context special emphasis is put on an analysis of the role of towns and cities as social agents. In view of the restricted amount of preliminary work and the chosen macro-level approach, this analysis can only outline some basic aspects of the urban mortality decline in Germany and in England and Wales, and provide the groundwork for further research.

To this end, the ten largest cities and towns in England and Wales (encompassing the population in the registration districts during the period 1901 to 1910) as well as in Germany (in the year 1910) are the object of investigation,[9] since on the one hand increasing urban size is often associated with a more rapid transmission of disease, and on the other hand only the larger towns had the political and financial potential and innovative power to apply often expensive public health measures on a large scale. In this sense, developments in the largest towns can be used as a paradigm for the situation in highly urbanized industrial societies. As population size is the crucial criterion for selection, and not administrative or political issues, the term 'town' instead of 'city' will be used in the following analysis; this also takes into account the fact that the German language does not differentiate between town and city in this sense. As the analysis focuses on the largest towns, the German term '*Großstädte*' (large towns) would be quite appropriate. The selected towns (in alphabetical order) in England and Wales were as follows: Birmingham, Bolton, Bradford, Bristol, Leeds, Liverpool, London, Manchester, Newcastle upon Tyne and Sheffield; in Germany: Berlin, Breslau, Cologne, Dresden, Düsseldorf, Frankfurt am Main, Hamburg, Leipzig, Munich and Nuremberg. With slightly more than nine million inhabitants, the English towns represented 26.5 per cent of the country's total population, and the German towns, with over seven million, 11.1 per cent of the total population. The potential influence of town size and regional location will be discussed later in the analysis. Their geographical distribution is shown in Figures 1 and 2. Due to different registration patterns in Scotland and Ireland, which require a different approach, the analysis focuses on England and Wales as most modern historical studies do, thus permitting the opportunity of drawing systematic comparisons. This criterion for selection is furthermore supported by the fact that England and Wales' share in the total population of the British Isles amounted to 72 per cent (in 1871), and even increased to 80 per cent (in 1911) (Mitchell, 1988). The selection of the German sample is based on the geographical area of the German Reich, founded in 1871. Unlike many other studies, it is not restricted to Prussia as the largest German state. A concentration on Prussia might have been acceptable as representative, if the focus of the investigation had been social or regional differences within Germany, but in the context of the present analysis this would have excluded five of the ten largest towns (Dresden, Hamburg, Leipzig, Munich and Nuremberg). At the same time, however, the specific developments in Prussia as a whole will serve as a platform for comparison (see Chapter 3).

Special emphasis is placed on the transition period leading to modern health conditions. Therefore the focus will be on the late nineteenth and early twentieth centuries (from 1870 to 1910), when the 'urban penalty' decreased substantially or

---

9 The relative ranking of the towns within the urban hierarchy, especially at the lower end of the scale, changed slightly during the period under investigation. Population size taken at the end of the timespan as a criterion for selection, includes those towns with a substantial rise during the previous decades. This fact would further facilitate the purpose of the study, as it hypothesizes an interrelationship between urbanization and mortality change. Compare Reulecke (1985), pp. 203–04 and the *Decennial Supplements to the Annual Reports of the Registrar-General of Births, Deaths, and Marriages in England and Wales*. See also Appendix 5.

disappeared entirely—accompanied by the rapid growth of the largest towns and cities during this period of urbanization.

England and Germany had a different timing, pace and level of urbanization. The population of England increased four-fold from about nine million in 1801 to 36.1 million in 1911 (Lawton, 1983, p. 181). Taking community size as a measure of urbanization, with 2,000 inhabitants as the cut-off point, England was one-third urbanized in 1800, one-half at mid-century and three-quarters by the end of the century (Law, 1967). By contrast, Prussia was not one-third urbanized until the second half of the century (Reulecke, 1985, p. 202). In Germany a significant relative increase in urban population was not achieved before 1871 (Laux, 1989, pp. 122–23), and overlapped with the period of high industrialization (Köllmann, 1974, p. 126; Matzerath, 1984, p. 85; 1985, pp. 241–83). Despite significantly higher

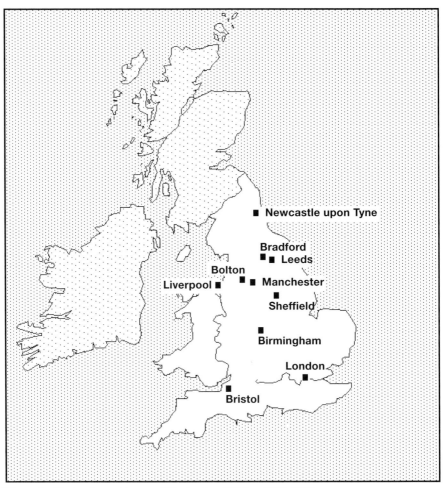

Figure 1: The ten largest towns of England and Wales, 1901–1910

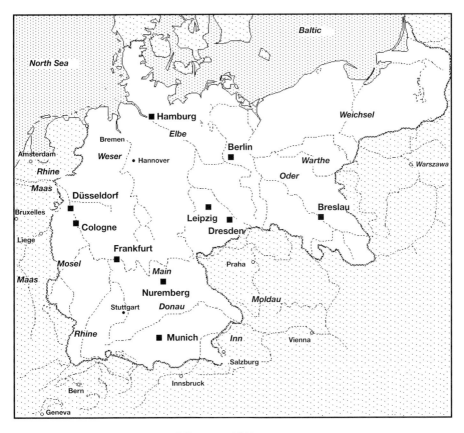

Figure 2: The ten largest towns of Germany, 1910

growth rates, Germany remained less densely urbanized than England (Weber, 1899, pp. 40–57 and 80–94). By 1910 three-fifths of the German population lived in communities of 2,000 or more, while in England the proportion was four-fifths (Kearns et al., 1989, p. 10). Urbanization spread regionally from Saxony and Berlin at the beginning of the nineteenth century to the industrial areas of the Rhineland and Westphalia. There was a clear east–west gradient in levels of urbanization. Urban growth was twice as high in the west as in the east, with the result that by 1910 population density was four times as high in the west (Matzerath, 1984, p. 90). Despite these differences, the largest cities in both countries registered their most rapid growth in the last decades of the nineteenth century (Law, 1967, p. 142; Matzerath, 1984, p. 90; Reulecke, 1985, p. 202).

In order to examine the two major issues of the project—the changing urban disease panorama and the measures undertaken to control major epidemics—it is important to establish a series of relevant indicators, including age-, sex- and cause-specific mortality, water supply, comparative sanitary conditions, housing density, number of hospitals and the overall extent of medical provision. In the first instance, statistical material for a broad sample of English and German cities has been collated and analysed. The methodological framework will involve a comparative temporal and spatial analysis. A comparison between the selected cities, as well as with the developments at the national level, will permit not only a reconstruction of urban mortality change, but also a comparative evaluation of various public health strategies. A direct comparison with rural areas, however, will have to be provided by other studies. Kearns' attempt to construct a rural sample which can be contrasted with the urban demographic development in nineteenth-century England may have shifted the focus too much towards population density as the sole crucial feature of urban–rural differences, implying that both towns and countryside were, in themselves, homogeneous units (Kearns, 1993). For Germany, age-specific cause-of-death data are available on the basis of Prussian *Stadt-* and *Landkreise* (politically defined urban and rural administrative units). Apart from the fact that Prussia is not conterminous with Germany, a source-specific problem in this context is that rural units also included rural communities of more than 20,000 inhabitants which often possessed an urban character.[10] This differentiation is similarly problematic as mortality rates, especially in Germany, followed a strong regional pattern with substantial variations over short distances, indicating a much more complex situation as a result of the immense diversity of occupational distribution, inheritance systems and land-holding patterns.[11] Certainly the impact of rural industry requires further exploration. Therefore a reasonable urban–rural comparison could only be obtained by investigating a specific town and its surrounding rural areas, using data on the level of larger registration areas. For the largest towns, however, this is not an adequate procedure as the areas directly surrounding the cities often had an urban character as well or were substantially influenced by central place functions of the neighbouring city. Furthermore, as the conditions in the largest towns acted as a role-model, the traditionally applied urban–rural dichotomy would underestimate their primary role within the context of the secular mortality decline. In Prussia, it was especially the large towns which benefited from this development, whereas the medium-sized towns lagged behind and registered higher death rates than rural areas or the big cities around the turn of the century (Ballod, 1899; Kruse, 1897; Spree, 1981a). This primary role of the large towns can be taken into account in the analysis as German urban mortality data allow a comparison of total death rates and mortality from selected diseases in the selected ten largest towns with the average for all towns with a population exceeding 15,000, whereas the age- and sex-specific disease panorama of the largest towns can be compared with Prussian aggregate rates as a substitute for non-compatible national aggregate figures referring to Germany as a whole (see Chapter 3). The English urban mortality data will be compared with aggregated rates for England and Wales.

10 See, for example, Vonde (1989), pp. 127–41.
11 See Evans and Lee (1986).

It has to be kept in mind, however, that a comparison of national figures essentially provides information on trends and levels rather than exact estimations as both countries became increasingly urbanized during the period under investigation, i.e. the urban component of the national sample changes over time. Furthermore, it has to be emphasized in this context that the analysis does not intend to provide a comprehensive direct comparison of the different overall health risks to which the populations in both countries were exposed. Their mortality profile was determined by a much broader range of factors than discussed here, including, for instance, the geographical contrast between England's island situation and Germany's continental location in Europe, which affected the transmission potential of disease. Differences in climate, in cultural behaviour and traditions may all have had their impact on health conditions and the way disease was handled. Therefore the analysis is restricted to a structural comparison of how the actual health conditions in the large towns of both countries manifested themselves and of how they developed within the framework of the specified socio-economic determinants. That implies that in many areas, where the cross-national comparison of urban mortality change is pursued, this investigation will concentrate on mortality trends rather than actual mortality levels. In order to avoid, to some extent, the risks of a deductive procedure, criticized in McKeown's work, the starting point for the second main theme, dealing with the determinants of mortality change, will not be the different diseases, but the prevalent living conditions, the various measures to fight disease and their potential impact on health. The viability of such a cross-national approach is, of course, very much dependent on the availability and comparability of the source material, which will be discussed in the following section.

Chapter 3

SOURCES

ENGLAND AND WALES

The Civil Registration Act of 1836 and the establishment of the General Register Office (GRO) in the following year provide the first comprehensive basis for a direct analysis of vital trends and causes of death in England and Wales.[1] Statistical material for registration districts and sub-districts is available from the *Annual Reports of the Registrar-General of Births, Deaths, and Marriages in England and Wales* since 1851, as well as from the *Decennial Supplements to the Annual Reports of the Registrar-General of Births, Deaths, and Marriages in England and Wales*. For the analysis of English urban mortality change, mortality data for the ten largest English cities, and for England and Wales as a whole, have been processed, taking annual mortality data for selected diseases from 1856 to 1910 from the Annual Reports, and age- and cause-specific mortality data for the two decades 1871–1880 and 1901–1910 from the *Decennial Supplements*. Unfortunately only material from the second period refers to age-specific mortality rates differentiated according to sex, whereas all registered causes of death broken down by age-group and the mean population are available for the two specified periods on a decennial average. In this classification 93 per cent of all deaths in the period 1871–1880 are specified, with the remainder grouped in the category 'other causes'. In the second period from 1901 to 1910 the explicitly specified causes are unfortunately reduced to 54 per cent of all deaths, with those remaining relegated to the category 'other causes'.

This central registration of the vital statistical material has the advantage of presenting a uniform disease nomenclature as well as a standard classification of the different age-groups, of the number of deaths and of the population at risk for the various towns and the national aggregate for any given time period (year or decade). Over time, disease classification underwent change. In the period 1871–1880 and 1901–1910 the diseases registered were as shown in Table 1, in the order listed.

In both periods registration focused on acute and chronic infectious diseases. Special emphasis was put on childhood infectious diseases, such as smallpox, measles, scarlet fever, diphtheria and whooping cough. In 1901–1910 the number of registered causes of death had diminished from 26 to 24 and changed substantially. Lung diseases and other tuberculous diseases were listed in greater detail, whereas the digestive disease complex had been reduced, with cholera, simple continued fever and diseases of the digestive system being omitted. That the selection of the registered causes of death did not necessarily reflect the importance of specific diseases

---

1 See Cullen (1974); Glass (1973). For the activities of the various superindendents and the GRO see Eyler (1979); Szreter (1991); Higgs (1993).

Table 1: Causes of death registered in England and Wales, 1871–1880 and 1901–1910

1877–1880		1901–1910	
a	Smallpox	a	Smallpox
b	Measles	b	Measles
c	Scarlet fever	c	Scarlet fever
d	Diphtheria	d	Typhus
e	Whooping cough	e	Influenza
f	Typhus	f	Whooping cough
g	Enteric fever	g	Diphtheria
h	Simple continued fever	h	Pyrexia
i	Puerperal fever	i	Enteric fever
j	Diarrhoea and dysentery	j	Diarrhoea and dysentery
k	Cholera	k	Pulmonary tuberculosis
l	Cancer	l	Phthisis (not otherwise defined)
m	Scrofula	m	Tuberculous meningitis
n	Tabes mesenterica	n	Tuberculous peritonitis
o	Phthisis	o	Tabes mesenterica
p	Hydrocephalus	p	Other tuberculous diseases
q	Diseases of nervous system	q	Cancer
r	Diseases of circulatory system	r	Septic diseases
s	Diseases of respiratory system	s	Rheumatic fever and rheum. of heart
t	Diseases of digestive system	t	Pneumonia
u	Diseases of urinary system	u	Bronchitis
v	Diseases of generative system	v	Childbirth and puerperal fever
w	Childbirth	w	Violence
x	Suicide	x	Other causes
y	Other violence		
z	Other causes		

Sources: *Decennial Supplements to the Annual Reports of the Registrar-General of Births, Deaths, and Marriages in England and Wales* (1871–1880 and 1901–1910).

is indicated by the omission of the important diseases of the digestive system, as well as of circulatory diseases, which remain a main modern cause of death. The predominance of the infectious diseases together with the neglect of the more modern disease groups may account for the limited number of cause-of-death categories listed in the period 1901–1910.

In the annual series from the *Annual Reports of the Registrar-General of Births, Deaths, and Marriages in England and Wales*, only a selection of diseases is presented, which cannot be differentiated according to age and sex. Coverage extends to about 63 per cent of all deaths on average. A special problem of the annual series is that not only does disease notation change, but also only a selection of diseases is presented, which also changed over time (see Appendix 3). This selective registration of causes of death seems to have been determined by the continued focus of contemporary statisticians, doctors and physicians on certain acute and chronic infectious diseases, rather than by the relative importance of the disease. For example, in the digestive disease group, there is an increase in mortality at the beginning of the 1880s which is a consequence of a new classification system, including 'digestive diseases', which previously had been noted in the 'other causes' group. This example highlights to some degree the shortcomings of the annual series.

GERMANY

Despite increasing debate concerning the need to establish an international causes of death classification system, such a project was still far from realization in the period under investigation. In fact, there was not even a standardized system used within the national borders of Germany. Due to the country's federalistic structure, health statistics, including statistics of causes of death, were to a large extent decentralized and a matter for the different states.[2] Even within those states, the methods of recording causes of death differed between the various statistical offices (Würzburger, 1909–1914, p. 45; Kasten, 1928, p. 131). In order to analyse causes of death differentiated according to age and sex for the towns constituting the sample, the material had to be put together from the different yearbooks of each town or state. In addition, classification changed over time. In Prussia, for example, major revisions were made in 1904.[3] Therefore available data are very heterogeneous concerning the specification of the diseases as well as the age-groups.[4] In addition, not all the towns offer age-specific causes of death differentiated according to sex. For example, in Leipzig for the year 1877 ninety different causes of death were registered, in contrast to fifty in 1912. However, in Dresden, only eleven causes of death were registered in 1876. For Nuremberg an age-specific disease panorama based on the age distribution of the population at risk was not available from the city's official statistical publications for the selected periods. In order to reconstruct changes in the disease panorama over time and to compare different towns and the development in England and Wales and Germany, the age-groups and the diseases had to be grouped together and standardized (see Appendices 1 and 3). This revised unified classification scheme was modelled on the Prussian registration system, as half of the towns in the German sample registered their causes of death according to this scheme, and the development in Prussia serves as a basis for comparison.[5] In those cases where a specific disease

2 A brief survey of the development of vital statistics and of attempts to create an international causes-of-death registration is offered by Tutzke (1969). Compare also Kintner (1993); Kohler (1991).

3 'Preußen. Erlaß, betr. die Neubearbeitung des Verzeichnisses der Krankheiten und Todesursachen', *Veröffentlichungen des Kaiserlichen Gesundheitsamtes*, **28** (1904), pp. 645–51.

4 For a synopsis of the different schemes in various German states and towns, see Würzburger (1909–1914), pp. 45–55.

5 Using source material for the large towns offers the opportunity to use a more detailed classification system than the scheme provided by Kintner, who arranges broad categories for Germany on the national level, derived from the various registration schemes of Saxony, Baden, Hamburg, Bremen, Prussia and Germany for the period 1878–1932. See Kintner (1986).

could not be subsumed in the selected categories, and the deaths from the specific disease constitute less than one per cent of the disease panorama, the disease has been grouped into the category 'other causes'. On average 85 per cent of all deaths in the ten largest towns could be attributed to specific diseases. This procedure led to the classification and registration of the diseases shown in Table 2. (For differences in the registration of the individual towns of the sample and changes over time, see Appendix 1.)

Table 2: Causes of death classification of the German sample

A	Weakness of life (*Lebensschwäche, Abzehrung*)
B	Childbirth
C	Infirmity (*Altersschwäche, akuter Gelenkrheumatismus*)
D	Smallpox
E	Scarlet fever
F	Measles and rubella
G	Diphtheria and croup
H	Whooping cough
I	Typhoid fever
J	Typhus
K	Dysentery
L	Digestive system
M	Scrofula
N+O	Tuberculosis (in most towns Tuberculosis, not otherwise defined, in some cases differentiated: pulmonary [N] and other tuberculosis [O])
P	Cancer
Q	Heart
R	Brain and nerves
S	Lungs
T	Urinary system
U	Influenza
V	Other communicable diseases
W	Violence
X	Other causes

Sources: See Appendix 2.

As in the case of the English registration system, the focus in Germany rests on acute and chronic infectious diseases—with a special emphasis on the childhood infectious disease complex (smallpox, measles and rubella, scarlet fever, diphtheria and croup,[6] whooping cough)—and increasingly on the more modern degenerative causes of death (heart/brain diseases). The latter might account for the increased

---

6 According to Rosen, croup was a popular term used for respiratory tract infections in young children characterized by stridulous breathing, and was often applied to cases of diphtheria. See Rosen (1973), p. 666, n. 86.

number of deaths covered by the German registration system after the turn of the century when compared with the English system. Of special importance for contemporary statisticians were the gastro-intestinal diseases, namely typhoid fever, dysentery and other diseases of the digestive system. In the registration of some towns cholera nostras, diarrhoea and convulsions formed separate additional categories, which have been subsumed under diseases of the digestive system for the sake of comparison as other towns already included them within this complex.[7] Similarly, most towns did not differentiate between pulmonary and other types of tuberculosis. From those which did, it becomes obvious that the latter only had a small share within the disease panorama so that, again for the sake of comparison, these two categories were combined in the specific towns. There are, however, two major problem groups in the various German classification systems, relating to deaths associated with weakness. The first refers to the childhood disease *Lebensschwäche*, which simply means 'too weak to live', and is often linked with *Abzehrung* (emaciation, atrophy), the latter most likely resulting from illness of the digestive system.[8] The second, even more obscure cause of death is weakness cf old age (*Altersschwäche*), in some few cases combined with rheumatism of the joints, categorized in the following as infirmity. As old age mortality on the national level fell when mortality from heart disease and cancer rose, a trade-off in reporting between these causes of death has been suggested (Kintner, 1993). This could well have been the case. Infirmity, however, was such a major cause of death, especially in areas with insufficient medical provision, that it might have been a standard cause proffered by medical laymen, referring to and including a wide range of various diseases. The combination with diseases of the joints in some registration schemes could also hint that cases of a major killer, tuberculosis, were also included. Overall, death from infirmity remains an unsolved problem.

In order to investigate changes in the age-specific disease pattern, the analysis for Germany has to refer to periods for which the precise age-specific composition of the population at risk is available for the individual towns. Whereas in some cities the absolute number of deaths is available for a wider range of years, the population composition is only available for selected single years, mostly census years, which started in Prussia in 1816. Most of the other states followed, yet uniform accounts began only in 1867, continued in 1871, and were held from 1875 onwards every five

---

7 Although 'convulsion' might not in all registration systems cover exclusively deaths from gastro-intestinal infections, according to contemporary judgement the majority did. See note 4 and H. Neumann (1906). H. J. Kintner confirmed this view, applying regression analysis on cause-specific infant mortality rates for various German administrative areas. See Kintner (1986).

8 The similar German terms *Auszehrung* and *Abzehrung* refer to completely different diseases. *Auszehrung* is a disease during adulthood and refers to consumption, whereas *Abzehrung* is an infant or childhood disease. Contemporary experts considered convulsions, emaciation, atrophy, and 'teeth' as causes of infant death following and resulting from sickness of the gastro-intestinal tract, and consequently subsumed those diseases under the digestive disease group. See Maier (1871), p. 175; Flügge (1894), p. 275; Prinzing (1900), pp. 636–37; Würzburg (1887/88), pp. 48–52.

years (Statistisches Bundesamt, 1972, p. 89). Data for the large towns, however, are
available from the official statistics only for an even more limited number of years
which are not completely congruent. In such cases the year closest to the selected
periods has been recorded (see Appendix 1). In order to be able to include as many
of the ten largest towns as possible, demographic and census data for the years 1877,
1885, 1900 and 1907 have been selected, which overlap with the sub-periods
selected for the English sample (1871–1880 and 1901–1910), and allows the location and analysis of changes over time more precisely. As only single years can be
analysed, the selection of four periods, of which two are always relatively conterminous (1877 and 1885, 1900 and 1907), is intended to reduce fortuitousness of any
results gained from a specific year. The year 1877 is congruent with the beginning of
the annual series of selected causes of death, while the selection of 1907 implies that
major changes in urban mortality which occurred at the beginning of the twentieth
century can also be included in the analysis.

The fact that one data set is decennial (for England) and the other annual (for Germany) has some implications which have to be taken into account in the analysis.
This is of special importance in the first period, when the impact of the major smallpox epidemic in the early 1870s is clearly evident in the English data, but not in the
German data of 1877. In general, it has to be kept in mind that the decennial periods
for England might reflect outbreaks of epidemics in the specific decade which might
not have been of importance in the selected year for the German period. In contrast,
the decennial average might smooth the death rates from diseases which were particularly prevalent in the selected single German years. On the whole, English data
cover a broader timespan than their German counterparts, including also the early
1870s and the late 1900s. As mortality change was not equally distributed within
these selected decades, there is no way of controlling for this difference in the data
used in the analysis. Therefore, once again, more emphasis should be put on trends
and levels than on the actual raw figures.

Furthermore, the German material does not allow an appropriate comparison of
developments in towns with national trends. Statistical data for the German Empire
were based on material from the *Regierungsbezirke* (larger administrative units) and
refer to only 10 out of 26 German states, although representing 93.8 per cent of the
population. By 1906 this number had increased to 24, but only from 1924 was the
whole of Germany included (*Reichsgesundheitsamt*, 1926, pp. 150–51). In addition,
until 1904 there is only a selection of 18 diseases available at this level (Würzburger,
1909–1914, p. 45). This registration is not differentiated according to sex, and refers
only to four age-groups (0–1, 1–15, 15–60, over 60). It is for this reason that developments in the age- and sex-specific disease panorama for the sample of towns will
be compared with the aggregate figures for Prussia, where the registration system
allows the required differentiation. That is, in this part of the analysis the Prussian
aggregate will form a substitute for a national aggregate covering Germany as a
whole. This should be considered to be legitimate for various reasons. First of all,
Prussia was the largest German state, representing slightly more than 60 per cent of
Germany's population in the period under consideration. The urban–rural population

distribution of both Prussia and Germany was quite similar, at least on the basis of a political definition of urban and rural areas. In Prussia 39.47 per cent of the population was living in urban areas (*Stadtgemeinden*) in 1890, while in the German Reich the percentage was 39.20 in the same year.[9] The percentage of population living in communities with fewer than 2,000 inhabitants in Prussia was 62.8 in 1871, 51.6 in 1890, and 38.4 in 1910; in Germany the corresponding rates were 63.9, 53.0, and 40.0 respectively.[10] In this respect Prussian aggregate data can be legitimately used as a substitute for a national aggregate for Germany as a whole for the age- and sex-specific analysis of the disease panorama.

The most explicit annual series of disease-specific mortality in German towns is available from the *Veröffentlichungen des Kaiserlichen Gesundheitsamtes* (Publications of the Imperial Health Office)[11] for the period 1877 to the First World War, where deaths from a selection of diseases in towns with more than 15,000 inhabitants are registered. Again, a comparison with national figures, covering the whole area of the German Empire, is not available for the corresponding selection of diseases. Indeed, the annual series for the towns provides the only cause of death registration for this period, where the whole of Germany is represented. An informative comparison, however, is offered by a yearly compilation of the average rates in all towns with over 15,000 inhabitants. The number of causes of death registered in this series is even smaller than in the English series, covering on average around 50 per cent of the disease panorama. A differentiation according to age and sex is not possible. As in the English annual series, the disease notation and the selection of diseases covered change over time. The focus was on acute infectious childhood diseases (e.g. measles and rubella, scarlet fever, diphtheria and croup) and puerperal fever, on acute infectious diseases (cholera, typhoid, diseases of the digestive system, acute diseases of the respiratory system), tuberculosis and violent deaths. There is, however, no classification of those diseases later incorporated into the category 'respiratory', including pneumonia, pleurisy, inflammation of the trachea (Dreyfuss, 1899, p. 169), and, at times, whooping cough (see Appendix 1). A very important missing element in the disease panorama is 'non-acute diseases of the digestive system'. Relying only on the annual series, therefore, runs the risk that major components of the urban mortality change might remain unrevealed. Furthermore, the category 'other causes' does not refer to unknown or unidentified causes of death, but to causes of death not taken into account by the publishers (Dreyfuss, 1899, p. 170).

SOURCE CRITICISM

The selection of registered diseases was generally restricted to 'the epidemiologically most important diseases required to follow the course of epidemics'

---

9 Source: *Statistisches Jahrbuch für das Deutsche Reich* (1896), pp. 2–3.

10 Source: Hohorst et al. (1975), p. 43.

11 The Imperial Health Office was founded in 1876 as a supervisory and statistical agency designed to monitor rather than intervene in public health matters. See *Das Kaiserliche Gesundheitsamt* (1886).

(*Reichsgesundheitsamt*, 1926, p. 148). This focus on infectious diseases, however, implies that other, maybe more implicit motives for this specific selection were also involved, including medical, political and military considerations. The following example of typhoid fever might illustrate this more clearly. The recording of an individual disease was of course dependent on medical knowledge and the ability to diagnose correctly. For example, the distinction between typhoid fever and typhus, two pathologically completely different diseases, the former a water-borne disease and the latter transmitted by the louse, was made from the beginning of the nineteenth century onwards.[12] Post-mortem examinations provided increased knowledge of pathological changes and formed the basis for a systematic differentiation between two independent diseases. The clinical differentiation was accomplished around the mid-nineteenth century, although the pathogenic agent of typhoid fever was discovered only in 1880 by Carl Eberth and Robert Koch, and isolated as bacilli-culture in 1884 by Georg Gaffky (Prausnitz, 1923, p. 563). Before that period, typhoid fever had often been considered to be a variant of typhus and described as fever of the nerves, mucous fever, in England as enteric fever and simple continued fever, or in Germany as typhoid fever (*typhoides Fieber*—in contrast to the later term *Abdominaltyphus*) (Lindemann, 1986; Rosen, 1973, pp. 629–41).

Soon typhoid fever together with cholera became the core issue in the disputes between supporters of miasmatic-localistic and bacteriological theories.[13] Proponents of the miasmatic theory postulated that infectious diseases were caused by an atmospherical state, corrupted by subterrestrial vapours; as a consequence they stressed the need for adequate sewerage in towns. By contrast, advocates of bacteriology focused on specific contagia, thereby prioritizing the provision of a filtered water supply. The result was that typhoid fever became a disease of political interest. In one camp, hygienists and bacteriologists centred on the disease to prove their theory of disease causation. On the other hand, towns invested large amounts of capital in improving their sanitary infrastructure, and this led to a close examination of typhoid fever mortality trends, either to justify or to criticize local expenditure. Whereas the epidemic nature of cholera excluded any long-term observation, endemic typhoid fever became the ideal object for demonstrating the success or failure of sanitary reform. Furthermore, typhoid fever together with cholera, dysentery, smallpox and typhus were amongst the most feared epidemics connected with war (Koch, 1888; 1902; Niedner, 1903; Prinzing, 1916; see also Chapter 12). Niedner wrote in 1903 that the fight against epidemics had become one of the most important

12 In the early nineteenth century the distinction between the two diseases became increasingly widespread. The clearest evidence was given by W. W. Gerhard in the United States in 1837 and by J. Schoenlein in Germany two years later. Schoenlein referred to the two diseases as typhus abdominalis and typhus exanthematicus. In England W. Jenner gave an analysis of the continued fevers in 1849 to 1851. The classic epidemiology of typhoid fever in the pre-bacteriologic era was given by W. Budd (1811–1880). See Lancaster (1990), pp. 70–74. For the works of Budd see the collection of his early studies in his famous monograph (Budd, 1873), and Winslow (1943), pp. 279–90.

13 For further details see Vögele (forthcoming b).

military questions (Niedner, 1903, p. 215). Their potential as a decisive element in times of war became increasingly a matter for concern, with the annual registration of deaths from those diseases forming the basis of substantial statistical interest. Despite the subordinate role of typhoid fever within the disease panorama at the beginning of the twentieth century—only three out of 1,000 deaths could be attributed to the disease—it retained the attention of various interest groups far beyond the point of its epidemiological importance. This leads to the question of disease classification in general, with particular respect to (a) its reliability and (b) its validity in terms of modern diagnosis.

(a) *Reliability of classification.* Although in England and Wales the Birth and Death Registration Bill of 1836 originally did not include provision for the cause of death to be recorded at death registration, the Bill was amended when it passed the House of Lords after successful lobbying by Edwin Chadwick and other public health promoters. As a consequence the Registrar-General has been able to collect and publish mortality information by cause of death since the Act came into operation on 1 July 1837 (Ashley and Devis, 1992, p. 22). The subsequent Births and Deaths Registration Act of 1874 made cause of death registration compulsory. The cause of death had to be certified by the attending physician, or, if there was no medical treatment during sickness, by a non-medically trained coroner (Prinzing, 1903, p. 441; 1906, p. 328). In England and Wales 91.8 per cent of all deaths in 1900 were certified by a doctor and 6.3 by coroners. Only 1.3 were not certified at all (63. Annual Report, XL, after Prinzing, 1906, p. 328). If the certified cause was unclear or ambiguous, the Registrar-General could return the certificate and ask for further clarification. After the turn of the century, for example, this occurred in about 4–5,000 cases a year (Prinzing, 1906, p. 321).

In Germany legislation differed from state to state. Official medical death certification (*Leichenschau*) was obligatory in Hamburg from 1820, Wurtemberg from 1822, Hesse from 1829, Bavaria from 1839 and Saxony from 1850, whereas there was no obligatory expert certification in Prussia, where the cause of death was certified by a relative (Prinzing, 1906, pp. 323–25; Heimann, 1906, pp. 20–21). Despite various political efforts to introduce mandatory post-mortem examinations, Prussia generally remained resistant, and although some Prussian cities required an examination by 1871,[14] even as late as 1926, only 70 per cent of its population lived in areas with such a requirement (Kintner, 1993). Post-mortem certifications were executed by physicians (mandatory in Hamburg), but also by surgeons, barbers and so-called laying-out women (*Leichenfrauen*). In the southern states of Germany the attending physician had to register the cause of death officially if the person received medical treatment during sickness, with the result that the number of deaths where a doctor was consulted during the final disease provides useful information about the reliability of the registered causes of death. In Wurtemberg 62.8 per cent of all deaths

---

14 Berlin, Breslau, Elberfeld, Königsberg, Stettin, Frankfurt am Main. Compare Kintner (1993), pp. 18–19.

were registered by medical personnel in the period 1899–1900, in Bavaria 63.4 per cent, in Baden 71.2 per cent and in Saxony 53.9 per cent in 1894–1898. In Hesse, where post-mortem examinations were carried out by physicians, the cause of death was medically certified in 87 per cent of all cases in 1898 (Prinzing, 1903, pp. 441–42). A very problematic case in this respect is infant mortality,[15] where doctors were normally not consulted during sickness and, consequently, the cause of death was often officially certified according to the information proffered by parents or relatives (Prinzing, 1900, p. 634). In Lower Bavaria in 1866–1867 a doctor was only consulted in 3 per cent of all cases of infant sickness (Maier, 1871, p. 193). In Wurtemberg only 38 per cent of all infants dying in 1900 received medical treatment, in comparison with 70 to 90 per cent in the higher age-groups (Prinzing, 1906, p. 322). Similarly, the rural population received less medical treatment. In Bavaria in areas locally referred to as on the right hand side of the Rhine, 80 per cent of the town population were treated by a doctor during their final illness in the last three decades of the nineteenth century, but only 45–57 per cent of the rural population received similar attention (Prinzing, 1906, p. 323). Finally, in periods of severe epidemics the reliability of official death certification most likely deteriorated. For example, the increase in typhoid fever during cholera epidemics might at least to some extent be the result of inadequate diagnosis. In the period under investigation the number of medically certified causes of death, however, was constantly increasing. In Saxony, where specific statistical information was recorded from 1873, the percentage of medically certified causes of all deaths rose from 37.1 in 1873 to 70.7 in 1910, and those of infants from 15.8 in 1875 to 39.5 in 1910. It was only in the 1920s that the number of medically certified infant deaths surpassed 50 per cent (Würzburger, 1930, p. 190).

(b) *Validity of diagnosis.* The use of a completely different classification system, often describing final symptoms (convulsions) or the period in life when death set in ('teeth' simply indicating that death occurred while the infant was teething; childbirth; infirmity), rather than the actual cause of death in a modern sense, makes a translation into present-day terminology at times impossible. Yet, a careful analysis of historical cause of death data is both feasible and legitimate, and provides important information. In contrast to the 999 official causes of death in modern death registration, we have only to deal with a relatively small number of causes for the period under consideration. The most important of these diseases were the classic infections so that a diagnosis was definitely not so taxing as it might be today, with the predominance of diseases of the heart and circulatory system as well as cancer. It was also commonplace for contemporary doctors and physicians to discuss and consider systems of disease classification, providing useful information about their concepts of disease and the actual diseases themselves. Seasonal and age-specific analysis gives further insights. Summer peaks in mortality of infants and young children, for instance, hint at gastro-intestinal disorders, whereas an accumulation of deaths in the

---

15 Infant mortality, by convention, refers to the number of deaths of infants under one year of age registered in a given year per 100 or per 1,000 live births registered in the same period.

cold winter months rather suggests diseases of the respiratory system. And finally, as this study does not intend to be a medical history of certain diseases, but rather a social history of urban mortality change and its determinants, it is sufficient to recognize the main disease categories. For example, if the digestive disease complex is taken as an indicator of urban environmental conditions, the question of whether the diagnoses of diarrhoea, dysentery, cholera, cholera nostras, enteric fever, simple continued fever and diseases of the digestive system were a hundred per cent accurate is only of secondary importance. The accuracy of the analysis might even be improved by referring to the broader disease complex. For instance, an increase in deaths from acute respiratory diseases combined with a decline in mortality from tuberculosis might be the result of differences in diagnosis over time, but would not affect mortality trends for the broader disease complex as a whole. The following analysis will therefore regularly refer to specific disease complexes, whereas in the data presented in the tables and figures the specific diseases will be kept separate and will be listed in the order in which they appear in the source material.

Another problem area is the definition of the population at risk, which is necessary to calculate relative mortality figures—a prerequisite for any synchronic or diachronic approach. English vital registration material from the Registrar-General is far from ideal for the analysis of urban mortality trends, since municipal limits or built-up urban areas and registration district boundaries are rarely congruent.[16] For larger towns very often several districts have to be taken into account, and particularly in the case of smaller towns, suburbs and rural areas might be included (Lawton, 1989, p. 153). In a more positive vein, this provides the chance to build up at least a rough inner-city differentiation by comparing mortality in the various registration districts of a town.

Further difficulties in analysing urban areas in the nineteenth century include boundary changes in the registration districts as well as the incorporation of adjacent municipalities by the cities. Such boundary adjustments influenced the size and composition of the population at risk, and may have substantially affected the demographic, economic and social structure of a city. In the English sample, the bulk of boundary changes fortunately involved the registration districts constituting an individual town (see Appendix 4); for example, there were several boundary changes between the registration districts of Bristol and Clifton (Barton). Even more important are the numerous territorial incorporations (*Eingemeindungen*) in the German sample,[17] which selectively had a substantial demographic impact on individual towns. In general, however, they did not affect the economic basis and structure

16 The following registration districts (in brackets) have been selected for the investigation: London (registration division); Bristol = (Bristol and Clifton/Barton); Birmingham = (Birmingham and Aston); Liverpool = (Birkenhead, Liverpool, Toxteth Park and West Derby); Bolton; Manchester = (Manchester, Chorlton, Salford and Prestwich); Bradford; Leeds; Sheffield = (Ecclesall Bierlow and Sheffield); Newcastle = (Gateshead and Newcastle upon Tyne). I am grateful to Naomi Williams for her help with this question.
17 See Matzerath (1980).

(Laux, 1989, p. 127). Large parts of the following analysis include an annual assess-ment of developments in urban health conditions as one way of minimizing this problem. As the dates of boundary changes and incorporations are known, and the annual population figures of the German towns are available from offical publica-tions, a temporal comparison of population growth and mortality development pro-vides some insight into whether changes in health conditions might be a result of changes in population composition. For the English data the exact total of the popu-lation at risk is only available for census years.[18] Here the population figures for the annual series have been either interpolated or extrapolated, taking into account mid-census boundary changes as far as they are registered in the Annual Reports of the Registrar-General (see Appendix 4).

It has to be kept in mind that the population census was held at a specific day of the year, in England at the beginning of April, in Germany at the beginning of December. In view of the strong population growth during the period of investiga-tion, this implies that the death rates, i.e. the number of deaths per 1,000 head of pop-ulation in one specific year, have to be calculated from population figures which slightly misrepresent the actual average population at risk in a specific year. As this growth was not equally distributed over the year, this remains a factor which cannot be controlled at the macro-level.[19]

In analysing the role of different public health strategies and types of medical intervention which were introduced during this time in individual cities in the two European states, a series of relevant indicators had to be established—with special reference to water supply and sanitation, housing conditions, number of hospitals and overall medical provision. Comparing these indicators with actual health condi-tions is also problematic given that infrastructural data taken from the published vol-umes of the census for England and Wales do not, unfortunately, present information on the basis of registration districts, but rather for sanitary districts or municipal bor-oughs, neither of which are congruent with the registration districts or even with the combined registration districts. The two problem cities in this respect are Bradford and Leeds, where there were numerous substantial boundary changes resulting in major differences between the population within these various administrative areas.

Finally, these problems are enlarged by using a cross-national comparative macro-level approach. The amount of material and the aspects to be dealt with increase immensely, and for this reason cannot be encapsulated fully by primary sources. From the discussion of differences in the source material it is clear that the number of prob-lems naturally increases with the size of the sample. Moreover, the existence of two different bureaucratic practices of recording these developments must be dealt with, stemming from and reflecting—in the broadest sense—various 'socio-cultural' dif-ferences between the two nations. At the same time, the macro-level approach does not allow an equally extensive discussion of the developments for each individual town in the sample. Otherwise, each chapter or each city in the sample would have

18 See also Lawton (1978).
19 See also Chapter 6 note 6.

deserved its own monograph. Similarly, an analysis completely balanced between both England and Germany or even selected English and German cities cannot always be sustained. This is largely the result of the different quality and quantity of the available source material, but also a consequence of analytical considerations. In many respects, the English path towards modern urban health conditions was the more 'straightforward' case, at least in demographic terms, whereas the German route was more uneven and complicated. Urban mortality in Germany has to be analysed within the framework of vast local or regional differences and particularities. The wide independence of the self-governing German towns and cities, together with Germany's federalistic structure, incorporating 26 states, reinforce the diversities in the German case. In contrast, despite England's traditional liberalism, allowing the medium-sized and large towns strong local autonomy, various strategies in the fight against disease, for example, with respect to sanitary reform, show strong elements of central government intervention and regulation.

Furthermore, individual parts of the analysis will only be presented for selected towns of the sample. Where the findings for the various towns were similar, this is in order not to bore the reader with unnecessary repetition. The criterion for selecting individual towns of the sample for further analysis was largely determined by the available source material. From the German sample Hamburg is repeatedly used as the outstanding example, particularly with respect to intra-urban differentiation, and Liverpool has a similar function in the English sample. Hamburg is marked by excellent long-running series of data, with respect to both the demographic and socio-economic indicators required for a detailed analysis. It is, furthermore, the city in the sample which allows the most detailed analysis of intra-urban structures. There is information available for various causes of death according to city districts as well as for various socio-economic indicators. Both can be accurately compared in Hamburg, as the districts the various investigations referred to were congruent. This is indeed rarely the case, and constitutes one major reason why Hamburg as a micro-level case study is explicitly covered by modern historical research, a factor a macro-level analysis is heavily reliant upon. Finally, due to the late appearance of typhoid fever and cholera epidemics in the 1880s and 1890s, Hamburg was the object of investigation of many nineteenth-century studies on death and disease (Evans, 1987; Wischermann, 1983). All this should out-weigh the one potential problem, and this is the question of how typical a German city Hamburg was in the nineteenth-century. In contrast, it has often been described as the most English of all German towns, and nineteenth-century Hamburg might indeed not be representative of German towns in relation to many aspects of its liberal policy, social composition and basic economic functions. From a broader demographic perspective, however, Hamburg was subject to a similar epidemiological regime to many other German towns in the sample. As Hamburg's mortality profile was less dominated by the high prevalence of digestive diseases in comparison with towns in the east and south-east (Munich, Nuremberg and Breslau), this makes it even more adaptable for an intra-urban analysis aimed at elaborating environmental and socio-economic determinants. As high mortality rates from digestive disease were connected with high infant mortality rates, their strong dependence on feeding patterns often obscures these other determinants. In the English sample a valid comparison can be made with another world harbour, the city of Liverpool, situated on the northern bank of the Mersey in the county of Lancashire. An effective intra-urban differentiation based on registration districts makes Manchester and Liverpool eligible examples, as both are compounds of four registration districts (RDs). In Manchester, however, there were major boundary revisions in the 1870s affecting the city centre, when the Prestwich RD was detached from Manchester RD on 1 October 1874, altering the size of the Manchester RD substantially, whereas the changes in Liverpool (Toxteth Park RD was created on 1 January 1881 from West Derby RD) were less significant, and left the inner district, the Liverpool RD, unchanged. Finally, as port-cities, both Hamburg and Liverpool constituted a highly mobile society, which left them particularly susceptible to the threats of endemic infectious diseases and epidemics. In this sense they are particularly suited to stand as representatives in an analysis of the health conditions in an industrialized society.

Despite this range of difficulties and problems, the sample of one registration division (London) and nineteen registration districts making up ten English towns, together with ten German towns, will provide a suitable basis for a critical evaluation of the different strategies and measures adopted in response to mortality conditions in the major urban centres of both states—an assessment often inadequately substantiated by individual case studies at the micro-level. Any analytical limitations resulting from the comparative cross-national approach are hopefully outweighed by the broader perspective that this study offers.

Chapter 4

CONCLUSION TO PART I

The analysis addresses the debates on the mechanisms which evoked the profound transition towards modern increased life expectancy and improved health conditions. Urban areas played a significant role within this process. Towns and cities in Western Europe, traditionally regarded as particularly unhealthy environments and having a so-called urban graveyard effect, registered a faster decline in death rates than rural areas or national units. In the late nineteenth and early twentieth centuries the 'urban penalty' became attenuated or disappeared entirely. The big cities especially were the forerunners on the path towards current health conditions. Obviously, they had the potential to overcome the stress created by industrialization and urbanization. Therefore, the analysis assesses the dramatic decline in mortality within an urban context on the basis of the developments in the ten largest towns in both Germany and England and Wales. In the next section (Chapters 5–7) urban mortality change will be analysed in terms of crude death rates, age-, sex- and disease-specific mortality. Variations in mortality between the towns and cities as well as within individual urban agglomerations will be described. The specific developments in urban mortality change will be compared with those on a larger aggregate level. In the German case this means mortality changes as an average for all towns with a population exceeding 15,000 and, as a compatible aggregate for Germany as a whole is lacking, with respect to the age- and sex-specific disease panorama in Prussia. Urban mortality change in England will be compared with aggregated rates for England and Wales. This serves as an essential prerequisite for the next section (III), in which the reasons for the mortality decline will be considered and evaluated (Chapter 8). Particular attention will be paid to the following determinants: economic growth (Chapter 9); in close connection, as largely dependent on the private sector, urban housing conditions (Chapter 10); environmental improvements through sanitary reform (Chapter 11), especially central water supply, sewerage systems and municipal milk supply; and finally, medical provision (including health education) and social security systems (Chapter 12). In order to delineate more general processes as well as ascertaining the truly distinctive national features of the European mortality decline, the analysis will adopt a comparative approach. Developments in the ten largest towns in England as the country of origin of the industrial revolution and in Germany provide a platform for comparison.

II URBAN MORTALITY CHANGE

Chapter 5

THE SETTING

The European mortality decline started in the seventeenth century and accelerated in the eighteenth and nineteenth centuries. English historical demographic research has emphasized the role of socio-economic determinants in this context (Flinn, 1974; 1981; Wrigley and Schofield, 1981; Kunitz, 1983). First, plague had disappeared from Central and Western Europe by the late seventeenth century for reasons still not satisfactorily explained. The timing of the last outbreaks, however, suggests a close relationship with efforts in quarantine enforcement. Second, decreasing military activities and changes in military organization first stabilized and then decreased mortality rates. Third, improvements in agriculture (for example, the spread of new crops, improvements in commercial organization) reduced crises caused by famine and may have led to better overall nutritional provision. Fourth, with growing population and improved communication networks, accompanied by increasing market integration, the so-called 'human-crowd diseases' (in particular smallpox, measles, scarlet fever and whooping cough) developed in the late eighteenth and early nineteenth century from non-age-specific to typical childhood diseases. This process was linked to the increasing importance of gastro-intestinal infectious diseases, primarily affecting infants and children. As this disease complex was particularly sensitive to socio-economic factors (working and housing conditions, income and nutrition), life expectancy was increasingly determined by class-specific differences (Spree, 1981a; Imhof, 1981a). High mortality patterns were associated with areas characterized by large estates worked on by an impoverished peasantry (Kunitz, 1983, p. 356), as for example in Eastern Prussia (Lee, 1984a; 1984b).

Rising industrialization and urbanization led to fundamental changes in living conditions. Whereas there was a substantial reduction in general mortality in England from 32 per 1,000 inhabitants in the early eighteenth century to 22 in the early nineteenth century (Lawton, 1983, p. 180), population growth slowed down from the 1830s onwards. Crude death rates changed little between 1841 and 1871. Unhealthy living conditions in urban industrial areas prevented general reductions in mortality rates. William Farr, Compiler of Abstracts to the Registrar-General, estimated that mortality rates between 1813 and 1830 ranged from 17.8 per 1,000 inhabitants in Suffolk to 30.3 in Middlesex for men and 16.7 in Cornwall to 25.3 again in Middlesex for women.[1] The poorest figures were for the big cities, particularly the industrial towns in the north; the 'urban penalty' was distinctly operating.[2] As general mortality

1 Farr (1974), p. 570. For further information about Farr see Eyler (1979).
2 For an introduction to English population development see Wrigley and Schofield (1981). For special reference to urban mortality conditions see Kearns (1988a); Woods and Woodward (1984); Woods and Hinde (1987).

began to decline from mid-Victorian times, the differential between best and worst widened, particularly due to very high infant mortality and deaths of older people in towns. E. H. Greenhow confirmed the dismal record of large towns in his study of mortality in 105 of the 623 registration districts of England and Wales, 1848–1854 (Greenhow, 1858). Urbanization brought about an immense accumulation of people in urban areas. With the prevalence of acute and chronic infectious conditions in the disease panorama, living in these densely populated places carried a high health risk. A central feature of mortality changes in England during the nineteenth and early twentieth centuries, however, is the attenuation and near removal of the urban penalty. In 1811, people in urban areas (towns over 10,000 inhabitants) had a life expectancy at birth of 31 years, in comparison with 41 in rural areas. By 1861 the ten-year gap had decreased to seven (38 and 45) and by 1911 to only three years (52 and 55) (Woods, 1985).

In Germany at the beginning of the nineteenth century mortality rates far surpassed those experienced in England. The crude death rate (CDR) in Prussia in 1821–1830, for example, was 28.0 deaths per 1,000 inhabitants (Vögele, forthcoming a). Mortality rates underwent some improvement during the late eighteenth and early nineteenth centuries.[3] The actual death rates, however, still remained at a high level, yet in many regions of Germany there was a decline in the number of years when deaths surpassed births in the late eighteenth century. Mortality crises increasingly disappeared, the intensity of variation in mortality decreased and the average crude death rate declined in most parts of Germany and in urban areas (Lee, 1980, p. 244; Vögele, 1991, p. 33). In numerous large towns the crude death rates tended to decline in the early nineteenth century (Kisskalt, 1922, p. 11; Vögele, 1991, p. 33). The actual crude urban death rates, however, increased in the 1830s, 1850s, 1860s and early 1870s (Vögele, 1991, p. 33), only interrupted by a decade of modest decline in the 1840s. From the late 1870s onwards urban mortality was characterized by a continuously declining trend. This fall was faster and stronger than in the national aggregate; the 'urban penalty' began to vanish. In order to be able to analyse the mechanism behind this development, the following chapter will focus on the character and course of urban mortality in this crucial period.

---

3 For an overview see Imhof (1981a); Imhof (1990); Kisskalt (1921), especially pp. 452–508; Kocka (1983), pp. 57–61; Lee (1980), especially p. 244; Marschalck (1984; 1987); Rürup (1984), pp. 28–29; Spree (1988), especially pp. 77–97; Vögele (1991); Wehler (1987), pp. 21–24. For a summary of the long-term patterns of the causes of death see Imhof (1985).

Chapter 6

URBAN MORTALITY IN ENGLAND AND GERMANY, 1870–1910

MORTALITY CHANGE—THE DEATH RATES

Crude Death Rates

In general the crude death rates (CDR) in Germany were consistently higher than the corresponding English figures (Table 3). After the middle of the nineteenth century (1851–1860), for example, England and Wales registered a mortality rate of about 22 deaths per 1,000 inhabitants, whereas the corresponding rate for Germany was about 27. In both countries, however, the aggregated urban mortality figures were above the average for the whole country, i.e. an 'urban penalty' can be clearly identified and, generally speaking, the verdict describing the towns as 'graveyards' is correct. In England all the towns in the sample registered death rates well above the national average (Fig. 3)[1], with especially high rates in the northern industrial and commercial towns, namely Manchester and Liverpool. Southern towns like Bristol and even metropolitan London registered comparatively lower death rates. By contrast, in Germany this penalty was not as obvious and coherent as in England. Amongst the ten largest German towns there was a much wider variation in crude death rates than amongst the English towns, and, in contrast to the latter, several German towns reported better figures than the average for the whole country, as well as for all towns with a population exceeding 15,000 inhabitants (Fig. 4). Frankfurt am Main, one of Germany's richest towns, registered very low death rates during the whole of the nineteenth century (Vögele, 1991, p. 33).[2] Amongst the healthier places was also the former residential and garrison town of Düsseldorf, which in the last quarter of the nineteenth century quickly developed into a modern industrialized town with an increasing component of bureaucratic and administrative functions, registering the strongest population growth amongst the ten largest towns. The capital Berlin, Dresden and the old commercial town of Leipzig were also relatively healthy places. Despite its exposed position as an international port, the city of Hamburg took some kind of intermediary, yet constantly improving position. The unhealthiest places were the old commercial town of Cologne, and especially the towns in the east and south-east, like Nuremberg, Munich and Breslau.

On the whole the connection between the size of a town and its mortality level is not as obvious in relation to the German towns as it has been demonstrated for English towns (Weber, 1899, p. 344)—even if infant mortality, strongly influenced by

---

1 Although the series for England and Germany cover different time spans, all the available data are given in the following graphic presentations of the annual developments in order to provide as much information as possible.
2 For a more detailed discussion of the economic base and occupational structure of the individual towns in the sample see Chapter 9.

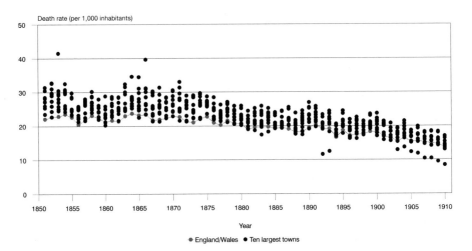

Figure 3: Crude death rate in English towns, 1851–1910 (per 1,000 inhabitants)
Source: *Annual Reports of the Registrar-General of Births, Deaths, and Marriages in England and Wales*, 1856–1910.

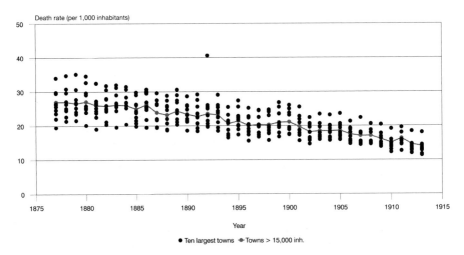

Figure 4: Crude death rate in German towns, 1877–1913 (per 1,000 inhabitants)
Source: *Veröffentlichungen des Kaiserlichen Gesundheitsamtes (Beilagen)* (1878–1914).

Table 3: Crude death rates in the ten largest German and English towns (per 1,000 inhabitants)

	1841–1850	1851–1860	1861–1870	1871–1880	1881–1890	1891–1900	1901–1910	Decline 1841/60– 1901/10	Decline Peak– 1901/10
Be	25	25	30	31	25	19	16	9	15
Br	33	35*	37*	34*	30	26	22	11	26
Co	29	28*	30*	30*	27	24	19	10	20
Dr	29	28	28	26	24	20	16	13	13
Du	23†	24	28	28	23	21	16	7	12
Fr	19	17	19	21	20	17	15	4	6
Ha	31	27	26	28	26	21	16	15	15
Le	28	24	25	25	22	21	16	12	12
Mu	32*	36	38	38	30	25	19	13	18
Nu	27	–	32	26‡	27	23	19	8	13
TO	–	–	–	27‡	25	21	18	–	9
Ge	27	26	27	27	25	22	19	8	8
EW	22	22	23	21	19	18	15	7	8
Bi	25	25	25	24	20	21	17	8	8
Bl	–	24	24	22	19	18	12	–	12
Bo	27	27	26	25	21	20	16	11	11
Br	25	26	26	24	21	19	16	9	10
Le	28	28	29	26	23	21	17	11	12
Li	34	27	31	26	24	23	19	15	15
Lo	–	24	25	23	20	19	15	–	10
Ma	32	28	29	28	24	23	19	13	13
Ne	27	27	27	26	22	20	17	10	10
Sh	26	27	27	25	22	20	17	9	10

Be=Berlin;   Br=Breslau;   Co=Cologne;   Dr=Dresden;   Du=Düsseldorf;   Fr=Frankfurt am Main;
Ha=Hamburg;   Le=Leipzig;   Mu=Munich;   Nu=Nuremberg;   TO=towns over 15,000 inhabitants;
Ge=Germany.
EW=England and Wales; Bi=Birmingham; Bl=Bristol; Bo=Bolton; Br=Bradford; Le=Leeds;
Li=Liverpool; Lo=London; Ma=Manchester; Ne=Newcastle upon Tyne; Sh=Sheffield.
* Includes still-births (1871–1880 for Breslau and Cologne: until 1875 includes still-births, 1876 is
missing, then without still-births).
† 1846 and 1850.
‡ 1877–1880.

Sources: Kisskalt (1922), p. 11; *Veröffentlichungen des Kaiserlichen Gesundheitsamtes (Beilagen)*
(1878–1911); *Medizinalstatistische Mitteilungen aus dem Reichsgesundheitsamte*, (1893) onwards;
Statistik des Deutschen Reichs NF **44** (1892), p. 6; *Preußische Statistik* **48, 2** (1879), p. 52; *Quellen zur
Bevölkerungs- Sozial- und Wirtschaftsstatistik* (1980), pp. 190–91, 226–27, 338–39; Statistisches
Bundesamt (1972), pp. 101–02; *Die Gesundheitsverhältnisse Hamburgs* (1901), pp. 106–07; Weyl (1904),
p. 12; *Die Entwicklung Münchens* (1899), p. 46; Brandlmeier (1942), p. 43; Fröhlich (1886), p. 728;
Prinzing (1930/31), p. 343; *Nürnberg* (1892), p. 171; *Statistisches Jahrbuch für die Stadt Dresden* (1902),
p. 20; *Statistisches Jahrbuch der Landeshauptstadt Düsseldorf* (1979/80), p. 11; *Düsseldorf* (1898), p. 67;
Annual Reports of the Registrar-General of Births, Deaths, and Marriages in England and Wales
(1851–1910); Dennis (1984), pp. 36–37.

Table 4: Crude death rates—infant mortality excluded—in selected German towns (per 1,000 inhabitants)

City/town	1877–1913	1877–1889	1890–1899	1900–1913
Breslau	17.8	20.3	17.7	15.5
Munich	15.8	19.3	15.2	12.9
Dortmund	15.4	19.3	14.8	12.1
Cologne	14.8	17.7	14.8	12.1
Hamburg	14.6	17.9	14.6	11.7
Essen	14.4	18.1	15.2	10.5
Nuremberg	14.3	17.3	14.5	11.3
Dresden	14.1	16.8	14.0	11.5
Berlin	13.7	16.4	12.9	11.9
Frankfurt	13.1	15.1	13.3	11.1
Düsseldorf	12.8	15.0	13.1	10.4
Leipzig	12.7	14.7	12.8	10.7
All towns over 15,000 inhabitants	14.5	17.1	14.3	12.2

Source: *Veröffentlichungen des Kaiserlichen Gesundheitsamtes (Beilagen)* (1878–1914).

regional patterns of feeding practices (Finkelnburg, 1882, p. 8), of child care (Imhof, 1981a) and of fertility levels (Kintner, 1987), is excluded (Tables 4 and 5).[3] Furthermore, urban death rates in Germany seem to have been influenced by two different regional demographic patterns. Towns in the less industrialized eastern parts showed extremely high rates reflecting, at least partly, demographic conditions in their rural hinterland, rather than being a specific urban penalty, whereas urban and rural mortality rates in the west were generally at a lower level (Kearns et al., 1989, p. 12). In fact, the large Westphalian peasant families with their low mortality rates were proclaimed as a national model (Salomon, 1923, pp. 218–19). Similarly, the new industrial towns in the western areas registered relatively low mortality rates. The reasons for this will be discussed during the analysis in the following chapters.

In terms of the general development of urban mortality, in Prussia and in most of the largest German towns—with the exception of Hamburg and Leipzig—the peak in urban death rates was reached in the 1860s and 1870s, corresponding with the beginning of Germany's main urbanization period. Prussian data permit an analysis of aggregate urban–rural mortality differentials from 1849 onwards.[4] In Prussia the

---

3 However, expressed as a coefficient of correlation of the number of population per hectare in 1871–1900 and the death rate from tuberculosis—the overcrowding disease par excellence—in 1877–1900 in the ten largest German towns, the connection is rather weak:

1870s: $r = -0.2498$, sig (two-tailed) $= 0.486$.

1900 : $r = -0.2425$, sig (two-tailed) $= 0.500$.

Sources: *Veröffentlichungen des Kaiserlichen Gesundheitsamtes (Beilagen)* (1878, 1901); Schott (1912), pp. 110–13.

4 In Prussia the differentiation between urban and rural mortality was based on administrative categories, not population size. See Prinzing (1931), p. 569.

Table 5: Town size, town growth, mortality and selected causes of death in the ten largest German towns

City/town	Population 1913	Growth % 1877–1913	CDR-I* 1877–1913 (per 1,000 inhabitants)	CDR 1900–1913	TB 1900–1913 (per 100,000 inhabitants)	Typhoid 1900–1913	IMR 1900–1913 (per 100 births)
Düsseldorf	401,734	476.4	12.8	15.7	153.0	3.0	16.9
Leipzig	616,776	455.2	12.7	16.0	204.5	3.9	19.8
Cologne	543,032	395.0	14.8	18.6	191.8	4.6	20.3
Nuremberg	353,145	370.7	14.3	18.1	248.7	1.5	21.9
Frankfurt	439,604	370.4	13.1	14.5	208.6	2.4	14.0
Munich	634,867	295.3	15.8	18.5	269.0	2.8	20.6
Hamburg	1,021,455	286.4	14.6	15.4	173.6	4.1	15.8
Dresden	561,865	273.7	14.1	15.6	207.9	4.2	16.3
Breslau	539,314	209.8	17.8	21.7	312.6	6.0	22.6
Berlin	2,079,662	209.1	13.7	15.8	213.5	3.8	18.1

* CDR without IMR

Source: *Veröffentlichungen des Kaiserlichen Gesundheitsamtes (Beilagen)* (1901–1914).

average urban mortality rate was above the rural average up to the beginning of the 1890s; subsequently the picture changed and urban areas showed lower mortality rates after the beginning of the twentieth century (Table 6).

For all German towns with a population exceeding 15,000 inhabitants, the situation improved at a slightly earlier date. At the end of the 1870s mortality rates were already lower in comparison with the total average for Germany and the rural areas of Prussia respectively. Despite remarkable urban population growth during the period under consideration—Table 5 shows the growth of the ten largest German towns in the period 1877 to 1913—average urban mortality declined and was well below the total average for the whole of Germany at the beginning of the twentieth century: 17.0 per 1,000 inhabitants in urban areas compared with a rate of 18.0 for the whole country.

In England and Wales the urban penalty basically showed a downward trend from the start of the period under investigation. English mortality figures also reveal a small peak in the 1860s, which is reflected as well in national aggregate data,[5] and therefore might not be attributable to the urban penalty, but may simply be an expression of the general economic crisis. An aggregated urban–rural comparison, available for the period 1847 to 1890, shows substantially higher death rates in the urban environment (Table 6). Differences between urban and rural death rates, however, tended to

5 It has to be kept in mind that due to the higher degree of urbanization, the English national aggregate represents urban conditions much more than the figures for Germany. See Chapter 2.

Table 6: The development of urban and rural mortality rates in Germany and England (per 1,000 inhabitants)

Prussia			German towns*	Prussia/ Germany†		England and Wales	
urban	rural					urban	rural
–	–	1816–1820	–	27.2		–	–
–	–	1821–1830	–	28.0		–	–
–	–	1831–1840	–	28.6		–	–
–	–	1841–1850	–	26.8	1847–1850	26.9	20.6
31.5	29.8	1851–1860	–	26.3	1851–1860	24.7	19.9
28.9	27.8						
30.8	27.8	1861–1870	–	26.8	1861–1870	24.8	19.7
31.4	28.3	1871–1880	26.9‡	27.2	1871–1880	23.1	19.0
28.9	26.3						
27.8	26.5	1881–1890	25.0	25.1	1881–1890	20.3	17.3
25.7	25.4						
24.1	24.3	1891–1900	21.4	22.3	1891–1900	18.9	16.7
22.2	22.2						
20.4	21.3	1901–1913	17.0	18.0		–	–
17.8	18.2						

Note: left-block periods are 1849–1855, 1856–1861, 1862–1870, 1871–1875, 1876–1880, 1881–1885, 1886–1890, 1891–1895, 1896–1900, 1901–1905, 1906–1908.

* German towns with more than 15,000 inhabitants.
† Prussia until 1840, then Germany.
‡ 1877–1880.

Sources: *Veröffentlichungen des Kaiserlichen Gesundheitsamtes (Beilagen)* (1878–1914); *Medizinalstatistische Mitteilungen aus dem Reichsgesundheitsamte* 1 (1893) onwards; *Statistik des Deutschen Reichs* NF**44** (1892), p. 6; *Preußische Statistik*, **48, 2** (1879), pp. 52, 61 and **200** (1906), p. 13; *Quellen zur Bevölkerungs-, Sozial- und Wirtschaftsstatistik* (1980), pp. 190–91, 226–27, 338–39; Statistisches Bundesamt (1972), pp. 101–02; Prinzing (1912), p. 503; Varrentrapp (1880), p. 548; Weber (1899), pp. 355, 63; *Annual Reports of the Registrar-General of Births, Deaths, and Marriages in England and Wales*, p. cxi.

converge towards the end of the nineteenth century, due to a stronger decrease in urban mortality. The maximum difference of 6.3 was recorded in the period 1847–1850, with a death rate of 26.9 in urban areas and 20.6 in rural areas. In the period 1891 to 1900 the aggregate urban death rate was 18.9, the rural death rate 16.7.

In the last decade of the nineteenth century all German towns with a population exceeding 15,000 and six of the ten largest towns reported lower mortality figures than the country as a whole, whereas in England none of the ten largest towns had lower figures than the average for the whole of England and Wales.[6] In both countries

---

6 In 1841–1850 none of the English towns and only two out of the ten largest German towns (Frankfurt am Main and Berlin) registered lower mortality figures than national aggregate data. Whether the low death rates of the two German towns can be primarily attributed to the role of local demographic or health factors cannot be answered within the context of an analysis of crude death rates. This would require a detailed investigation of age- and sex-specific death rates as well as of the disease panorama which cannot be provided in this volume.

the urban mortality decline was accompanied by diminishing local variations in the crude death rates. At the beginning of the twentieth century the crude mortality rates of the ten largest German and English towns were very similar, with a slight advantage to the English towns, whereas the figures for the whole of Germany were still much higher than for England and Wales. In the German sample the strongest decline in mortality was registered in towns with a high death rate. Breslau registered a decline in mortality from a peak in the period 1861–1870 to 1901–1910 of 26 per 1,000, and Cologne and Munich of 20 and 18 respectively in the same period. Similarly, in England the strongest decline occurred in unhealthy Liverpool and Manchester, 15 and 13 respectively in 1841–1850 to 19 in both towns in 1901–1910. Relatively healthy Bristol was also amongst towns with a strong improvement of 12 per 1,000 between 1851–1960 and 1901–1910.

In conclusion, it can be stated that although German data suggest at least a temporary correlation between urbanization and mortality, the 'urban penalty' in Germany was not so unequivocal, and became attenuated and disappeared earlier than in England. German towns recovered rather more quickly from the 'urban penalty' and recovered more successfuly from their higher death rates than the country as a whole, so that the towns in both countries registered similar mortality rates towards the end of the period under investigation.

Standardized Mortality Rates

Comparing the absolute crude death rates in both countries has indicated that average urban mortality was well above the rates for national aggregates and that England and the English towns of the nineteenth century enjoyed much better health conditions than Germany. Crude death rates, however, offer only a very rough picture of the actual health conditions. As the risk of dying is unevenly distributed between men and women and very strongly dependent on age, the age- and sex-composition of the population at risk plays a crucial role in determining the actual level of the crude death rate in a specific population. Correspondingly, the improvements in average crude mortality rates during the period under investigation do not inevitably lead to the conclusion that there was any dramatic improvement in health conditions within the towns. Rather, migration into urban areas may have had a profound effect on the age-structure of both sending and receiving areas.

The emerging industrial society was extremely mobile and therefore significantly marked by migration.[7] Population growth in the towns during the period under

7 This migration movement included both in-migration and out-migration. In Berlin between 1880 and 1890, for example, population growth was 34.4 per cent, 24 per cent of which was the result of in-migration. In the same period in-migration was 119.4 per cent of the average population, out-migration 95.4 per cent. The actual population growth by migration was therefore only 11.2 per cent of the total migration movement. See Langewiesche (1979), p. 70; Langewiesche (1977). As the age-structure of both in-migrants and out-migrants was similar, with the highest mobile group being aged between about 20 and 30 (Langewiesche, 1979), the study in this context can be limited to the analysis of how the gains by in-migration affected the age-structure of the population at risk, and through this the actual mortality rates. There are, however, two effects which should be kept in mind. First of all, such a highly mobile society

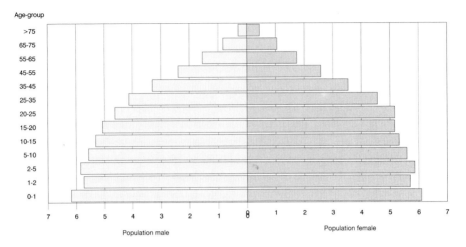

Figure 5: Age-structure of the population in England and Wales, 1901–1910 (%)
Source: *Decennial Supplement to the Annual Reports of the Registrar-General of Births, Deaths, and Marriages in England and Wales* (1901–1910).

investigation was substantially determined by in-migration, especially of younger 'healthy' age-groups. As German towns in this period registered a stronger in-migration than English towns (Weber, 1899, p. 240), this might be a key to explaining why differences in urban and rural mortality were not so distinctive and pronounced in Germany. Whereas in England over the period 1851–1911 natural growth exceeded net migration (Lawton, 1989, p. 157), in Prussia in the last quarter of the nineteenth century 54 per cent of the total increase in urban population was due to net in-migration, in comparison with 31 per cent which was attributable to natural increase and about 14 per cent to territorial incorporations (Laux, 1989, p. 135). An impression of how strongly the age-structure of the population at risk in the towns of the two samples was influenced by migration can be gauged from Figures 5–8. In Germany in the early twentieth century differences in the age-structures of the sample of towns and Prussia were still more pronounced than the corresponding English figures. Yet there were also substantial differences between the various towns. Amongst the largest German towns, around two-thirds of the population were born

facilitates the spread of the prevalent infectious diseases and epidemics. Second, migration followed a specific seasonal pattern, reaching its high in spring and autumn, and its low in December, when the population accounts in Germany were actually held. In this respect, the total population at risk during the year in an individual town was under-represented, neglecting the highest mobile groups, with the consequence that the death rates overestimate the actual risk of dying in that specific town. This is a factor which cannot be controlled at the macro-level. However, this should not bias the analysis in any substantial way, as the problem addresses particularly the low-mortality age-groups, and is counterbalanced by the reverse effect that a census held in December includes the net population gains of the year, thus over-estimating the actual population at risk, particularly at the beginning of a specific year.

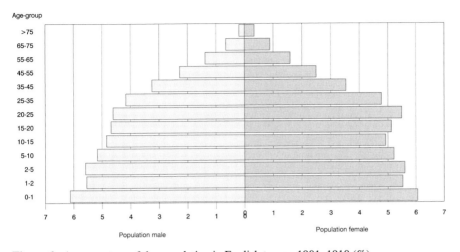

Figure 6: Age-structure of the population in English towns, 1901–1910 (%)
Source: *Decennial Supplement to the Annual Reports of the Registrar-General of Births, Deaths, and Marriages in England and Wales* (1901–1910).

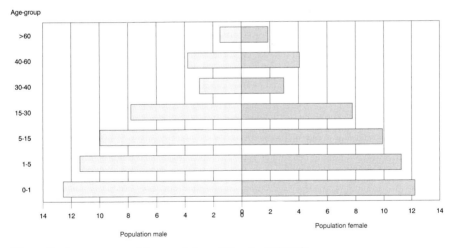

Figure 7: Age-structure of the population of Prussia, 1907 (%)
Sources: See Appendix 2.

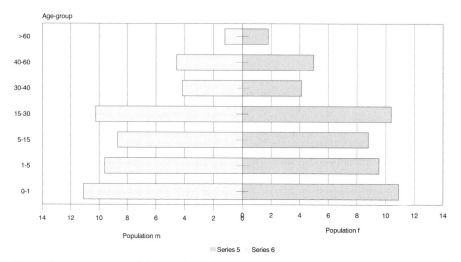

Figure 8: Age-structure of the population in German towns, 1907–1910 (%)
Sources: See Appendix 2.

outside the town in Leipzig, Frankfurt am Main and Munich, almost 60 per cent in Dresden, Berlin and Breslau, and around 50 per cent in Düsseldorf, Hamburg, Nuremberg and Cologne (Brückner, 1890, p. 179). In 1885 almost two-thirds of these in-migrants were in the low-mortality age-group between 15 and 30 years of age (Brückner, 1890, p. 630), with a slight predominance of the male sex (Brückner, 1890, p. 183; Langewiesche, 1979, pp. 78–79). The only exception is Frankfurt am Main, where the female:male ratio was 1:0.9 between 1880 and 1890 (Bleicher, 1895, p. 6).

In order to compensate for these influences the crude death rates have to be related to a single specific population at risk, either a theoretical or historical one. In the following case the structure of the population of England and Wales 1871–1880 has been selected as a basis to calculate the so-called standardized mortality rates (SMR). The calculation of SMRs is designed to adjust CDRs to reflect differences in the age-structure based on the mortality rates of different age-groups derived from a specific population. Correspondingly, the following standardized mortality rates represent the mortality of the inhabitants of various locations, assuming the structure of their population at risk was the same as that of England and Wales in 1871–1880.

The impact of differences in the age distribution becomes immediately obvious. Standardized mortality rates in the towns of both countries were well above the crude death rates in the 1870s (Table 7). The English towns registered an SMR of 25.3 (per 1,000 inhabitants) in comparison with a crude death rate of 24.0 (per 1,000 inhabitants), whereas the German towns' SMR was 28.0, in comparison to a CDR of 26.8. That is, urban health conditions were even worse during this period than assumed by analysing solely the crude death rates. The differences between the towns of the two countries, however, remain stable. This pinpoints the fact that urban existence in both countries most likely posed a great threat to life for the whole urban population.

Table 7: Crude death rates (CDR) and standardized mortality rates (SMR) in England and Wales and Germany (per 1,000 inhabitants)

	CDR	SMR England/Wales 1871–1880		CDR	SMR Prussia 1877	SMR England/Wales 1871–1880
England/Wales 1871–1880	21.3	–	Prussia 1877	25.7	–	25.2
England/Wales 1901–1910	15.4	16.1	Prussia 1907	18.0	18.8	18.3
Ten largest English towns 1871–1880	24.0	25.3	Ten largest German towns 1877	26.8	29.1	28.0
Ten largest English towns 1901–1910	16.8	18.5	Ten largest German towns 1907	15.7	18.4	18.0

Sources: See Appendix 2; *Decennial Supplements to the Annual Reports of the Registrar-General of Births, Deaths, and Marriages in England and Wales* (1871–1880 and 1901–1910).

After the turn of the century urban health conditions in England were still much worse when compared with the whole of England and Wales, with an SMR of 18.5 for the urban sample and 16.1 nationwide. By contrast, the German towns registered better rates than the corresponding Prussian figures (18.0 against 18.3), although the improvement was not as strong as the crude death rates indicated. On the whole, the results of the previous chapter can be sustained; urban health conditions improved faster and to a greater degree than those of the whole nation, and the disadvantage of the towns became further attenuated in England and disappeared entirely in Germany. The death rates of the German towns improved relatively more strongly than their English counterparts, starting, however, from a higher level. Urban mortality rates tended to converge in both countries, with a slight advantage for the English towns in terms of standardized mortality rates. National figures, however, still reveal noticeably better health conditions in England and Wales in 1901–1910, with an SMR of 16.1, in contrast to 18.3 for Prussia in 1907.

THE RISK GROUPS—AGE-SPECIFIC MORTALITY

The investigation can be carried into greater depth by analysing age-specific mortality rates, that is by calculating mortality from the number of deaths in a specific age-group related to the population at risk of the same age-group. This will provide information about the special risk groups in terms of disease and death. A comparison between aggregated rates on the national level and the urban figures will also facilitate an analysis of the specific periods in the life-cycle when urban health conditions were most threatening. This, again, provides further insight into major differences in the health conditions of the two countries under examination.

In the 1870s the higher mortality of Germany and the German towns, compared with the English experience, was evident in relation to children, young adults and especially infants (Fig. 9).[8] In the German towns infant mortality rates (IMR) clearly surpassed those in the English towns, even if one excludes the towns in the east and south-east of Germany, where high infant mortality rates were predominant, arguably because of a general absence of breast-feeding (Beetz, 1882; *Nürnberg*, 1892).[9] For those between the ages of 20 and 35, German towns offered better health conditions than their English counterparts; thereafter both countries recorded almost equal rates, with a slight advantage for German towns.

Although in German towns mortality in all age-groups improved after the turn of the century (Fig. 10),[10] the main changes can be found in the younger age-groups, and

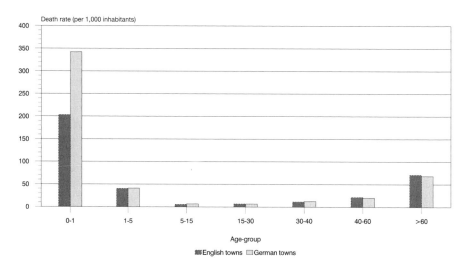

Figure 9: Age-specific mortality in English towns,1871–1880 and German towns, 1877
Sources: *Decennial Supplement to the Annual Reports of the Registrar-General of Births, Deaths, and Marriages in England and Wales* (1871–1880); *Preußische Statistik* (1879) and statistical yearbooks of the various towns.

8 The figure represents the situation in the largest towns in England and Wales as well as in Germany.
9 Concerning infant mortality, still-births have been excluded from the analysis of the German material, except where otherwise indicated. It has to be kept in mind that still-birth registration was differently practised. Whereas in some Catholic areas of Germany the Nottaufe (i.e. any person was allowed to baptize the infant in an emergency) reduced the number of registered still-births, in areas with the Civil Code all infants who died before the three days mandatory registration period was over were counted as still-births. See Mayr (1870), p. 203; Maier (1871), p. 156. In the English statistics still-births were not registered. In view of the fact that still-birth registration even nowadays differs from country to country due to varying definitions of still-births, it has to be emphasized that this is even more the case in statistics supplied by a sample of nineteenth-century cities. For frequencies and causes of late nineteenth-century still-births see Prinzing (1914).
10 The figure represents the situation in the largest towns in England and Wales as well as in Germany.

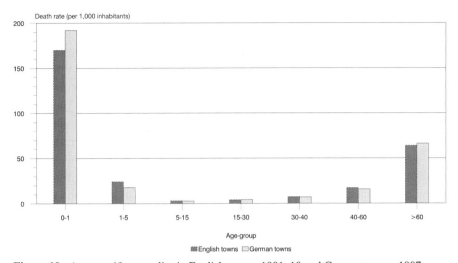

Figure 10: Age-specific mortality in English towns, 1901–10 and German towns, 1907
Sources: *Decennial Supplement to the Annual Reports of the Registrar-General of Births, Deaths and Marriages in England and Wales* (1901–1910); *Preußische Statistik* (1908) and statistical yearbooks of the various towns.

especially amongst infants. Young adults in the towns registered the strongest relative improvement in relation to rural areas; in absolute terms, however, it was infant mortality which improved most. In English towns improvements occurred amongst infants and in the age-group 20 to 25, whereas health conditions for the higher age-groups actually deteriorated.

Concerning relative urban–rural differences, almost all age-groups recorded a markedly higher mortality rate in towns at the beginning of the period under investigation (Fig. 11);[11] in both countries, however, the high urban risk groups during the second phase of the epidemiologic transition were infants, young children and men in the higher age-groups over 40 (Spree, 1986, pp. 79–83; Kearns, 1991; Vögele, forthcoming a).

In England, urban infant mortality began to decline in the 1870s, whereas the decline at the national level occurred only after the turn of the century (Laxton and Williams, 1989, pp. 111–16; Williams, 1989, pp. 42–46). A particularly distinctive feature, distinguishing England and Wales from many other European countries, is the fact that infant mortality in both urban and rural areas deteriorated again in the 1880s and 1890s, followed by a rapid downturn after 1900 (Woods et al., 1988/9, pp. 348–59).[12] However, infant mortality, commonly seen as one of the most sensitive indicators of changes in the environment and economic development, was almost consistently higher in an urban environment (*Forty-Second Annual Report*, 1913, p.

11 The figure represents the situation in the largest towns in England and Wales as well as in German towns over 20,000 inhabitants.

12 For a detailed analysis of infant mortality change in England see Woods et al. (1988/89); Williams (1989); Woods et al. (1993); Williams and Mooney (1994).

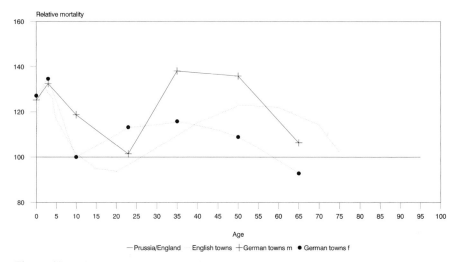

Figure 11: Relative age- and sex-specific mortality in urban areas, in England and Wales, 1871–1880 and Prussia, 1867
Sources: *Decennial Supplement to the Annual Reports of the Registrar-General of Births, Deaths and Marriages in England and Wales* (1871–1880); *Preußische Statistik* (1869) p. 17.

3; Prinzing, 1900, p. 630; Woods et al., 1993, pp. 41–44). In England the relative standing of towns in the higher age-groups did not improve significantly despite the fact that age-specific mortality improved in line with national rates (Kearns, 1991).

In German towns after the turn of the century relative improvements were registered amongst infants, as well as in the 5 to 20 age-group; in particular, women in an urban environment benefited and recorded better rates than in rural areas (Fig. 12).[13] On the other hand, the 'urban penalty' became even more severe in the older male age-groups. Here the cumulative effects of urban life even led to a relative deterioration in mortality for both sexes, but especially for males. In these groups the gap in mortality between the sexes was much more obvious than in England.

For Prussia 1876–1910 it has been demonstrated that changes in age-specific mortality were in favour of the larger cities rather than medium-sized towns (Tables 8, 9 and 10; see also Spree, 1981a; Kearns et al., 1989, pp. 12–13). By the 1880s adult mortality was worst in medium-sized towns between 20,000 and 100,000 inhabitants (Ballod, 1899, pp. 112–13; Kruse, 1897, p. 138). After the turn of the century (1900–1901) average life expectancy for men and women in the 22 largest Prussian towns was in almost all age-groups equal to or higher than in medium-sized towns, while female life expectancy in the large towns was even higher than in small towns with less than 20,000 inhabitants (Ballod, 1906, p. 11). Infants in the large towns, however, were still disadvantaged in terms of life expectancy.

13 The figure represents the situation in the ten largest towns in England and Wales as well as in the largest towns in Prussia.

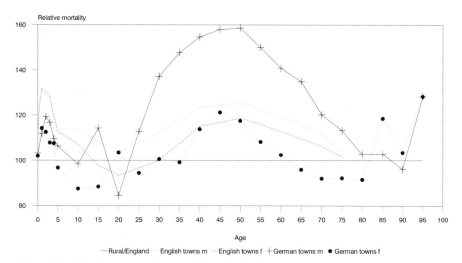

Figure 12: Relative age- and sex-specific mortality in urban and rural areas, in England and Wales, 1901–1910 and Prussia, 1905–1906
Sources: *Decennial Supplement to the Annual Reports of the Registrar-General of Births, Deaths and Marriages in England and Wales* (1901–1910); Ballod (1913), p. 48.

Table 8: Age-specific death rates in Prussia, 1895–1896 (per 1,000 inhabitants)

Age	Six eastern large towns		Twelve western large towns		Medium-sized towns		Small towns		Rural communities	
	m	f	m	f	m	f	m	f	m	f
2–3	26.8	–	23.7	23.7	24.4	22.9	22.0	22.2	22.2	21.3
3–4	18.3	–	14.9	13.5	15.1	13.8	13.9	13.7	14.4	14.1
4–5	12.8	–	9.7	9.2	10.3	9.8	9.8	10.2	10.1	10.1
5–10	6.5	–	4.6	4.5	5.2	5.0	5.4	5.4	5.4	5.6
10–15	2.9	–	2.4	2.4	2.5	2.8	2.7	3.1	2.9	3.3
15–20	4.6	–	2.2	3.1	4.6	3.5	4.5	4.3	4.1	3.8
20–25	5.2	–	4.7	3.8	5.2	4.8	6.4	5.5	6.4	5.0
25–30	6.5	–	5.8	5.1	6.8	5.9	6.9	6.6	5.3	6.0
30–35	9.7	–	8.0	6.3	8.6	7.3	8.7	7.2	5.9	7.0
35–40	12.4	–	10.0	7.5	12.6	8.9	11.0	8.3	7.4	8.1
40–45	17.5	–	14.3	9.4	15.9	9.9	14.2	9.6	9.6	8.6
45–50	21.5	–	19.0	11.4	20.9	11.6	18.4	10.9	12.9	9.6
50–55	27.2	–	25.9	14.9	26.6	15.4	24.0	14.6	16.8	13.3
55–60	36.5	–	33.4	29.1	34.9	20.9	31.8	20.6	23.8	19.7
60–65	49.8	–	46.4	33.1	48.8	32.5	43.5	30.6	34.2	31.8
65–70	69.4	–	64.9	48.2	64.0	48.2	62.6	48.4	52.4	50.4
70–75	89.6	–	92.7	68.4	102.4	80.8	86.3	75.9	79.8	79.1
75–80	139.5	–	138.9	128.1	135.1	114.6	129.0	112.0	122.6	121.3
80–85	198.1	–	195.2	165.7	194.1	147.7	183.1	172.5	186.4	180.6
85–90	247.1	–	304.2	253.7	279.0	268.1	285.8	241.4	275.4	250.3
90–95	–	–	500.0	380.8	–	–	–	–	365.3	347.8

Source: Ballod (1899), p. 113.

Table 9: Average life expectancy for men and women in Prussia, 1900–01

Age	Prussia		Urban		Rural		Twenty-two big cities		Medium-sized towns* 20,000–100,000		Small towns <20,000	
	m	f	m	f	m	f	m	f	m	f	m	f
0	42.07	45.84	39.85	44.92	43.72	46.48	39.19	44.78	39.95	48.87	40.45	45.05
1	52.69	55.22	50.52	54.77	54.34	55.55	50.27	55.17	50.00	54.18	51.00	54.59
2	54.38	56.91	52.33	56.67	55.97	57.10	52.20	57.23	51.88	56.26	52.70	56.24
3	54.48	57.02	52.48	56.85	56.03	57.17	52.38	57.45	52.05	56.53	52.83	56.37
4	54.19	56.74	52.21	56.61	55.72	56.86	52.13	57.25	51.85	56.35	52.49	56.06
5	53.69	56.26	51.71	56.16	55.22	56.37	51.65	56.82	51.40	55.92	51.96	55.58
10	49.95	52.64	47.94	52.55	51.52	52.75	47.85	53.18	47.74	52.41	48.19	51.96
15	45.61	48.40	43.55	48.25	47.20	48.54	43.45	48.84	43.34	48.13	43.82	47.70
20	41.53	44.27	39.45	44.09	43.14	44.43	39.26	44.61	39.27	43.98	39.76	43.61
25	37.67	40.27	35.45	40.09	39.43	40.43	35.19	40.55	35.21	39.95	35.98	39.74
30	33.69	36.42	31.53	36.25	35.40	36.57	31.20	36.63	31.27	36.09	32.16	36.00
35	29.75	32.57	27.70	32.42	31.32	32.71	27.36	32.74	27.37	32.24	28.33	32.25
40	26.01	28.77	24.12	28.64	27.41	28.89	23.78	28.93	23.76	28.45	24.76	28.51
45	22.47	24.93	20.81	24.84	23.65	25.01	20.48	25.11	20.45	24.68	21.38	24.71
50	19.12	21.07	17.72	21.09	20.07	21.07	17.42	21.36	17.31	20.91	18.24	20.98
55	15.97	17.40	14.84	17.52	16.69	17.32	14.59	17.75	14.44	17.39	15.28	17.42
60	13.03	14.01	12.18	14.20	13.53	13.67	12.00	14.47	11.83	14.09	12.49	14.06
65	10.33	10.96	9.77	11.18	10.63	10.80	9.70	11.46	9.37	11.06	9.98	11.02
70	7.97	8.39	7.62	8.59	8.16	8.25	7.60	8.85	7.30	8.46	7.73	8.46
75	6.01	6.27	5.82	6.44	6.11	6.15	5.87	6.66	5.49	6.31	5.86	6.34
80	4.48	4.71	4.38	4.82	4.54	4.64	4.52	5.02	4.18	4.68	4.39	4.74
85	3.37	3.54	3.27	3.56	3.43	3.53	3.39	3.69	3.26	3.54	3.24	3.48
90	2.57	2.89	2.50	2.90	2.65	2.88	2.50	2.83	2.50	2.92	2.62	2.92
95	2.50	2.51	–	2.49	2.53	2.49	–	2.49	–	2.50	2.57	2.50

* Includes rural communities with 20,000–100,000 inhabitants.

Source: Ballod (1906), p. 11.

As has been demonstrated, the most substantial differences in the urban death rates between England and Germany concerned infants, with much higher rates in the German sample. Although in Germany infant mortality remained high throughout the nineteenth century, it differed widely between towns and was not invariably higher than in rural areas or in the national aggregate.[14] In areas with high infant

---

14 For a comprehensive account of the development of infant mortality in Germany see Kintner (1982); Vögele (1994). For an attempt to explain areal variations see: Imhof (1981a). With special reference to social inequality see Spree (1988; 1995). An explicit regional approach is offered by Stöckel (1986).

Table 10: Average life expectancy for men and women in Prussia, 1905–1906

Age	Prussia		Rural		Small towns <20,000		Medium-sized towns 20,000–100,000		Large towns >100,000	
	m	f	m	f	m	f	m	f	m	f
0	44.81	48.50	46.32	48.90	43.56	47.84	42.58	47.64	42.71	48.35
1	54.75	57.16	56.52	57.58	53.16	56.46	52.07	56.15	52.43	57.12
2	56.17	58.58	57.92	58.90	54.46	57.82	53.78	57.85	53.92	58.75
3	56.03	58.46	57.76	58.74	54.31	57.71	53.75	57.88	53.85	58.70
4	55.60	58.04	57.32	58.31	53.85	57.29	53.34	57.53	53.46	58.31
5	55.01	57.47	56.73	57.72	53.25	56.72	52.77	57.02	52.88	57.75
10	51.09	53.65	52.81	53.91	49.34	52.86	48.92	53.22	48.95	53.91
15	46.68	49.36	48.41	49.64	44.96	48.66	44.47	48.90	44.50	49.54
20	42.57	45.21	44.27	45.50	40.86	44.60	40.44	44.71	40.40	45.29
25	38.64	41.21	40.47	41.50	37.02	40.69	36.31	40.70	36.32	41.23
30	34.62	37.29	36.39	37.58	33.17	36.86	32.32	36.78	32.24	37.25
35	30.61	33.38	32.26	33.65	29.25	33.01	28.39	32.87	28.29	33.31
40	26.71	29.48	28.21	29.74	25.47	29.17	24.62	29.02	24.52	29.38
45	23.03	25.58	24.34	25.78	21.93	25.33	21.08	25.17	21.82	25.55
50	19.57	21.67	20.65	21.77	18.64	21.49	17.87	21.36	17.81	21.75
55	16.34	17.97	17.17	17.98	15.57	17.86	14.92	17.79	14.90	18.18
60	13.35	14.51	13.95	14.45	12.73	14.46	12.22	14.46	12.23	14.79
65	10.63	11.42	11.02	11.33	10.21	11.40	9.81	11.46	9.80	11.77
70	8.22	8.77	8.44	8.66	7.94	8.73	7.63	8.84	7.74	9.11
75	6.20	6.61	6.33	6.52	6.04	6.60	5.81	6.67	5.96	6.89
80	4.61	4.92	4.65	4.86	4.53	4.86	4.40	4.96	4.57	5.14
85	3.41	3.74	3.39	3.72	3.48	3.68	3.36	3.75	3.34	3.83
90	2.58	2.86	2.52	2.86	2.86	2.93	2.50	2.84	2.62	2.78

Source: Ballod (1913), p. 58.

mortality, the rates were lower in an urban environment, while in low infant mortality regions the opposite was the case. In Bavaria, Wurtemberg and Baden, i.e. in non-breast-feeding areas, IMR was consistently lower in urban areas compared with rural areas (Maier, 1871, p. 181; Prinzing, 1900, p. 633). In the last three decades of the nineteenth century urban–rural differences in infant mortality were predominantly marked by a higher risk of dying after the initial month (post-neonatal mortality) in towns (Prinzing, 1900, pp. 610–12). Still-births and neonatal mortality were consistently higher in rural areas, yet urban–rural differences were much less pronounced (Bleicher, 1895, pp. 476–77; Prinzing, 1900, pp. 602–09; Knodel, 1977, p. 373). Taking account of all German towns with over 15,000 inhabitants, infant mortality declined in the last decades of the nineteenth century (Fig. 13), whereas the decline for the whole of Prussia did not begin before the first decades of the twentieth century (Rothenbacher, 1982, pp. 343–47, 396–97). In the course of the twentieth century the situation changed and infant mortality rates in towns dropped below those in rural areas (Kuczynski, 1897, pp. 198–214; Vögele, 1991, p. 26): for example, in Berlin infant mortality was 90.1 (per 1,000 births) in 1924–1926, compared with 103.8 in Prussia as a whole (Prinzing, 1930/31, p. 569). Even the death rate of illegitimate infants—traditionally very high—declined in an urban environment, whereas they increased in the countryside (Prinzing, 1900, p. 613).[15]

This might partly be attributed to an earlier onset and faster decline of urban birth rates. The specific interrelationship between the birth rate and infant mortality, however, is still far from clear, both with respect to the strength of the relationship and the direction of the influences (Knodel, 1974, pp. 148–87; 1977, pp. 367–71; Woods et al., 1989, pp. 121–26). A decline in infant mortality may lead to more extended birth intervals, either by a conscious limitation of reproductive behaviour, through birth control, or by lactation-amenorrhoea during the period of breast-feeding. In this sense, intensive breast-feeding reduces not only infant mortality, but also fertility (Knodel, 1988, pp. 393–405). A smaller number of children again might have a positive influence on the survival chances of infants, in that greater spacing between births might lead to more intensive care of already existing children. For Germany,

---

15 The percentage of total births which were illegitimate remained fairly constant in Germany over time, ranging between 8 and 12 per cent between 1867 and 1939. The potential impact of the legitimacy composition of births on the mortality decline can therefore be neglected. There were, however, vast local and regional differences in illegitimacy, accounting in some cases for 20 per cent of total births in south-eastern Germany, Thüringen and Saxony in contrast to 3 to 4 per cent in the western parts of Prussia. In the German urban sample the percentage of illegitimate births from all live births in 1907 was 27.7 in Munich, 19.7 in Dresden, 18.9 in Breslau, 18.4 in Berlin, 18.1 in Leipzig and Nuremberg, 13.8 in Frankfurt, 13.2 in Hamburg, 11.9 in Cologne, and only 7.6 in Düsseldorf. Source: *Statistisches Jahrbuch Deutscher Städte*, **16** (1908), p. 29. Unfortunately, these comparisons rest on this illegitimate ratio, rather than on a more refined index relating illegitimacy to the specific age-groups of unmarried women.

The legitimacy composition of births, however, had only minor effects on the infant mortality rate. H. Kintner gives an illustrative example in this respect. Supposing that two administrative areas had the same mortality rates of illegitimate and legitimate infants as Germany in 1875–1877 (23.2 per 100 births) and 20 per cent of all live births were illegitimate in one area in contrast to 4 per cent in the other, the infant mortality rates would be 24.8 and 22.7 respectively. This comparison even over-estimates the impact of the legitimacy composition as differences in mortality rates were lower in areas with a high percentage of illegitimates. Bearing this in mind, differences in the illegitimate rates of infants in Germany and Britain, with rates around one per cent, cannot satisfactorily explain the immense differences in the levels of infant mortality between the two nations. See Kintner (1982), pp. 55–56; Knodel (1974), p. 76.

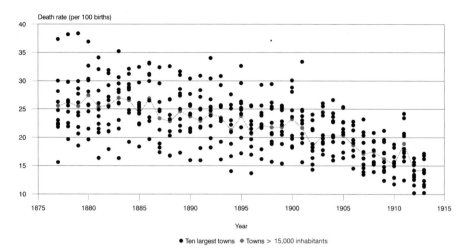

Figure 13: Infant mortality rate 1877–1913 in German towns (per 100 births)
Sources: *Veröffentlichungen des Kaiserlichen Gesundheitsamtes (Beilagen)* (1878–1914).

at the end of the nineteenth century, a strong statistical association between the birth rate and infant mortality can be established in some areas (Mayr, 1870, p. 230). In Bavaria during the period 1871 to 1910, for example, the coefficient of correlation between the birth rate and infant mortality was up to 0.7777 (sig=0.001, n=40),[16] i.e. a high birth rate went along with high infant mortality, or as a contemporary commentator expressed it, 'mass births provoke mass deaths of infants, and these again provoke mass births' (G. Mayr quoted in Burgdörfer, 1914, p. 97). In the urban milieu there was no direct association in both countries (Ballod, 1899, pp. 41–42; *Forty-Second Annual Report*, 1913, p. 57). A reduced birth rate did not lead obviously to a decline in infant mortality. Nor is there any direct verification of the plausible argument that a decline in infant mortality brought about lower birth rates. A correlation between the birth rate and infant mortality in 19 German towns with over 15,000 inhabitants (amongst which are the ten largest) suggests a figure of only 0.3657 between 1877 and 1913 (sig.=0.001; n=691).[17] Using fertility rates for the ten largest towns in selected years, the analysis provides a similarly low coefficient.[18] This is at least partly the result of regional particularities. F. Prinzing hinted that high birth rates in the Rhineland were accompanied by low infant mortality rates (Prinzing, 1900, p. 640): the towns of this region, amongst them Düsseldorf, registered low infant mortality and were frontrunners in the general overall decline in infant mortality after the turn of the century. Obviously, infants benefited to a large degree from the improving urban health conditions. The following analysis of the predominant disease panaroma will provide a further insight into health conditions in the period under consideration.

16 Source: Burgdörfer (1914), pp. 102–03.
17 Source: *Veröffentlichungen des Kaiserlichen Gesundheitsamtes (Beilagen)* (1878–1914).
18 R = 0.3694, sig. (two-tailed) = 0.045. Selected years and sources see Table 3.

THE URBAN DISEASE PANORAMA—CAUSES OF DEATH

During the period when the gap between urban and rural mortality began to close, the main causes of death in both countries were diseases of the respiratory and digestive systems, although 'modern' causes of death (diseases of the heart and of the circulatory system as well as cancer) were already on the increase. Correspondingly, in England and Wales, as well as in Germany, the urban disease panorama was predominantly characterized by respiratory (tuberculosis and acute respiratory disease) and digestive diseases (diarrhoea, dysentery, typhoid fever, enteric fever, simple continued fever, convulsions).[19]

In the English towns of the period 1871–1880, the disease panorama was marked by a high prevalence of respiratory conditions, with these and phthisis (tuberculosis) accounting for 73.7 deaths per 10,000 inhabitants. The main single killers were diseases of the respiratory system, with 48.2 deaths a year per 10,000 inhabitants, followed by 'other causes' (41.7), diseases of the nervous system (28.2), phthisis (25.5), diseases of the circulatory system (12.8) and diarrhoea and dysentery (12.34) (for more detail see Table 20). The latter, combined with the rate for diseases of the digestive system, enteric and simple continued fever, formed a total of 26.1 deaths from gastro-intestinal diseases. These main killers are followed by the group of childhood infectious diseases, the most prominent of which were scarlet fever (8.5) and whooping cough (7.8). Violent deaths played an important part in the cause of death panorama, with 7.9 annual deaths per 10,000 inhabitants. Cancer, with 5.0 deaths, was not yet among the predominant diseases.

In the German towns of 1877 the outstanding killers were diseases of the digestive system, with a death rate of 61.3 per 10,000 inhabitants.[20] Considering that 'weakness' (27.3) also refers mainly to digestive diseases, this underlines the paramount importance of this disease complex. Together with typhoid fever (4.7) and dysentery (1.4) this produces a total of 94.7 deaths per 10,000 inhabitants, caused by the gastro-intestinal disease complex. The second main killer in German towns was the respiratory disease complex, accounting for 67.3 deaths per 10,000 inhabitants, with 38.1 deaths from tuberculosis and 29.2 from lung disease. These were followed by 'other causes' (26.3) and diseases of the brain and nerves (21.5). Within the childhood disease complex, diphtheria (and croup) played an outstanding role, responsible for 9.1 deaths. Further important causes of death were infirmity (9.9), heart diseases (9.4), cancer (6.9) and violence (6.1).

19 For an approach drawing largely on contemporay reports and articles on health conditions in nineteenth-century cities see Rosen (1973); Smith (1979). For a detailed analysis based on primary sources see Kearns (1988a).
20 Compare Spree's analysis of the disease panorama for various Prussian *Regierungsbezirke* and towns (Spree, 1981b; 1986).

When compared with the national disease panorama, in England almost all important diseases showed higher death rates in an urban context (Fig. 14),[21] with 'other diseases' as the only substantial exception. This might be the result of inferior medical provision in rural areas, leading to uncertainty over diagnosis. The main differences between urban and national mortality, however, can be attributed to the two main disease complexes. Death rates from respiratory diseases, tuberculosis, whooping cough, but also, in second place, from digestive disease were substantially to the disadvantage of urban areas.

The situation in Germany was more complex (Table 11; Fig. 15; Vögele, 1991, p. 29). Almost exclusively responsible for the higher overall death rates in towns were the main killers of the period, namely respiratory and digestive diseases. Death rates from cancer were also substantially higher in urban areas. By contrast, death rates from most childhood infectious diseases (especially diphtheria), childbirth, typhoid fever and 'other causes' were lower in urban areas, when compared with the aggregate figures for Prussia in 1877. The main advantage of the towns, however, was in the death rate from infirmity, which was more than twice as high in the Prussian aggregate (towns 9.9 per 10,000 inhabitants; Prussia 25.4). Although there is no statistical evidence available, the high rates in Prussia might be the result of strong migration effects. Younger people moved into the towns in order to find work, while older individuals may have tried to leave the expensive city and moved back to their places of birth. This led to a stronger representation of the higher age-groups in rural areas, which finds expression in the aggregate figures for Prussia. In the absence of obligatory death certification by medical personnel in Prussia and a low doctor: population ratio in rural areas, infirmity was a regular cause of death, diagnosed by the family or relatives of the victim.

By 1907 the picture had changed in some crucial respects. Overall mortality was lower in the sample of German towns when compared with Prussia. Although the urban advantage in the childhood disease complex had completely disappeared, this was counterbalanced by the elimination of the urban disadvantage with respect to mortality from respiratory diseases and 'weakness', a substantial reduction in the higher urban mortality from digestive diseases, and much lower death rates from 'other causes' (Fig. 15). Substantially higher death rates in urban areas were now registered with respect to cancer, heart disease and tuberculosis.

Correspondingly, the urban disease panorama was predominantly marked by these diseases (for more detail, see Table 18). The main single killer was still mortality from digestive diseases, with 23.2 deaths per 10,000 inhabitants, followed by tuberculosis (21.7) and lung diseases (21.2). These were followed by degenerative diseases, heart diseases (18.7) and cancer (12.5). Of similar importance were diseases of the brain and nerves with 12.7 deaths, 'other causes' (10.6) and 'weakness' (9.4). From an epidemiological point of view, the acute childhood infections played only a minor part in the disease panorama of early twentieth century German towns.

---

21 As relative figures would unnecessarily emphasize the role of epidemiologically less important diseases,
    Figures 14 and 15 simply show the result of the subtraction of the national death rates from the urban rates.

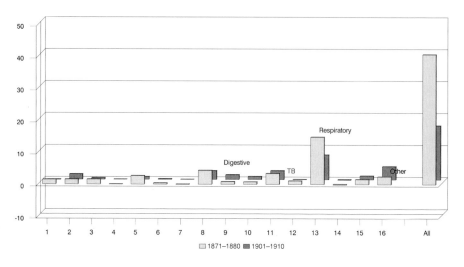

Urban death rate – death rate for England and Wales

Figure 14: Differences in standardized mortality in English and Welsh towns, 1871–1880 and 1901–1910, and SMR in England and Wales, 1871–80

1=Smallpox; 2= Measles; 3=Scarlet fever; 4=Diphtheria; 5=Whooping cough; 6=Typhus; 7=Enteric fever and simple continued fever; 8=Diarrhoea and dysentery, diseases of the digestive system and cholera; 9=Cancer; 10=Other tuberculous diseases; 11=Phthisis and pulmonary tuberculosis; 12=Diseases of the circulatory system; 13=Diseases of the respiratory system, pneumonia, bronchitis; 13=Childbirth and puerperal fever; 15=Violence; 16=Other causes; All causes.

Sources: *Decennial Supplements to the Annual Reports of the Registrar-General of Births, Deaths, and Marriages in England and Wales* (1871–1880 and 1901–1910).

In England, urban death rates still surpassed the national average, due to substantially higher urban mortality from respiratory diseases, tuberculosis and digestive diseases (Fig. 14). The reduction in the gap between urban and national mortality resulted from a slightly reduced urban disadvantage with respect to respiratory diseases, whooping cough and scarlet fever.

In the urban disease panorama of English towns most deaths from specified causes resulted from respiratory diseases, namely pneumonia (15.8 per 10,000 inhabitants), bronchitis (14.2), pulmonary tuberculosis (7.4) and phthisis (7.4) (for more detail see Table 22). Further important killers were cancer (9.8), diarrhoea and dysentery (7.9) and violence (6.6).

In both countries the contribution of the individual diseases towards the overall decline in urban mortality was distributed differently (see Table 11). In urban England the major contribution was due to tuberculosis which accounted for a 14.9 per cent fall in mortality, followed by respiratory diseases (11.4 per cent), scarlet fever (9.9 per cent), diarrhoea and dysentery (6.1 per cent), whooping cough (6.0 per cent) and smallpox (5.3 per cent). Whereas in the English towns the lung disease complex as a whole played a major role with an overall contribution of 26.3 per cent (tuberculosis and respiratory dis-

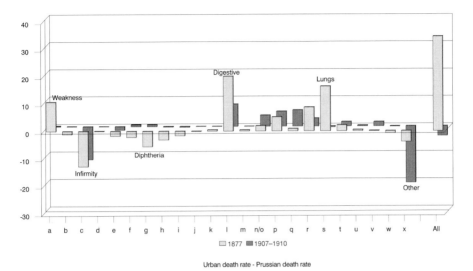

Figure 15: Differences in standardized mortality in Prussian towns, 1877 and 1907–1910, and SMR in Prussia, 1877

A=Weakness of life; B=Childbirth; C=Infirmity; D=Smallpox; E=Scarlet fever; F=Measles and rubella; G=Diphtheria and croup; H=Whooping cough; I=Typhoid fever; J=Typhus; K=Dysentery; L=Digestive system; M=Scrofula; N=Tuberculosis; P=Cancer; Q=Heart; R=Brain and nerves; S=Lungs; T=Urinary system; U=Influenza; V=Other communicable diseases; W=Violence; X=Other causes; All causes. Sources: See Appendix 2.

eases) to the decline, in the German towns it was the digestive diseases that played an overwhelming role in the urban mortality decline, accounting for 34.5 per cent of the registered fall, followed by the related 'weakness' (16.2 per cent). An essential role was also played by the respiratory disease complex, accounting for 14.9 (tuberculosis) and 7.2 per cent (respiratory diseases) respectively of the overall fall in mortality. The decline in diphtheria (6.0 per cent) was the most predominant factor in relation to the childhood infectious diseases. The overall decline in urban mortality was substantially counterbalanced by an increase in deaths from cancer and heart disease.

Summing up so far, the predominant causes of death in the urban disease panorama in both countries were respiratory diseases, including tuberculosis, and digestive diseases. Both played key roles in determining the level of urban mortality. The contribution of the respiratory disease complex to the decline was of similar magnitude in both urban samples (in English towns 26.3 per cent; in German towns 22.1 per cent). However, whereas the respiratory complex played a more outstanding part in the decline of urban mortality in England,[22] the digestive disease complex

---

22 The substantial contribution of respiratory diseases towards the level and decline of overall mortality in Britain might well have been exceptional, when compared with other Western European countries or the United States. See Meeker (1972); Condran and Crimmins-Gardner (1978); Higgs (1979); Condran and Cheney (1982).

played a substantial role in the reduction of mortality in German towns. Therefore, in both countries special emphasis has to be put on the development of the two diseases.

In the towns of England and Wales during the 1870s, the tuberculosis death rate was lower than in German towns. However, if the rates for all the respiratory diseases are analysed, the figures were similar, with a slight advantage for the German towns (73.6 deaths per 10,000 inhabitants in the ten largest English towns, 67.3 in the ten largest German towns). From the 1870s to the first decade of the twentieth century the absolute fall in the death rate from all respiratory diseases was sharper in the largest English towns (28.9) than in the whole of England and Wales (23.0) or in the German towns (24.4). The decline for the whole of Germany was even less (5.5), so that urban and rural mortality rates from respiratory diseases tended to converge, although the urban figures remained higher. In Prussia, for example, in 1876 35.8 persons (per 10,000 inhabitants) died from tuberculosis in towns (*Stadtgemeinden*), as against 28.4 in rural areas (*Landgemeinden*); by 1926 the tuberculosis death rate was 11.4 in urban areas, and 8.3 in rural areas (Fränkel, 1911, p. 534; Prinzing, 1930/31, p. 573). In both countries the decline in the tuberculosis death rate was more constant than the development of the death rate from respiratory diseases, which even increased in England and Wales until the beginning of the 1890s (Figs 16–19). Again town size seems not to be so crucial in Germany: whereas in England the death rates from tuberculosis and respiratory diseases were above the average for the whole country, in Germany only the death rates from tuberculosis were largely above the average of all towns with more than 15,000 inhabitants, whereas the urban death rates from respiratory diseases differed widely, so that the rates of the ten largest towns were almost equally distributed above and below the national average. In England and Wales, the urban mortality figures were uniformly above the national rates, while in Germany the situation was more complex.

In England during this period (1871–1880) mortality from diseases of the digestive system, including diarrhoea and dysentery as well as enteric and simple continued fever, was higher in the large towns than in the country as a whole (26.2 deaths per 10,000 inhabitants in urban areas, 23.2 in England and Wales), whereas the rates for typhoid fever alone were relatively similar (4.2 deaths per 10,000 inhabitants in urban areas compared with 4.3 deaths in England and Wales). The decline of the whole disease complex from the 1870s to the end of the nineteenth century was slightly more modest in the largest towns (2.5)[23] than in England and Wales (3.6), so that mortality remained higher in urban areas (23.7 deaths per 10,000 inhabitants in urban areas compared with 20.2 deaths in England and Wales). The decline in mortality from diarrhoea and dysentery between the 1870s and the first decade of the twentieth century was stronger in urban areas (4.4) than nationwide (3.4). Mortality from typhoid fever alone, however, still showed similar rates in the first decade of the twentieth century (0.9 deaths per 10,000 inhabitants in both urban areas and England and Wales).

23 For the digestive diseases the period 1891–1900 has been selected, because this is the last decade when diarrhoea and dysentery as well as diseases of the digestive system were recorded; after the turn of the century only the diarrhoea and dysentery categories were retained.

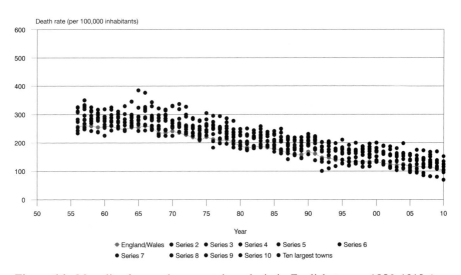

Figure 16: Mortality from pulmonary tuberculosis in English towns, 1856–1910 (per 100,000 inhabitants)
Sources: *Annual Reports of the Registrar-General of Births, Deaths, and Marriages in England and Wales* (1856–1910).

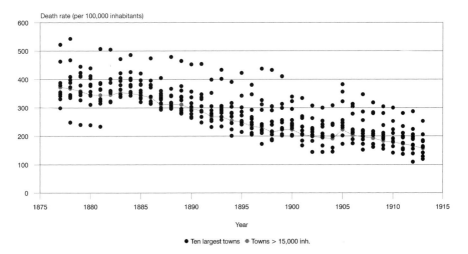

Figure 17: Mortality from tuberculosis in German towns, 1877–1913 (per 100,000 inhabitants)
Sources: *Veröffentlichungen des Kaiserlichen Gesundheitsamtes (Beilagen)* (1878–1914).

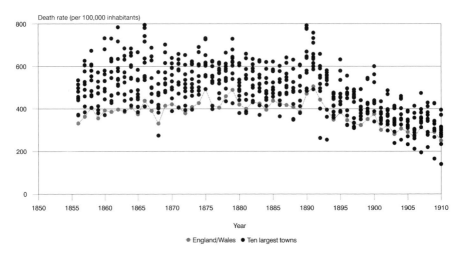

Figure 18: Mortality from respiratory diseases in English towns, 1856–1910 (per 100,000 inhabitants. Respiratory diseases: diseases of the respiratory system, influenza, pneumonia, bronchitis, whooping cough.

Sources: *Annual Reports of the Registrar-General of Births, Deaths, and Marriages in England and Wales* (1856–1910).

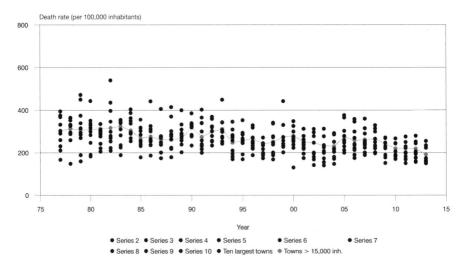

Figure 19: Mortality from acute respiratory diseases in German towns, 1877–1913 (per 100,000 inhabitants)

Respiratory diseases: see Appendix 1.

Sources: *Veröffentlichungen des Kaiserlichen Gesundheitsamtes (Beilagen)* (1878–1914).

The higher mortality rates in German towns of the 1870s were to a large degree determined by differences in mortality from digestive diseases: average rates were almost three times as high in German towns and more than twice as high in Prussia in 1877, when compared with England and Wales 1871–1880. In German towns the decline of this disease complex was stronger than in England (38.5). The rates fell more sharply in urban areas than in the country as a whole: (33.8), so that the urban–rural ratio became more balanced with slightly lower rates in the national aggregate.[24] It should be noted that a major part of the decline was furnished by the non-acute digestive diseases. Taking typhoid fever alone, the rates for the largest German towns showed lower values than those for Prussia in 1877 and 1907. Following the annual development of the death rate from digestive diseases in the English case is more problematic (Fig. 20), as the apparent increase in the 1880s and 1890s and the subsequent decline were to a substantial degree the results of changes in disease registration (see Chapter 3, Table 11 and Appendix 3). In any case, however, the 'urban penalty' was quite obvious with the largest towns reporting higher mortality rates than the national aggregate. The health conditions in German towns again were more independent of population size as the rates are distributed above and below the average for all towns with a population exceeding 15,000 inhabitants (Fig. 21).

AGE-SPECIFIC CAUSES OF DEATH

As diseases affected people differently depending on their age and sex, and urban and rural areas were characterized by a different population composition, the disease panorama has to be differentiated in more detail. Particularly in relation to the largest German towns, the highest mortality rates in 1877 occurred in the age-group under one year dying from diseases of the digestive system (1,717.12 per 10,000), followed by deaths from 'weakness' (too weak to live) in the same age-group (Table 12). In the age-group 1–5 years, mortality from digestive diseases stood at 75.9, followed by respiratory diseases (69.1) and diphtheria (60.0). The next age-group 5–15 was mainly affected by mortality from diphtheria and croup (15.1), scarlet fever (11.6), as well as tuberculosis (8.4), whereas the digestive diseases played a less important role. The following age-groups were marked by an increasing death rate from tuberculosis and other diseases of the respiratory system. In the last age-group (over 60) infirmity (*Altersschwäche*, i.e. weakness of old age) was the biggest single category, followed by diseases of the lungs and of the brain and nerves. In comparison with Prussia in 1877 the following major differences were apparent (see Tables 12 and 13):

(1) In Prussia the death rate from diseases of the respiratory system was lower in almost all age-groups, whereas the tuberculosis death rate was higher in the over-60 age-group.

(2) The death rates from digestive diseases and weakness amongst infants were lower in Prussia.

---

24 Mortality from digestive diseases is much higher if different sources are taken into account. See the age- and cause-specific mortality data in Tables 12–19.

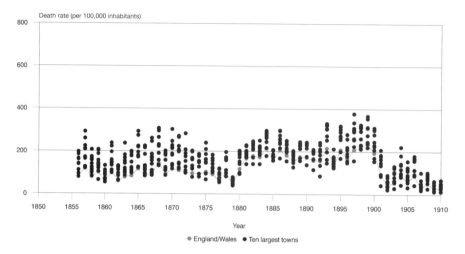

Figure 20: Mortality from digestive diseases in English towns, 1856–1910 (per 100,000 inhabitants). Digestive diseases: diarrhoea, dysentery and diseases of the digestive system; see Appendix 3.

Source: *Annual Reports of the Registrar-General of Births, Deaths, and Marriages in England and Wales* (1856–1910).

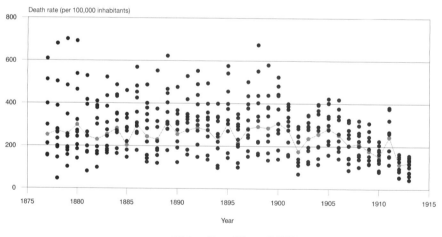

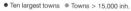

Figure 21: Mortality from acute digestive diseases in German towns, 1877–1913 (per 100,000 inhabitants)

For the classification of the diseases see Appendix 1.

Sources: *Veröffentlichungen des Kaiserlichen Gesundheitsamtes (Beilagen)* (1878–1914).

Table 11: Cause-specific mortality decline in German and English towns, absolute (related to death rates per 10,000 inhabitants) and relative figures

	Decline 1877–1907 in German towns			Decline 1871/80–1901/10 in English towns	
Cause of death	absolute	relative	Cause of death	absolute	relative
Weakness of life	17.9	16.2			
Childbirth	0.5	0.5	Childbirth+puerperal	0.7	1.0
Infirmity	4.4	4.0			
Smallpox	0.1	0.1	Smallpox	3.8	5.3
Scarlet fever	4.2	3.8	Scarlet fever	7.1	9.9
Measles and rubella	0.4	0.4	Measles	0.9	1.3
Diphtheria and croup	6.6	6.0	Diphtheria	−0.7	−1.0
Whooping cough	1.2	1.1	Whooping cough	4.3	6.0
Typhoid fever	4.4	4.0	Enteric+simple fever	3.2	4.4
Typhus	0.0	0.0	Typhus	0.9	1.3
Dysentery	1.4	1.3	Digestive+ diarrhoea/dysentery	0.7	1.0*
Digestive system	38.1	34.5	Diarrhoea/dysentery only	4.4	6.1
Scrofula	0.9	0.8			
Tuberculosis	16.4	14.9	Phthisis+pulm. tb	10.7	14.9
			Tabes mesenterica	3.2	4.4
Cancer	−5.6	−5.1	Cancer	−4.8	-6.7
Heart	−9.3	−8.4			
Brain and nerves	8.8	8.0			
Lungs	8.0	7.2	Respiratory+pneumonia +bronchitis	8.2	11.4
Urinary system	−1.4	−1.3			
Influenza	−0.8	−0.7			
Other communicable diseases	−1.2	−1.1			
Violence	−0.5	−0.5	Suicide+violence	2.1	1.39
Other causes	15.7	14.2	Other causes	−34.9	−48.5
All causes	110.4	100.0	All causes	72.0	100.0

* Diarrhoea and dysentery, 1901–1910 + diseases of the digestive system, 1891–1900. The period 1891–1900 is the last decade when both diarrhoea and dysentery as well as diseases of the digestive system were recorded; thereafter only data on diarrhoea and dysentery were included.

Sources: See Appendix 2; *Decennial Supplements to the Annual Reports of the Registrar-General of Births, Deaths, and Marriages in England and Wales* (1871–1880 and 1901–1910).

(3) Mortality from the so-called childhood infectious diseases, such as scarlet fever, measles and rubella, diphtheria and croup as well as whooping cough, was higher amongst infants and young children until the age of five in Prussia.

(4) Mortality from infirmity in the highest age-group was higher for Prussia. This not only reflected urban–rural differences in the age-structure of the population at risk—as can be seen from the SMR—but might also be attributed to urban–rural differences in the quality of diagnosis, as a function of much better medical provision in urban areas (see Chapter 12).

(5) For almost all higher age-groups death rates from violence were similar in Prussia and in the largest towns. This implies that urban-industrial and rural-agricultural working lives obviously bore similar risks. In the highest age-group (over 60) Prussian rates surpassed those in the largest towns—maybe a reflection of the prolonged working life in rural areas. The main difference, however, occurred amongst infants, with death rates from violence of 8.2 per 10,000 in urban areas and 3.5 in rural areas. It remains doubtful, however, whether this is the result of higher illegitimate rates in urban areas, as there is no statistical evidence.[25]

In the ten largest German towns mortality had declined by 1885 in almost all age-groups (except 1–5) and in 15 of the 23 disease categories. In contrast, diphtheria, influenza and diseases of the urinary system registered an increase of between one and three per 10,000; measles and rubella, cancer, scrofula, violence and 'other communicable diseases' registered a more marginal rise (Table 14). The figures for Prussia as a whole, on the other hand, remained almost stable (Table 15). The biggest change in the ten largest towns occurred in the digestive diseases group (especially affecting infants) with a fall in mortality from 61.3 to 48.6 per 10,000. This was followed by an improvement in mortality from typhoid and from scarlet fever, especially in the age-group 1–5, and from 'weakness'—also affecting mainly infants. Improvements in the other age-groups were more equally distributed over the whole disease panorama. Mortality rates from tuberculosis and from diseases of the lungs only showed a slight improvement.

By 1900 this trend had clearly become more obvious with major improvements in mortality rates (between 5 and 10 per 10,000) from digestive diseases, diphtheria, 'other causes', tuberculosis, 'weakness', and diseases of the brain and nerves (Table 16). This improvement, however, was accompanied by an increase in the death rate from degenerative diseases (cancer, diseases of the heart and circulatory system). Furthermore, the death rate from diseases of the respiratory system, excluding tuber-

---

25 According to Prinzing the higher death rates of illegitimate infants operated mainly through digestive diseases. The disease panorama he referred to, however, did not include violent deaths. See Prinzing (1906), p. 289. The correlation coefficient between the ratio of illegitimate live births and infant deaths from violence, from digestive diseases, and from weakness in 1907 are:

Violence: $r = -0.0014$, sig. (two-tailed) = 0.997;
Digestive diseases: $r = -0.1719$, sig. (two-tailed) = 0.658;
Weakness: $r = 0.4115$, sig. (two-tailed) = 0.271.
Sources: See Tables 18 and 19, and *Statistisches Jahrbuch Deutscher Städte*, **16** (1908), p. 29.

culosis, remained almost stable. In Prussia as a whole the situation had improved slightly, with the age-groups 5 to 40 benefiting in particular, whereas the death rate of infants and people over 40 years of age actually increased (Table 17). These trends continued during the first decade of the twentieth century (Table 18), although there was an improvement in the situation of infants in Prussia (Table 19). A disease group that remained remarkably stable was deaths from violence, with about six cases per 10,000 inhabitants, both in the large towns and in Prussia as a whole.

In England the urban disease panorama was differently distributed (Tables 20 and 21). Infant mortality was much lower in comparison with German towns. Consequently digestive diseases did not play as important a part as they did in Germany. In contrast there was a higher urban risk in England of dying from diseases of the respiratory system, both as an infant and especially over 45 years of age, and from phthisis with increasing age. Diseases of the nervous system, which especially affected infants and the elderly, also played an important role: the death rate was 27.92 per 10,000 inhabitants in the English towns and 21.46 in the German towns. The English death rates were generally higher in an urban context as far as almost all causes of death in all age-groups were concerned, yet the 'urban penalty' in the 1870s was predominantly marked by diseases of the respiratory system.

By the beginning of the twentieth century mortality had improved substantially (Table 22). The infectious diseases affecting mainly children (smallpox, measles, scarlet fever) had been conquered to a larger extent, mortality from diseases of the respiratory system had fallen, yet, with pneumonia, bronchitis and tuberculosis (including phthisis), they remained predominant in the disease panorama. Together with the digestive diseases they were decisively responsible for the persistence of an 'urban penalty', although almost all causes of death were still higher in urban areas than in England and Wales as a whole (with the exception of smallpox, influenza and childbirth) (Table 23). For infants the 'urban penalty' consisted mainly in the digestive disease complex, followed by pneumonia and violence. The latter might be a consequence of the larger number of illegitimate children in urban areas—which in a puritan context might have been more disadvantaged than in Germany.[26] In the following age-groups pneumonia and infectious diseases were the main killers, which remained especially threatening in an urban context. In the higher age-groups diseases of the respiratory system and cancer were predominant, and again living in the towns involved a major risk of dying from those diseases. The differences with Germany were still marked particularly in terms of the high continental mortality in the digestive disease group.

---

26 It remains difficult to estimate the extent to which this risk group had reduced chances of survival. In areas and countries (like Germany) with a high proportion of illegitimate infants they were most likely to be socially accepted to a larger degree and correspondingly found better living conditions than in areas with a low proportion (like England).

Table 12: Age- and cause-specific mortality (per 10,000 inhabitants) in the largest German towns (both sexes), 1877

Causes of death		All ages	0–1	1–5	5–15	15–30	30–40	40–60	>60	SMR*	SMR†
A	Weakness of life	27.3	828.4	21.4	1.0	0.0	0.0	0.0	0.0	31.0	27.0
B	Childbirth	1.8	0.0	0.0	0.1	2.9	4.3	0.7	0.2	1.3	1.5
C	Infirmity	9.9	0.3	0.3	0.5	0.4	1.1	1.1	171.0	12.5	13.5
D	Smallpox	0.1	0.8	0.3	0.0	0.0	0.0	0.1	0.3	0.1	0.1
E	Scarlet fever	5.0	8.2	29.4	11.6	0.3	0.3	0.1	0.0	6.0	6.1
F	Measles and rubella	2.2	22.8	14.3	0.6	0.0	0.1	0.0	0.1	2.5	2.3
G	Diphtheria and croup	9.1	27.9	60.0	15.1	0.5	0.2	0.3	0.5	10.9	10.8
H	Whooping cough	2.9	52.6	13.6	0.3	0.0	0.0	0.0	0.0	3.3	3.1
I	Typhoid fever	4.7	2.9	6.9	3.8	5.4	4.4	3.2	5.0	4.3	4.6
J	Typhus	0.0	0.0	0.0	0.0	0.0	0.0	0.0	0.0	0.0	0.0
K	Dysentery	1.4	18.6	3.9	0.8	0.2	0.2	0.7	2.1	1.6	1.5
L	Digestive system	61.3	1,717.1	75.9	2.0	1.1	2.0	3.3	10.2	69.5	61.3
M	Scrofula	0.9	10.7	5.6	0.3	0.0	2.4	0.0	0.1	1.4	1.3
N+O	Tuberculosis	38.1	40.3	21.4	8.4	33.1	55.7	60.0	50.9	34.0	35.4
P	Cancer	6.9	0.3	0.2	0.2	0.5	3.9	19.4	51.3	7.8	7.9
Q	Heart	9.4	16.1	3.9	3.4	2.2	5.3	17.8	63.4	10.5	10.8
R	Brain and nerves	21.5	131.4	46.9	6.2	2.7	8.3	24.7	102.2	24.2	24.1
S	Lungs	29.2	293.9	69.1	3.3	4.5	11.3	25.9	102.4	32.5	31.6
T	Urinary system	3.1	6.6	2.7	1.5	1.0	2.4	5.4	14.4	3.3	3.4
U	Influenza	0.4	4.0	1.1	0.0	0.0	0.0	0.1	2.7	0.5	0.5
V	Other communicable diseases	0.1	0.7	0.0	0.0	0.0	0.0	0.1	1.1	0.1	0.1
W	Violence	6.1	8.2	4.3	1.8	5.4	7.3	9.6	8.5	5.5	5.7
X	Other causes	26.3	226.6	26.9	6.1	6.5	15.8	34.9	95.7	28.5	27.9
All causes		267.7	3,417.9	408.0	66.8	66.8	124.5	207.3	681.8	291.2	280.4

* SMR Prussia 1877.

† SMR England and Wales 1871.

For the classification and grouping of the diseases in the individual towns during the recorded years see Appendix 1.

Sources: See Appendix 2.

Table 13: Age- and cause-specific mortality (per 10,000 inhabitants) in Prussia (both sexes), 1877

	Causes of death	All ages	0–1	1–5	5–15	15–30	30–40	40–60	>60	SMR*	SMR†
A	Weakness of life	20.4	464.2	32.7	4.2	0.0	0.0	0.0	0.0	–	18.2
B	Childbirth	2.4	0.0	0.0	0.0	3.7	8.1	2.1	0.0	–	2.7
C	Infirmity	25.4	0.1	0.1	0.3	0.4	0.5	0.9	353.3	–	27.3
D	Smallpox	0.0	0.0	0.0	0.0	0.0	0.0	0.0	0.0	–	0.0
E	Scarlet fever	7.8	28.7	41.3	10.2	0.8	0.1	0.0	0.0	–	7.8
F	Measles and rubella	4.6	38.1	24.8	2.7	0.1	0.0	0.0	0.0	–	4.4
G	Diphtheria and croup	16.4	94.2	91.0	15.0	0.4	0.2	0.2	0.2	–	16.0
H	Whooping cough	6.4	108.0	23.2	0.9	0.0	0.0	0.1	0.2	–	5.9
I	Typhoid fever	5.9	4.4	6.1	4.7	5.6	5.6	7.3	7.8	–	6.3
J	Typhus	0.1	0.0	0.0	0.0	0.1	0.1	0.2	0.2	–	0.1
K	Dysentery	1.1	11.7	3.4	0.6	0.2	0.2	0.4	0.9	–	1.0
L	Digestive system	49.5	1,131.6	78.0	3.4	1.3	1.8	2.5	5.2	–	44.0
M	Scrofula	0.9	7.1	4.8	0.8	0.0	0.0	0.0	0.0	–	0.9
N+O	Tuberculosis	32.0	21.7	11.8	5.3	28.3	41.2	57.3	81.1	–	33.8
P	Cancer	2.7	0.2	0.1	0.1	0.2	1.4	7.3	15.3	–	2.7
Q	Heart	9.6	5.6	5.2	2.6	2.5	5.3	17.1	55.0	–	9.9
R	Brain and nerves	15.6	88.8	21.3	5.1	3.2	7.0	17.5	59.5	–	15.5
S	Lungs	16.3	74.4	23.3	2.9	4.4	9.6	23.4	56.0	–	16.3
T	Urinary system	1.2	1.4	1.1	0.5	0.5	1.0	1.6	5.0	–	1.2
U	Influenza	–	–	–	–	–	–	–	–	–	–
V	Other communicable diseases	–	–	–	–	–	–	–	–	–	–
W	Violence	6.3	3.5	6.0	2.3	5.4	6.9	9.4	11.1	–	6.4
X	Other causes	32.3	243.9	43.2	8.5	8.6	15.5	38.5	85.2	–	31.7
	All causes	256.8	2,327.7	417.3	70.2	65.5	104.4	185.6	736.1	–	252.0

* SMR Prussia 1877.

† SMR England and Wales 1871.

For the classification and grouping of the diseases see Appendix 1.

Sources: See Appendix 2.

Table 14: Age- and cause-specific mortality (per 10,000 inhabitants) in the largest German towns (both sexes), 1885

Causes of death		All ages	0–1	1–5	5–15	15–30	30–40	40–60	>60	SMR*	SMR†
A	Weakness of life	25.1	871.8	19.5	0.2	0.0	0.0	0.0	0.0	32.1	27.9
B	Childbirth	1.4	0.0	0.0	0.0	2.1	3.8	0.8	0.0	1.1	1.2
C	Infirmity	9.0	0.1	0.2	0.4	0.2	0.4	0.7	147.9	10.7	11.6
D	Smallpox	0.1	0.9	0.1	0.0	0.0	0.1	0.1	0.3	0.1	0.1
E	Scarlet fever	3.0	5.7	19.0	5.9	0.3	0.1	0.0	0.0	3.6	3.6
F	Measles and rubella	3.1	38.7	22.1	0.8	0.1	0.0	0.1	0.2	3.9	3.7
G	Diphtheria and croup	11.7	34.0	83.2	19.5	0.4	0.2	0.2	0.2	14.5	14.4
H	Whooping cough	2.4	44.0	14.3	0.1	0.0	0.0	0.0	0.0	3.1	2.9
I	Typhoid fever	2.2	1.2	2.0	1.7	2.9	2.5	1.5	2.6	2.0	2.2
J	Typhus	0.0	0.0	0.0	0.0	0.0	0.0	0.0	0.0	0.0	0.0
K	Dysentery	0.3	3.4	1.1	0.2	0.1	0.0	0.2	0.7	0.4	0.4
L	Digestive system	48.6	1,542.3	59.0	1.6	1.1	1.9	3.3	9.1	61.5	54.1
M	Scrofula	1.2	12.5	9.2	0.3	0.0	0.0	0.0	0.0	1.5	1.4
N+O	Tuberculosis	37.0	37.6	23.3	8.6	32.1	58.9	55.9	46.8	33.3	34.7
P	Cancer	7.6	0.3	0.2	0.1	0.4	3.8	19.7	55.8	8.1	8.3
Q	Heart	9.3	10.6	2.0	2.6	2.3	6.1	16.6	63.1	9.9	10.2
R	Brain and nerves	20.2	96.0	39.3	6.5	2.9	8.2	24.0	112.5	22.9	23.0
S	Lungs	29.0	298.5	83.6	3.2	4.0	10.1	23.5	105.7	33.8	32.8
T	Urinary system	4.1	4.4	4.8	1.8	1.4	3.2	6.7	19.4	4.3	4.4
U	Influenza	2.3	56.9	9.3	0.0	0.0	0.0	0.0	0.2	3.0	2.7
V	Other communicable diseases	0.2	3.0	0.2	0.0	0.1	0.0	0.1	0.7	0.2	0.2
W	Violence	6.2	5.2	4.3	1.7	5.7	7.8	9.5	11.3	5.7	6.0
X	Other causes	24.8	208.5	30.1	5.7	6.2	16.4	33.1	85.9	27.1	26.6
	All causes	249.5	3,275.4	426.9	60.9	62.3	123.5	196.1	662.4	282.6	272.2

* SMR Prussia 1877.

† SMR England and Wales 1871.

For the classification and grouping of the diseases in the individual towns during the recorded years see Appendix 1.

Sources: See Appendix 2.

Table 15: Age- and cause-specific mortality (per 10,000 inhabitants) in Prussia (both sexes), 1885

Causes of death	All ages	0–1	1–5	5–15	15–30	30–40	40–60	>60	SMR*	SMR†
A Weakness of life	19.7	526.8	25.2	3.3	0.0	0.0	0.0	0.0	21.5	19.0
B Childbirth	2.3	0.0	0.0	0.0	3.3	8.2	1.9	0.0	2.1	2.3
C Infirmity	25.0	0.1	0.1	0.3	0.3	0.4	1.0	321.7	23.0	24.8
D Smallpox	0.1	1.4	0.3	0.1	0.1	0.1	0.1	0.1	0.1	0.1
E Scarlet fever	6.2	22.4	32.3	9.3	0.4	0.1	0.0	0.0	6.3	6.3
F Measles and rubella	5.6	46.1	33.1	3.4	0.1	0.0	0.0	0.0	5.9	5.7
G Diphtheria and croup	18.8	94.8	106.6	20.7	0.8	0.3	0.2	0.2	19.4	19.1
H Whooping cough	4.8	90.1	17.1	0.7	0.0	0.0	0.1	0.3	5.1	4.7
I Typhoid fever	3.4	2.4	2.9	2.8	3.7	3.4	3.7	4.7	3.2	3.4
J Typhus	0.0	0.0	0.0	0.0	0.0	0.0	0.0	0.0	0.0	0.0
K Dysentery	0.6	6.8	1.8	0.4	0.1	0.1	0.2	0.6	0.6	0.6
L Digestive system	46.2	1,193.0	70.7	3.3	1.0	1.4	1.9	3.6	50.3	44.6
M Scrofula	1.0	9.8	5.3	0.7	0.0	0.0	0.0	0.0	1.1	1.0
N+O Tuberculosis	30.8	23.6	12.2	6.1	27.4	41.9	53.7	70.8	29.2	30.5
P Cancer	3.5	0.2	0.2	0.1	0.2	1.7	9.2	20.7	3.5	3.5
Q Heart	8.7	4.5	3.3	2.4	2.3	4.5	15.1	51.0	8.4	8.7
R Brain and nerves	16.2	78.6	21.2	6.3	3.5	7.2	18.6	65.8	16.0	16.0
S Lungs	21.9	114.9	36.5	4.1	5.5	11.4	28.4	75.5	21.8	21.7
T Urinary system	1.9	1.9	1.9	1.0	0.7	1.6	2.7	7.4	1.8	1.9
U Influenza	–	–	–	–	–	–	–	–	–	–
V Other communicable diseases	–	–	–	–	–	–	–	–	–	–
W Violence	6.2	3.7	5.5	2.2	5.7	7.1	9.7	11.5	5.9	6.1
X Other causes	27.5	212.9	32.5	7.2	7.4	14.7	34.5	78.1	27.6	27.1
All causes	250.4	2,433.9	408.6	74.1	62.5	104.0	181.1	712.0	252.9	247.1

* SMR Prussia 1877
† SMR England and Wales 1871
For the classification and grouping of the diseases see Appendix 1.
Sources: See Appendix 2.

Table 16: Age- and cause-specific mortality (per 10,000 inhabitants) in the largest German towns (both sexes), 1900

	Causes of death	All ages	0–1	1–5	5–15	15–30	30–40	40–60	>60	SMR*	SMR†
A	Weakness of life	18.7	746.3	4.8	0.1	0.0	0.0	0.0	0.0	26.2	22.6
B	Childbirth	0.9	0.0	0.0	0.0	1.4	2.3	0.5	0.0	0.7	0.8
C	Infirmity	8.4	0.2	0.1	0.5	0.2	0.3	0.5	106.3	7.8	8.4
D	Smallpox	0.0	0.0	0.0	0.0	0.0	0.0	0.0	0.1	0.0	0.0
E	Scarlet fever	1.7	2.0	11.6	3.7	0.2	0.1	0.0	0.0	2.2	2.2
F	Measles and rubella	2.7	38.9	19.4	0.7	0.0	0.0	0.0	0.0	3.6	3.4
G	Diphtheria and croup	2.1	10.5	15.3	3.3	0.1	0.1	0.0	0.1	2.8	2.7
H	Whooping cough	1.9	39.9	10.6	0.2	0.0	0.0	0.0	0.0	2.6	2.4
I	Typhoid fever	0.6	0.2	0.5	0.4	0.8	0.6	0.6	0.3	0.5	0.6
J	Typhus	0.0	0.0	0.0	0.0	0.0	0.0	0.0	0.0	0.0	0.0
K	Dysentery	0.0	0.2	0.1	0.0	0.0	0.1	0.0	0.1	0.0	0.0
L	Digestive system	38.5	1,367.8	34.6	1.4	1.0	1.4	2.9	7.5	52.5	46.0
M	Scrofula	1.5	25.3	9.6	0.1	0.0	0.0	0.0	0.0	1.9	1.8
N+O	Tuberculosis	28.0	53.7	28.4	8.7	23.4	34.0	39.3	36.0	25.6	26.6
P	Cancer	10.8	0.5	0.7	0.2	0.9	4.6	23.9	68.0	10.1	10.3
Q	Heart	12.4	12.5	1.9	2.5	2.6	5.7	20.4	78.0	11.6	12.0
R	Brain and nerves	14.9	102.8	22.1	3.9	1.7	4.4	17.0	71.6	15.8	15.7
S	Lungs	28.9	331.6	64.6	2.5	3.2	7.4	22.5	115.9	32.8	31.7
T	Urinary system	5.1	6.1	1.9	1.1	1.4	2.5	9.9	25.8	4.9	5.0
U	Influenza	0.5	0.3	0.1	0.0	0.0	0.1	0.4	3.1	0.3	0.4
V	Other communicable diseases	0.2	8.0	0.1	0.0	0.0	0.0	0.0	0.0	0.3	0.3
W	Violence	6.2	7.8	5.2	2.2	5.1	6.1	8.9	12.3	5.6	5.9
X	Other causes	15.7	144.6	7.6	2.9	5.0	9.0	21.4	55.2	16.4	16.1
	All causes	199.6	2,899.0	239.1	34.4	47.2	78.6	168.5	580.3	224.1	214.4

* SMR Prussia 1877.
† SMR England and Wales 1871.
For the classification and grouping of the diseases in the individual towns during the recorded years see Appendix 1.
Sources: See Appendix 2.

Table 17: Age- and cause-specific mortality (per 10,000 inhabitants) in Prussia (both sexes), 1900

Causes of death		All ages	0–1	1–5	5–15	15–30	30–40	40–60	>60	SMR*	SMR†
A	Weakness of life	18.5	559.7	12.4	1.0	0.0	0.0	0.0	0.0	20.8	18.1
B	Childbirth	1.2	0.0	0.0	0.0	1.8	4.3	1.0	0.0	1.1	1.2
C	Infirmity	24.8	0.1	0.1	0.3	0.2	0.3	0.8	325.6	23.2	25.1
D	Smallpox	0.0	0.2	0.0	0.0	0.0	0.0	0.0	0.0	0.0	0.0
E	Scarlet fever	3.6	12.1	18.8	5.5	0.3	0.1	0.0	0.0	3.7	3.7
F	Measles and rubella	2.0	22.9	11.5	0.7	0.0	0.0	0.0	0.0	2.2	2.1
G	Diphtheria and croup	4.8	33.7	25.8	4.8	0.2	0.1	0.1	0.1	5.1	4.9
H	Whooping cough	4.0	86.5	12.3	0.3	0.0	0.0	0.0	0.1	4.4	4.0
I	Typhoid fever	1.4	0.9	0.9	1.1	2.0	1.6	1.2	1.1	1.3	1.4
J	Typhus	0.0	0.0	0.0	0.0	0.0	0.0	0.0	0.0	0.0	0.0
K	Dysentery	0.2	2.6	0.6	0.1	0.0	0.1	0.1	0.3	0.2	0.2
L	Digestive system	49.0	1,369.0	58.4	2.7	0.8	0.9	1.2	2.0	54.6	48.0
M	Scrofula	1.3	16.2	6.5	0.6	0.0	0.0	0.0	0.0	1.4	1.3
N+O	Tuberculosis	21.1	23.0	9.5	5.5	21.5	27.4	34.1	38.8	19.9	20.9
P	Cancer	6.1	0.3	0.2	0.1	0.5	2.6	15.0	39.0	6.0	6.1
Q	Heart	8.7	7.8	1.9	1.8	2.3	4.4	14.8	53.7	8.4	8.7
R	Brain and nerves	15.0	69.4	15.9	5.0	2.9	5.5	17.8	73.5	14.9	15.0
S	Lungs	31.0	198.5	48.9	4.7	6.0	11.3	32.7	133.1	31.1	30.9
T	Urinary system	2.8	3.8	2.3	1.1	1.0	1.8	4.6	12.1	2.7	2.8
U	Influenza	–	–	–	–	–	–	–	–	–	–
V	Other communicable diseases	–	–	–	–	–	–	–	–	–	–
W	Violence	6.3	4.2	5.3	2.4	5.6	6.7	10.0	12.5	5.9	6.2
X	Other causes	21.1	171.1	14.9	3.6	5.8	10.9	27.8	75.4	21.2	20.9
All causes		223.1	2,582.2	246.2	41.2	51.0	78.0	161.1	767.2	227.9	221.1

* SMR Prussia 1877.
† SMR England and Wales 1871.
For the classification and grouping of diseases see Appendix 1.
Sources: See Appendix 2.

Table 18: Age- and cause-specific mortality (per 10,000 inhabitants) in the largest German towns (both sexes), 1907

Causes of death	All ages	0–1	1–5	5–15	15–30	30–40	40–60	>60	SMR*	SMR†
A Weakness of life	9.4	428.8	0.0	0.0	0.0	0.0	0.0	0.0	14.8	12.7
B Childbirth	1.3	0.0	0.0	0.0	2.0	3.3	0.6	0.0	0.9	1.0
C Infirmity	5.5	0.0	0.0	0.0	0.0	0.0	0.0	87.6	6.2	6.7
D Smallpox	0.0	0.0	0.0	0.0	0.0	0.0	0.0	0.0	0.0	0.0
E Scarlet fever	0.8	1.4	5.9	1.7	0.1	0.0	0.0	0.0	1.1	1.1
F Measles and rubella	1.8	27.0	15.5	0.7	0.0	0.0	0.0	0.0	2.7	2.6
G Diphtheria and croup	2.5	9.0	17.7	4.7	0.3	0.1	0.1	0.2	3.3	3.3
H Whooping cough	1.7	41.7	10.0	0.1	0.0	0.0	0.0	0.0	2.5	2.3
I Typhoid fever	0.3	0.1	0.1	0.2	0.5	0.4	0.3	0.2	0.3	0.3
J Typhus	0.0	0.0	0.0	0.0	0.0	0.0	0.0	0.0	0.0	0.0
K Dysentery	0.0	0.0	0.0	0.0	0.0	0.0	0.0	0.0	0.0	0.0
L Digestive system	23.2	725.4	17.8	2.6	2.7	4.7	10.9	28.4	32.6	29.3
M Scrofula	0.0	0.0	0.0	0.0	0.0	0.0	0.0	0.0	0.0	0.0
N+O Tuberculosis	21.7	43.2	26.3	6.1	20.2	25.7	28.3	28.0	20.2	21.0
P Cancer	12.5	1.5	0.8	0.5	1.2	5.4	28.0	89.8	12.6	12.9
Q Heart	18.7	35.5	3.5	2.1	3.1	6.6	26.6	159.7	19.6	20.3
R Brain and nerves	12.7	87.0	14.4	1.9	1.6	3.8	16.2	81.0	14.4	14.4
S Lungs	21.2	268.5	46.1	1.9	2.5	5.4	16.2	107.7	26.3	25.6
T Urinary system	4.5	7.4	1.5	0.7	1.3	2.9	8.3	25.3	4.5	4.6
U Influenza	1.2	2.7	0.5	0.1	0.1	0.3	1.2	11.6	1.2	1.3
V Other communicable diseases	1.3	34.5	1.0	0.6	0.4	0.5	0.8	0.6	1.7	1.6
W Violence	6.6	7.6	5.5	2.3	5.4	6.4	9.8	16.4	6.2	6.5
X Other causes	10.6	195.3	12.4	1.8	2.1	4.2	10.8	26.7	13.3	12.5
All causes	157.3	1,916.7	178.9	27.8	43.5	69.8	157.9	663.1	184.4	179.9

* SMR Prussia 1877.

† SMR England and Wales 1871.

For the classification and grouping of the diseases in the individual towns during the recorded years see Appendix 1.

Sources: See Appendix 2.

Table 19: Age- and cause-specific mortality (per 10,000 inhabitants) in Prussia (both sexes), 1907

	Causes of death	All ages	0–1	1–5	5–15	15–30	30–40	40–60	>60	SMR*	SMR†
A	Weakness of life	11.7	420.9	0.0	0.0	0.0	0.0	0.0	0.0	14.5	12.5
B	Childbirth	1.0	0.0	0.0	0.0	1.6	3.4	0.8	0.0	0.9	1.0
C	Infirmity	19.6	0.0	0.0	0.0	0.0	0.0	0.0	258.5	18.2	19.7
D	Smallpox	–	–	–	–	–	–	–	–	–	–
E	Scarlet fever	2.2	7.3	11.0	3.8	0.2	0.1	0.0	0.0	2.3	2.3
F	Measles and rubella	1.8	22.4	10.3	0.6	0.0	0.0	0.0	0.0	2.0	1.9
G	Diphtheria and croup	2.5	13.0	13.4	3.0	0.2	0.1	0.0	0.0	2.6	2.6
H	Whooping cough	2.3	54.3	7.6	0.2	0.0	0.0	0.0	0.1	2.7	2.5
I	Typhoid fever	0.6	0.3	0.3	0.4	0.8	0.7	0.6	0.4	0.5	0.6
J	Typhus	–	–	–	–	–	–	–	–	–	–
K	Dysentery	–	–	–	–	–	–	–	–	–	–
L	Digestive system	21.0	484.0	20.3	2.4	2.4	3.8	10.1	26.3	24.0	21.9
M	Scrofula	–	–	–	–	–	–	–	–	–	–
N+O	Tuberculosis	17.2	27.3	10.2	5.2	19.0	22.0	25.0	25.2	16.2	17.0
P	Cancer	7.4	1.1	0.4	0.2	0.6	2.8	17.1	49.5	7.2	7.3
Q	Heart	14.1	33.1	3.3	1.9	3.2	6.7	21.3	91.3	13.7	14.1
R	Brain and nerves	11.4	50.6	10.9	3.4	2.4	4.6	14.2	58.3	11.4	11.5
S	Lungs	25.6	226.1	42.1	3.7	4.7	9.1	24.5	98.7	26.6	26.1
T	Urinary system	3.0	5.0	1.8	0.9	1.1	2.2	5.0	13.5	2.9	3.0
U	Influenza	1.5	3.4	0.5	0.2	0.2	0.4	1.5	11.9	1.4	1.5
V	Other communicable diseases	0.7	8.3	1.5	0.6	0.3	0.2	0.2	0.2	0.7	0.7
W	Violence	6.3	4.8	5.5	2.1	5.8	6.8	9.6	12.9	5.9	6.2
X	Other causes	29.8	648.1	34.3	3.4	2.9	4.9	14.1	47.9	33.9	31.0
	All causes	179.6	2,010.0	173.5	31.9	45.3	67.6	144.0	694.8	187.9	183.3

* SMR Prussia 1877.
† SMR England and Wales 1871.
For the classification and grouping of the diseases see Appendix 1.
Sources: See Appendix 2.

Table 20: Age- and cause-specific mortality (per 10,000 inhabitants) in the largest English towns (both sexes), 1871–1880

Causes	All ages	0-1	1-2	2-3	3-4	4-5	5-10	10-15	15-20	20-25	25-35	35-45	45-55	55-65	65-75	>75
A	3.9	17.1	7.0	6.5	6.8	7.2	4.8	2.3	3.2	4.5	3.7	2.5	1.6	1.0	0.6	0.5
B	5.3	36.9	77.9	36.2	20.1	11.0	2.5	0.2	0.1	0.1	0.1	0.0	0.0	0.0	0.0	0.0
C	8.5	16.1	48.0	57.2	54.4	44.3	18.3	3.4	1.0	0.6	0.5	0.2	0.1	0.1	0.0	0.0
D	1.2	3.4	6.3	5.8	6.4	6.1	2.6	0.6	0.2	0.2	0.2	0.2	0.1	0.2	0.2	0.2
E	7.8	96.7	95.4	42.8	23.3	12.4	2.4	0.1	0.0	0.0	0.0	0.0	0.0	0.0	0.0	0.0
F	0.9	0.2	0.3	0.4	0.6	0.5	0.6	0.6	0.8	1.0	1.0	1.3	1.6	1.4	1.2	0.6
G	3.0	2.4	4.3	5.1	4.8	4.7	3.5	2.9	3.6	3.3	2.5	2.3	2.3	2.6	2.6	2.3
H	1.1	1.8	2.9	3.1	3.3	2.9	1.5	0.7	0.6	0.5	0.5	0.8	1.0	1.5	2.0	2.5
I	0.8	0.0	0.0	0.0	0.0	0.0	0.0	0.0	0.4	2.0	2.2	1.5	0.1	0.0	0.0	0.0
J	12.3	270.5	82.8	13.6	4.1	2.2	0.8	0.2	0.2	0.3	0.5	0.9	1.8	4.8	13.3	35.4
K	0.4	5.1	1.8	0.5	0.3	0.2	0.1	0.0	0.0	0.1	0.1	0.2	0.3	0.6	0.7	0.7
L	5.0	0.1	0.1	0.2	0.2	0.2	0.1	0.1	0.2	0.4	1.6	6.6	15.7	26.1	33.8	32.2
M	1.5	15.2	10.9	4.5	2.7	2.1	1.1	0.8	0.7	0.4	0.4	0.4	0.4	0.7	0.8	0.3
N	3.7	63.1	35.6	11.6	4.8	2.7	1.4	0.8	0.4	0.2	0.2	0.2	0.2	0.2	0.2	0.1
O	25.5	14.4	13.4	7.3	4.7	4.3	4.4	6.8	19.6	29.5	40.1	48.2	43.0	31.8	16.9	5.8
P	4.2	49.6	41.3	18.3	10.9	8.3	3.4	1.1	0.4	0.2	0.1	0.1	0.1	0.1	0.0	0.0
Q	28.2	308.9	81.4	33.3	20.5	13.7	6.7	3.3	3.3	3.4	5.8	12.8	26.5	59.9	132.5	231.1
R	12.8	2.0	1.1	0.7	0.8	1.0	2.0	3.1	3.8	3.9	7.4	15.8	27.1	51.6	89.3	112.6
S	48.2	386.4	234.5	82.7	39.7	23.5	7.3	2.4	3.3	5.0	9.9	22.7	51.7	119.9	239.9	410.2
T	9.7	45.2	8.8	4.0	2.8	2.5	1.9	1.6	2.1	2.6	4.8	10.0	19.0	32.8	48.1	61.6
U	4.4	1.2	2.0	1.9	2.2	1.9	1.3	0.9	1.3	1.7	3.0	5.5	9.0	15.1	24.5	33.3
V	0.7	0.1	0.1	0.0	0.0	0.0	0.0	0.0	0.1	0.3	0.7	1.2	1.8	2.1	2.7	2.8
W	0.9	0.0	0.0	0.0	0.0	0.0	0.0	0.0	0.4	1.3	2.3	2.5	0.1	0.0	0.0	0.0
X	0.8	0.0	0.0	0.0	0.0	0.0	0.0	0.0	0.3	0.5	0.8	1.3	2.0	2.7	0.0	1.8
Y	7.9	54.9	12.3	10.0	8.3	7.1	4.6	3.4	3.7	3.9	4.8	6.5	9.1	12.0	15.3	30.1
Z	41.7	640.6	116.2	37.8	21.8	15.7	7.0	4.2	3.8	3.9	5.7	9.7	16.1	37.3	145.5	736.3
All	240.2	2,031.8	884.3	383.6	243.3	174.4	78.3	39.4	53.4	69.6	98.5	153.3	230.4	404.2	772.8	1,700.3

A=Smallpox; B=Measles; C=Scarlet fever; D=Diphtheria; E=Whooping cough; F=Typhus; G=Enteric fever; H=Simple continued fever; I=Puerperal fever; J=Diarrhoea and dysentery; K=Cholera; L=Cancer; M=Scrofula; N=Tabes mesenterica; O=Phthisis; P=Hydrocephalus; Q=Diseases of nervous system; R=Diseases of circulatory system; S=Diseases of respiratory system; T=Diseases of digestive system; U=Diseases of urinary system; V=Diseases of generative system; W=Childbirth; X=Suicide; Y=Other violence; Z=Other causes; All causes.

Source: *Decennial Supplement to the Annual Reports of the Registrar-General of Births, Deaths, and Marriages in England and Wales* (1871–1880).

Table 21: Age- and cause-specific mortality (per 10,000 inhabitants) in England and Wales (both sexes), 1871–880

Causes	All ages	0-1	1-2	2-3	3-4	4-5	5-10	10-15	15-20	20-25	25-35	35-45	45-55	55-65	65-75	>75
A	2.4	10.7	3.9	3.5	3.6	4.0	2.8	1.4	2.0	3.0	2.4	1.7	1.1	0.7	0.5	0.4
B	3.8	27.7	54.1	24.7	13.9	7.8	2.1	0.2	0.1	0.1	0.1	0.0	0.0	0.0	0.0	0.0
C	7.2	14.1	39.7	45.4	42.9	34.7	15.2	3.2	1.0	0.6	0.5	0.2	0.1	0.1	0.0	0.0
D	1.2	2.9	4.9	4.8	5.8	5.5	2.9	0.9	0.3	0.2	0.2	0.2	0.1	0.2	0.2	0.1
E	5.1	73.9	60.4	24.4	12.8	6.6	1.4	0.1	0.0	0.0	0.0	0.0	0.0	0.0	0.0	0.0
F	0.6	0.1	0.2	0.3	0.4	0.5	0.5	0.5	0.7	0.7	0.6	0.7	0.7	0.7	0.7	0.4
G	3.2	2.5	4.2	4.7	4.4	4.3	3.4	3.1	4.1	3.8	2.9	2.5	2.5	2.7	2.9	2.2
H	1.1	1.4	2.4	2.6	2.6	2.2	1.4	0.8	0.7	0.6	0.6	0.6	0.8	1.2	1.9	2.4
I	0.7	0.0	0.0	0.0	0.0	0.0	0.0	0.0	0.4	1.9	2.3	1.6	0.1	0.0	0.0	0.0
J	9.1	195.1	55.4	9.7	3.2	1.8	0.6	0.2	0.2	0.3	0.5	0.8	1.4	3.7	11.4	34.5
K	0.3	3.1	1.1	0.3	0.2	0.1	0.1	0.0	0.0	0.0	0.1	0.1	0.2	0.4	0.5	0.6
L	4.7	0.1	0.1	0.1	0.2	0.1	0.1	0.1	0.2	0.3	1.3	5.3	12.6	22.1	31.2	33.3
M	1.3	11.9	7.5	2.9	1.7	1.3	0.8	0.7	0.8	0.7	0.5	0.5	0.5	0.7	0.9	0.5
N	3.2	53.3	29.7	8.9	3.6	2.2	1.3	0.8	0.6	0.4	0.3	0.2	0.2	0.2	0.2	0.1
O	21.2	14.1	11.7	5.4	3.4	3.0	3.6	6.6	20.4	31.2	36.2	37.5	31.3	24.5	14.8	4.9
P	3.2	36.8	30.1	12.5	7.6	5.9	3.0	1.2	0.5	0.2	0.2	0.1	0.1	0.0	0.0	0.0
Q	27.7	308.8	66.8	26.2	15.9	10.8	5.7	3.3	3.6	3.8	6.0	12.0	22.5	49.1	114.3	212.8
R	13.1	1.8	0.8	0.5	0.6	0.7	1.4	2.4	3.0	3.4	6.2	13.1	22.7	48.1	94.8	120.9
S	37.6	317.9	169.8	55.8	27.3	16.4	5.6	2.0	3.0	4.5	7.8	16.2	32.5	74.3	160.8	302.4
T	9.8	43.5	7.9	3.7	2.7	2.4	1.8	1.5	2.1	2.6	4.4	9.0	16.7	30.1	48.4	56.9
U	3.9	1.4	1.7	1.5	1.5	1.4	0.9	0.7	1.0	1.5	2.5	4.3	6.6	12.0	22.1	33.1
V	0.6	0.1	0.0	0.0	0.0	0.0	0.0	0.0	0.1	0.3	0.5	0.9	1.5	1.7	2.2	1.9
W	0.9	0.0	0.0	0.0	0.0	0.0	0.0	0.0	0.5	1.6	2.6	3.0	0.2	0.0	0.0	0.0
X	0.7	0.0	0.0	0.0	0.0	0.0	0.0	0.0	0.3	0.5	0.7	1.1	1.7	2.4	0.0	1.8
Y	6.6	26.3	10.2	9.3	7.2	6.1	3.9	3.5	4.2	4.5	5.0	6.1	7.5	9.4	12.2	23.7
Z	43.8	626.7	96.5	30.1	18.5	13.4	6.1	3.7	3.7	3.8	5.2	8.3	13.4	30.5	126.1	783.1
All	212.7	1,774.1	659.2	277.1	180.0	131.1	64.4	37.0	53.3	70.4	89.3	126.2	177.2	314.9	648.5	1,615.9

A=Smallpox; B=Measles; C=Scarlet fever; D=Diphtheria; E=Whooping cough; F=Typhus; G=Enteric fever; H=Simple continued fever; I=Puerperal fever; J=Diarrhoea and dysentery; K=Cholera; L=Cancer; M=Scrofula; N=Tabes mesenterica; O=Phthisis; P=Hydrocephalus; Q=Diseases of nervous system; R=Diseases of circulatory system; S=Diseases of respiratory system; T=Diseases of digestive system; U=Diseases of urinary system; V=Diseases of generative system; W=Childbirth; X=Suicide; Y=Other violence; Z=Other causes; All=All causes.
Source: *Decennial Supplement to the Annual Reports of the Registrar-General of Births, Deaths, and Marriages in England and Wales (1871–1880).*

Table 22: Age- and cause-specific mortality (per 10,000 inhabitants) in the largest English towns (both sexes), 1901–1910

Causes	All ages	0–1	1–2	2–5	5–10	10–15	15–20	20–25	25–35	35–45	45–55	55–65	65–75	>75
A	0.1	0.4	0.1	0.1	0.0	0.0	0.0	0.1	0.1	0.1	0.1	0.1	0.1	0.0
B	4.4	41.4	86.6	20.8	2.0	0.1	0.0	0.0	0.0	0.0	0.0	0.0	0.0	0.0
C	1.4	2.6	7.9	10.1	3.5	0.8	0.3	0.2	0.1	0.1	0.0	0.0	0.0	0.0
D	0.0	0.0	0.0	0.0	0.0	0.0	0.0	0.0	0.0	0.1	0.0	0.0	0.0	0.0
E	1.7	2.9	1.2	0.4	0.3	0.2	0.4	0.5	0.7	1.3	2.5	5.3	12.2	26.5
F	3.5	63.3	52.3	11.5	1.0	0.0	0.0	0.0	0.0	0.0	0.0	0.0	0.0	0.0
G	1.9	5.4	14.7	12.4	5.1	0.7	0.2	0.1	0.1	0.1	0.0	0.1	0.1	0.0
H	0.0	0.1	0.0	0.0	0.0	0.0	0.0	0.0	0.0	0.0	0.0	0.0	0.0	0.0
I	0.9	0.1	0.2	0.4	0.5	0.8	1.1	1.3	1.4	1.2	0.8	0.6	0.3	0.1
J	7.9	248.5	57.7	3.8	0.4	0.1	0.1	0.1	0.2	0.3	0.5	1.5	4.3	12.1
K	7.4	4.4	5.9	2.3	1.2	1.4	4.2	6.2	8.9	13.3	14.8	12.3	8.3	3.7
L	7.4	1.3	1.5	0.8	0.8	1.4	4.6	7.1	9.7	13.8	14.9	12.4	7.6	3.3
M	2.2	22.3	21.7	9.0	3.2	1.1	0.6	0.3	0.2	0.2	0.1	0.1	0.0	0.0
N	1.1	14.7	8.3	2.5	1.0	0.6	0.5	0.3	0.3	0.3	0.3	0.3	0.3	0.1
O	0.5	13.6	4.5	0.8	0.2	0.1	0.0	0.0	0.0	0.0	0.0	0.0	0.0	0.0
P	1.9	15.2	10.8	3.7	1.7	1.3	1.2	1.0	1.0	1.1	1.1	1.2	1.3	1.4
Q	9.8	0.4	0.5	0.5	0.3	0.3	0.4	0.6	1.9	8.1	24.5	49.3	72.9	81.1
R	1.2	8.3	1.4	0.4	0.3	0.4	0.6	0.7	0.7	1.0	1.6	2.5	4.0	7.1
S	0.7	0.2	0.1	0.3	0.9	1.1	0.8	0.6	0.6	0.7	0.8	0.9	1.2	1.2
T	15.8	157.4	115.9	22.8	4.0	1.6	2.3	3.1	5.0	9.4	15.2	25.9	42.0	69.4
U	14.2	132.7	42.5	5.5	0.6	0.2	0.2	0.3	0.8	3.1	11.2	38.5	104.9	255.0
V	1.0	0.0	0.0	0.0	0.0	0.0	0.3	1.8	2.9	2.3	0.1	0.0	0.0	0.0
W	6.6	50.3	10.5	8.6	3.5	1.8	2.2	2.6	3.6	5.6	8.3	11.2	14.7	32.2
X	76.6	914.2	110.9	23.8	10.5	9.4	10.7	11.0	16.8	38.4	80.3	170.7	375.4	969.4
All causes	168.2	1,699.7	555.3	140.2	41.0	23.4	30.8	37.8	55.0	100.4	177.4	332.9	649.2	1,462.9

A=Smallpox; B=Measles; C=Scarlet fever; D=Typhus; E=Influenza; F=Whooping cough; G=Diphtheria; H=Pyrexia; I=Enteric fever; J=Diarrhoea and dysentery; K=Pulmonary tuberculosis; L=Phthisis (not otherwise defined); M=Tuberculosis meningitis; N=Tuberculosis peritonitis; O=Tabes mesenterica; P=Other tuberculosis; Q=Cancer; R=Septic diseases; S=Rheumatic fever and rheumatism of heart; T=Pneumonia; U=Bronchitis; V=Childbirth and puerperal fever; W=Violence; X=Other causes; All causes.

Source: *Decennial Supplement to the Annual Reports of the Registrar-General of Births, Deaths, and Marriages in England and Wales* (1901–1910).

Table 23: Age- and cause-specific mortality (per 10,000 inhabitants) in England and Wales (both sexes), 1901–1910

Causes	All ages	0–1	1–2	2–5	5–10	10–15	15–20	20–25	25–35	35–45	45–55	55–65	65–75	>75
A	0.1	0.5	0.2	0.1	0.1	0.1	0.1	0.1	0.1	0.2	0.2	0.1	0.1	0.1
B	3.1	30.1	58.3	14.1	1.7	0.1	0.1	0.0	0.0	0.0	0.0	0.0	0.0	0.0
C	1.1	1.9	5.5	7.1	2.7	0.7	0.3	0.2	0.1	0.1	0.0	0.0	0.0	0.0
D	0.0	0.0	0.0	0.0	0.0	0.0	0.0	0.0	0.0	0.0	0.0	0.0	0.0	0.0
E	2.1	4.4	1.6	0.6	0.3	0.2	0.5	0.6	0.9	1.5	2.6	5.7	13.3	29.3
F	2.8	57.5	38.4	8.0	0.7	0.0	0.0	0.0	0.0	0.0	0.0	0.0	0.0	0.0
G	1.8	3.6	10.1	11.4	5.5	0.9	0.2	0.1	0.1	0.1	0.1	0.1	0.1	0.1
H	0.0	0.1	0.1	0.0	0.0	0.0	0.0	0.1	0.1	0.1	0.1	0.1	0.1	0.0
I	0.9	0.1	0.2	0.4	0.6	0.8	1.2	1.4	1.4	1.1	0.8	0.6	0.3	0.1
J	5.7	180.0	36.9	2.5	0.3	0.1	0.1	0.1	0.2	0.3	0.5	1.4	3.9	11.4
K	4.8	3.1	3.7	1.4	0.9	1.2	3.5	5.4	6.9	8.1	8.1	6.8	4.4	1.8
L	6.8	1.5	1.6	0.7	0.8	1.6	5.3	8.3	10.2	11.7	11.9	9.9	6.5	2.6
M	1.8	17.6	15.7	6.5	2.7	1.2	0.7	0.4	0.3	0.2	0.1	0.1	0.0	0.0
N	1.0	13.5	7.4	2.0	0.9	0.6	0.6	0.4	0.4	0.4	0.3	0.3	0.2	0.1
O	0.5	12.5	4.3	0.7	0.2	0.1	0.0	0.0	0.0	0.0	0.0	0.0	0.0	0.0
P	1.7	12.5	8.0	2.4	1.3	1.1	1.3	1.2	1.2	1.1	1.1	1.2	1.2	1.1
Q	9.0	0.3	0.3	0.3	0.2	0.2	0.3	0.5	1.4	6.4	19.5	41.7	66.7	78.9
R	0.9	6.3	0.8	0.3	0.2	0.3	0.4	0.4	0.5	0.8	1.2	1.8	3.1	5.5
S	0.7	0.2	0.1	0.2	0.7	1.0	0.9	0.6	0.6	0.7	0.8	1.0	1.2	1.2
T	12.5	130.4	85.3	16.8	3.1	1.2	2.1	2.8	4.1	7.2	11.3	19.4	32.2	50.2
U	11.7	121.3	37.3	4.8	0.5	0.2	0.2	0.2	0.5	1.9	6.8	24.7	72.1	185.7
V	1.1	0.0	0.0	0.0	0.0	0.0	0.3	1.9	3.2	2.7	0.1	0.0	0.0	0.0
W	5.7	28.2	8.3	6.6	2.8	1.7	2.7	3.2	3.9	5.4	7.6	9.9	12.3	24.2
X	77.8	876.0	94.0	21.2	9.4	7.9	9.4	10.3	15.5	33.4	69.8	156.4	370.0	135.8
All causes	153.6	1,501.7	417.8	108.3	35.6	21.1	29.9	38.2	51.3	83.1	142.9	281.2	587.7	1,428.1

A=Smallpox; B=Measles; C=Scarlet fever; D=Typhus; E =Influenza; F=Whooping cough; G=Diphtheria; H=Pyrexia; I=Enteric fever; J=Diarrhoea and dysentery; K=Pulmonary tuberculosis; L=Phthisis (not otherwise defined); M=Tuberculosis meningitis; N=Tuberculosis peritonitis; O=Tabes mesenterica; P=Other tuberculosis; Q=Cancer; R=Septic diseases; S=Rheumatic fever and rheumatism of heart; T=Pneumonia; U=Bronchitis; V=Childbirth and puerperal fever; W=Violence; X=Other causes; All causes.

Source: *Decennial Supplement to the Annual Reports of the Registrar-General of Births, Deaths, and Marriages in England and Wales* (1901–1910).

AGE- AND SEX-SPECIFIC CAUSES OF DEATH

The previous discussion of age-specific mortality rates has already revealed substantial differences between the sexes. An analysis of the age-specific disease panorama differentiated according to sex provides further insight. The German sample allows an age- and sex- specific differentiation of the disease panorama for most of the towns,[27] whereas for England this is, unfortunately, only possible for the second selected period, 1901–1910.

Considerable amounts of research have been undertaken with respect to changes in female mortality during the nineteenth century. W. R. Lee demonstrated the impact of agrarian change on the health of mothers and children in Prussia (Lee, 1984b). Based on an analysis of three rural areas and one small town in Germany, A. E. Imhof registered an excess mortality of married women between the ages 15 and 49 during the whole nineteenth century, even after the deduction of deaths in childbirth. He attributes this to the manifold burdens weighing on women as spouse, mother and worker (Imhof, 1979; 1981c). In general, however, the industrialized world seems to have reduced excess female mortality in several European countries and in North America.[28] For Germany, R. Spree pinpointed the excess male mortality during adulthood, particularly in the large towns, as a result of a higher mortality from tuberculosis (Spree, 1986). Again, however, little attention has been paid to the actual changes in the disease panorama in the large towns.

In the ten largest German towns the female death rate in 1877 was lower in all age-groups (when compared with male mortality), even in those age-groups which were burdened with a high death rate from childbirth mortality (the sex-specific disease panorama for the towns of the sample, for Prussia as well as for England and Wales, is reported in Appendix 6). Consequently the death rates for females were lower in relation to almost all diseases—with the significant exception of (naturally) childbirth and (more surprisingly) infirmity. The male population, on the other hand, registered relatively higher mortality rates from tuberculosis and violence, especially with increasing age. This indicates that in an urban environment men were to a higher degree exposed to health-damaging factors often caused by the nature of the labour market. Consequently gender differences in mortality were lower for Prussia as a whole, yet there was still an obviously higher risk for men. The main villain, however, was mortality from digestive diseases under one year of age, and only in second place mortality from tuberculosis. Female mortality surpassed the rates for men with respect to infirmity and, of course, childbirth, the latter bearing a risk for the age-group 30–40 which was more than twice as high as in the urban world.

---

27 Exceptions are Hamburg and Dresden for the first selected period, Dresden for 1900, and Dresden and Munich for the last. For these towns the age-specific disease panorama is only available for the sexes combined.

28 See Imhof (1981c); Johansson (1984; 1991).

Whereas the situation for Prussia as a whole remained almost stable, urban death rates showed major improvements by 1885. The death rates for the female population improved at a slightly faster rate (female: 269.22–224.08=45.14; male: 313.54–275.92=37.62) as a result of stronger decrease in the incidence of most diseases, with the exception of the gastro-intestinal disorders. Infants of both sexes benefited similarly from the decline of the digestive diseases, and 'weakness'. Mortality from diseases of the respiratory system decreased in the female population, although it increased among males; the death rates from cancer increased in both sexes, particularly, however, in the male population. The reduction in male tuberculosis mortality affected the very young and the very old. It remained almost stable in the middle age-groups or even rose in the age-group 30–40. Women also benefited from a reduction in mortality from this disease complex, the decline, however, predominantly affecting the higher age-groups.

Until 1900 the urban situation continued to improve. Male death rates registered an accelerated decline (275.92–221.69=54.23) in comparison with the rates for females (224.08–181.50=42.58) so that the gap in mortality between the sexes became slightly attenuated. Improvements started to become more visible in relation to Prussia as a whole, affecting both sexes in a similar manner. In the first decade of the twentieth century male urban mortality continued to improve faster than female mortality (male: 221.69–171.38=50.31; female: 181.50–149.96=31.45), with a fall in male infant mortality from digestive diseases and weakness underpinning this trend most intensively.

In England and Wales in 1901–1910 male mortality surpassed female mortality in all age-groups except between 5 and 15. Higher female death rates within these years cannot be attributed to specific diseases, but rather resulted from a higher mortality risk from a variety of diseases. By contrast, young males up to five years of age suffered especially from respiratory and digestive diseases. Beyond the age-groups 5–15 higher male mortality was particularly caused by respiratory diseases, including tuberculosis.

SPATIAL VARIATIONS

Corresponding to the relative consistency in the 'urban penalty' in the sample of English towns, variations in the health conditions between the towns of the sample were not as distinct as in the German case (a brief description of the mortality profile and the prevailing disease panorama in the towns constituting the sample in both countries can be found in Appendix 7). In England spatial variations, expressed as a coefficient of variation (which is the standard deviation of the variable divided by the mean), were more equally distributed over the whole disease complex. Focusing on the development of the two main disease complexes, respiratory and digestive diseases, the latter continued to be responsible for inter-city variations to a larger degree (Fig. 22). Whereas mortality rates from tuberculosis and respiratory diseases constituted a high background mortality in cities and towns in general, death rates from typhoid fever and digestive diseases showed a higher degree of local variation. The wide variation in typhoid fever mortality reflects local epidemic outbreaks that occurred in

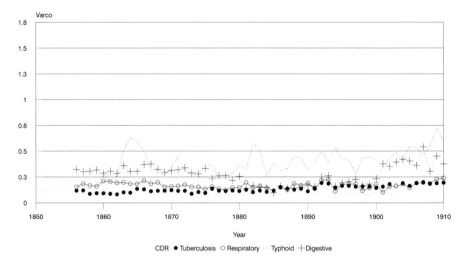

Figure 22: Inter-urban variations in mortality from selected diseases in English towns, 1851–1910
Sources: *Annual Reports of the Registrar-General of Birth, Deaths, and Marriages in England and Wales* (1856–1910).

addition to the endemic prevalence of this disease. Growing market integration obviously had a levelling effect only with respect to some diseases, whereas others—especially in the digestive disease group[29]—remained very much determined by local conditions, so that spatial variations remained stable or even increased over time. The level of mortality from digestive diseases was strongly dependent on the extent of breast-feeding and the quality and quantity of the sanitary infrastructure. As in England as a whole, breast-feeding was not universal, but it was general in urban areas (Woods et al., 1989, p. 116; Fildes, 1992, pp. 55–64)—in London only 3.9 per cent of the mothers had never breast-fed their infants (Prinzing, 1906, p. 293). This therefore indicates that local public health measures which aimed to improve the environment still differed both in quantity and quality. By transmission via polluted waterways, trade-routes or migration in general, typhoid fever could spread from city to city. Improvements in the urban infrastructure could have interrupted this chain and served to provide a quarantine for the city adequately supplied with public health facilities. Those towns with an insufficient public health infrastructure were still, to a certain extent, exposed to the risk of infection (see, however, Chapter 11, 'The Impact of Central Water Supply and Sewerage Systems on Urban Health').

In Germany the patterns of inter-city variations in mortality from the selected diseases were much more strongly pronounced (Figure 23). As with England, however, major spatial variations in a sample of 19 German towns (including the ten largest)

---

29 The lower coefficients of variation concerning digestive diseases in the last two decades of the nineteenth century might be a result of changes in registration (see Chapter 7).

were primarily the result of regional differences in the death rates from typhoid fever and acute digestive diseases; in contrast, mortality from tuberculosis and respiratory diseases was more equally distributed across the towns. Low spatial variation in mortality from respiratory diseases and tuberculosis pinpoints again the subordinate role of local factors in determining the death rates from these diseases.

As mentioned earlier, regional differences in the frequency of intestinal diseases in Germany were, to a substantial extent, due to wide regional variations in infant feeding practices.[30] Even within the different German states, breast-feeding varied substantially. In Baden, for example, the percentage of infants not breast-fed ranged from 10 to 52 per cent (Knodel and van de Walle, 1967, p. 120). In general, breast-feeding was relatively uncommon in the eastern regions of Germany (Kintner, 1985).

Artificial feeding was associated with high infant mortality, and extensive breast-feeding with low infant death rates. A substantial survival advantage of breast-fed infants over artificially nourished infants, particularly in the first months of life, has been noted for historical populations as well as for contemporary less developed countries (Böckh, 1887a; 1887b; Prinzing, 1906, pp. 290–94; Knodel and Kintner, 1977). In Sweden at the beginning of the nineteenth century, for example, low infant mortality rates were linked with legislative coercion to breast-feed infants (Selter,

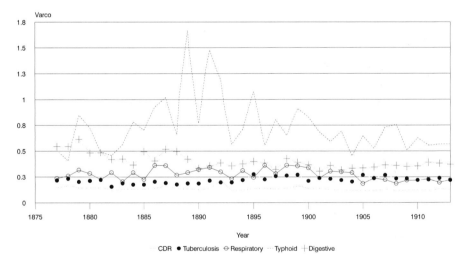

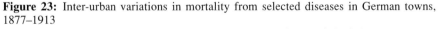

Figure 23: Inter-urban variations in mortality from selected diseases in German towns, 1877–1913

Source: *Veröffentlichungen des Kaiserlichen Gesundheitsamtes (Beilagen)* (1878–1914).

30 Compare Kintner's map of regional breast-feeding patterns (Kintner, 1982 p. 220). Investigations about the duration of breast-feeding, however, are few and far between. For some late nineteenth- and early twentieth-century reports, see the works of Kintner and Knodel.

1902, p. 389).[31] The potential impact of breast-feeding on the survival chances of infants becomes obvious when a homogeneous social group is analysed, in this case 628 women who gave birth in the Cologne maternity asylum (*Wöchnerinnen-Asyl*). Only poor married women were admitted, and the municipal welfare committee had to confirm their indigence. Amongst this group in 1900–1901 infant mortality fluctuated between 8 deaths per 100 live births—when breast-feeding was practised for over three months—and 37 deaths per 100 births for infants who were either not breast-fed at all or only for a period shorter than three months (Dietrich, 1902, p. 48). Early twentieth-century German surveys, carried out in the Regierungsbezirk Düsseldorf and in Hanover and Linden, indicate that feeding practices outweighed social class as a major determinant of infant mortality. Breast-fed infants from the lower classes had a substantially higher survival chance than artificially-fed infants from wealthier families (Baum, 1912, p. 313). Breast-feeding minimizes the chances both of malnutrition and of the acquisition of infectious diseases. Breast milk is not only considered to be nutritionally ideal, it is also clean and transmits immunities from the mother to the child. In contrast, artificial food promotes bacterial infection, especially when prepared with milk, water or, as was customary in some areas, with food pre-chewed by an adult. In the non-breast-feeding areas of Bavaria and Swabia artificial feeding was especially predominant in urban areas, whereas breast-feeding at least accompanied artificial nourishment in the countryside (Maier, 1871, p. 189). Infants were nourished with meal-pap and sugar water, often prepared in the morning and warmed up three to four times a day. Chicory-coffee was given to babies from birth. The dummy was filled with pre-chewed bread and sugar, and dipped in beer (Maier, 1871, pp. 190–93; Seidlmayer, 1937, p. 29). Prinzing reports that in both southern Germany and England it was not uncommon to use opiate additives in artificial food to pacify the infants (Prinzing, 1906, p. 291). Contemporaries in both countries often complained of the widespread use of beer, gin and spirits (*Branntwein*) to 'nourish' the infant or child. Even at the beginning of the twentieth century parental guidelines for infant care felt obliged to explicitly point out that alcohol might damage the infant's health.[32]

The wide spatial variation in mortality from diseases of the digestive system, however, cannot be attributed solely to differences in infant feeding practices (see also Kintner, 1987); it also reflects the role of local environmental factors. Feeding practices, for example, cannot explain the extensive mortality differences in the western towns, where feeding patterns were essentially similar, with deaths from intestinal diseases per 10,000 ranging from 29.15 in Frankfurt am Main, 58.15 in Düsseldorf, to 78.88 deaths in Cologne (1877). The infant mortality rate in Cologne was actually

31 As there are no statistics on breast-feeding habits available for nineteenth-century Sweden, it remains unclear how effective this procedure was. According to quantitative reports requested by the National Board of Health from provincial doctors in 1869, there were wide spatial variations between breast-fed and partly breast-fed children. There were, however, only a few areas where children were exclusively artificially nourished. See Brändström (1993), p. 30.

32 See, for example, Langstein and Rott (1918).

higher than in the non-breast-feeding area of Breslau, although both towns had sim-ilar birth rates. Here environmental factors may have played a more important role. This is supported by the fact that the biggest variations in the death rate from intesti-nal diseases did not occur amongst infants (coefficient of variation in 1877, 0.33), but increased with age and reached a maximum for the age-group over 60 (coefficient of variation in 1877, 1.37).

What is even more important, the decline in urban infant mortality occurred at the same time as breast-feeding declined in the large towns of Germany (Selter, 1902, pp. 382–85; Hohlfeld, 1905, p. 1392; Prinzing, 1906, p. 294; Kintner, 1985, pp. 169–72). In Cologne, for example, 40 per cent of all mothers breast-fed their infants in 1902, whereas one generation earlier the rate was 94 per cent (Selter, 1902, p. 384). For Berlin, regularly published surveys proffer explicit information about breast-feeding habits (Böckh, 1887a; 1887b). In the city 55.5 per cent of all infants were exclusively breast-fed in 1885, 4.0 per cent additionally fed with animal milk, and 33.9 per cent solely raised on animal milk. In 1900 only 31.4 per cent were breast-fed, 0.7 per cent supplied with additional animal milk, whereas 54.8 per cent relied on animal milk (Neumann, 1902, p. 795). In the traditional non-breast-feeding areas the percentage of infants artificially nourished grew even higher. According to material from the Munich children's hospital the number of infants never breast-fed was 78.3 per cent in 1861–1869, and increased in the following decades to 82.3 (1870–1878) and 86.4 (1879–1886) (Büller, 1887, p. 320; Escherich, 1887, p. 233; Seidlmayer, 1937, p. 29 and graph 12). It was only after the turn of the century that breast-feeding again became more widespread, but, as questionnaires carried out during vaccination against smallpox reveal, 56 to 60 per cent were still artificially fed (Seidlmayer, 1937, p. 30). In view of decreasing breast-feeding in the last quar-ter of the nineteenth century, environmental improvements must have played a more important role in determining urban mortality change. Improved hygiene conditions not only restricted outbreaks of severe epidemics of typhoid fever that were still all too prominent in the 1880s and early 1890s, but the nutritional adequacy of artificial food was also improved, thereby reducing the survival advantage of breast-fed infants over those artificially nourished (Wray, 1978, pp. 213–19). In Berlin, for example, in 1885 the death rate of artificially nourished infants of married families was almost seven times higher than the rate for breast-fed infants (Böckh, 1887a, p. 18); by 1910 the rate for the artificially fed was 4.4 times higher (*Statistisches Jahrbuch der Stadt Berlin*, 1913, p. 212). In poor and inappropriate sanitary condi-tions, however, breast-feeding was of paramount importance. Declining variations in the digestive disease group in Germany indicate that the expansion of health-related infrastructural measures may have had a profound impact on the control of the diges-tive disease complex, an issue which will be discussed in more detail in Chapter 11.

Comparing the disease-specific death rates of the various towns and cities, it becomes clear that an unhealthy city was a health hazard in every respect, i.e. health-damaging factors had a uniformly negative effect on all age-groups, both sexes and with respect to all diseases. In England, Manchester and Liverpool registered by far the highest death rates in the period 1871–1880 (Manchester 28.4; Liverpool 26.1

per 1,000 inhabitants). This was the result of not only a strong prevalence of the major killers in these cities, but also relatively high death rates from almost all diseases in comparison with the other towns.

Furthermore, it was not the 'healthy' localities that developed the more modern disease panorama, with high mortality rates from degenerative diseases. On the contrary, towns like Liverpool and Manchester registered high death rates from cancer (8.84 and 9.06 per 10,000 inhabitants respectively), which were only surpassed by London, Bradford and Leeds. In the German sample the case of Breslau clearly supports this view: it was the unhealthiest town in the sample due to very high death rates from intestinal diseases and weakness, affecting predominantly infants, and from tuberculosis and diseases of the respiratory system in all age-groups. In addition there was also a high death rate from degenerative diseases. After the turn of the century mortality from digestive diseases and from weakness was reduced substantially. Breslau, however, remained an unhealthy town. The high death rates from tuberculosis and respiratory diseases were now accompanied by extraordinarily high death rates from diseases of the circulatory system.

MORTALITY PATTERNS INSIDE THE CITY

Variations in mortality within the city, where particularly poor conditions were prevalent in the inner-city, even surpassed inter-city differences. The second half of the nineteenth century brought about increasing social segregation of residential areas. People moved from the inner-city areas to the new suburbs, and new business centres were created and set up in the urban core. Complementary to this outward movement of a city's internal population, the central zones often received large numbers of low-status in-migrants (Lawton and Pooley, 1976, pp. 85–91; Carter, 1983, pp. 190–99; Dennis, 1984, pp. 200–49). Furthermore, in a number of English cities these high density areas were inhabited by culturally and economically distinctive ethnic groups, among which the Irish predominated. In Liverpool, for example, almost a quarter of the population was Irish-born (Lawton, 1989, p. 164). The strong link between migrant-origin and occupational and social status is reflected in the fact that members of the Irish community were mainly engaged in casual and unskilled work (Taylor, 1976, p. 101). Poor living conditions in these central areas and a high birth rate among the Irish population, associated with high infant mortality rates, found their expression in appallingly high mortality rates in the inner-city, whereas the healthiest suburban districts compared well with most parts of the country. During mortality crises these intra-urban mortality differences increased even further (Taylor, 1976, p. 209). Basic vital statistics for the different city districts (wards), provided regularly by the Health Department of the City of Liverpool, indicate that disease was still rampant in the inner-city districts after the turn of the century (Figs. 24–27). In Liverpool in 1900, crude death rates were highest in the core of the city, with particularly high mortality in the densely inhabited districts of Exchange (36.5 per 1,000 inhabitants) and Scotland (34.5), followed by Abercromby (24.7), Everton (23.9), Toxteth (23.5), Kirkdale (22.4) and West Derby-West (21.4). The surrounding districts of West Derby-East, Walton, Wavertree and Sefton Park registered death rates substantially below the city's

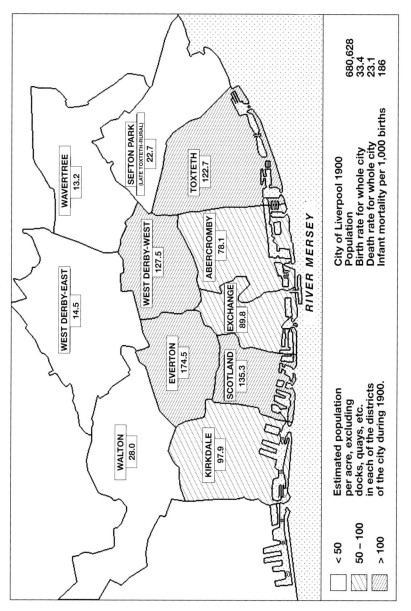

Figure 24: The population of Liverpool districts, 1900
Source: Health Department (1901).

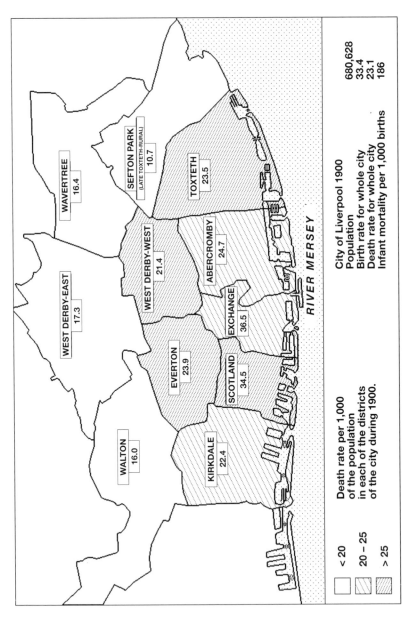

Figure 25: Crude death rates in Liverpool districts, 1900
Source: Health Department (1901).

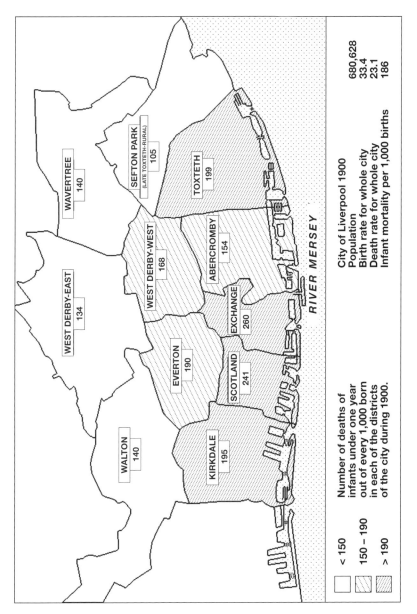

Figure 26: Infant mortality in Liverpool districts, 1900
Source: Health Department (1901).

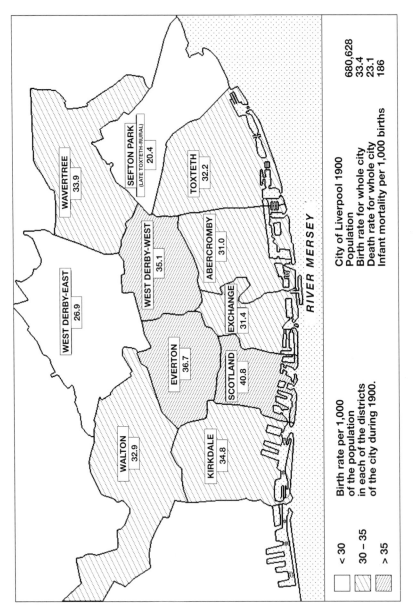

Figure 27: Birth rates in Liverpool districts, 1900
Source: Health Department (1901).

average of 23.1. Infant mortality rates showed a similar distribution over the city, with extremely high rates in Exchange (260 per 1,000 births) and Scotland (241), followed by Toxteth (199) and Kirkdale (195). Despite relatively high birth rates in Wavertree and Walton, the surrounding districts again registered relatively low infant mortality rates. Similar findings have been registered for other towns. In Bradford, for example, the three central wards (Exchange, South and West), which contained the most disadvantaged social groups living in poor housing conditions, registered the city's highest infant mortality rates in 1882–1900 (Thompson, 1984, pp. 134–35); in 1906 crude death rates ranged from 11.0 (per 1,000 inhabitants) in Heaton to 20.4 in North Bierley East ('Cost of Living of the Working Classes', 1908, p. 109). In nineteenth-century Manchester, the highest death rates were recorded in the inner residential areas, while low mortality rates were registered around the periphery (Pooley and Pooley, 1984, pp. 161–67). According to the Medical Officer's Report for 1905, infant mortality in Sheffield was 27.9 (per 100 births) in the oldest and most depressed part of the city, in Sheffield North, whereas the average for the city as a whole was 17.4 ('Cost of Living of the Working Classes', 1908, p. 412).

More detailed information about the devastating effects of different diseases can be obtained if we return to the larger registration areas, contained in the Reports of the Registrar-General, and compare the mortality statistics of the various registration districts (RDs) of the City of Liverpool, namely Liverpool, West Derby, Birkenhead and, later, Toxteth Park. In 1871–1880 the Liverpool registration district registered an average annual death rate of 33.6 per 1,000 inhabitants in contrast to much better rates in West Derby (23.4) and Birkenhead (20.4). Infant mortality in the Liverpool RD was 27.3 and surpassed the rates in suburban West Derby (18.9) and Birkenhead (16.0) by far. Almost all registered diseases contributed to the unhealthy conditions in the Liverpool RD. Particularly high death rates were recorded from typhus, diarrhoea and dysentery, diseases of the nervous system, phthisis, violence and 'other causes'. A very high mortality rate was due to diseases of the respiratory system. This was only comparable with the inner-city of Manchester, represented by the Manchester RD. The death rate from diseases of the respiratory system in the Liverpool RD stood at 70.53 per 10,000 inhabitants (1871–1880), in comparison with 61.23 (1871–1873) and 71.59 (1874–1880) respectively in the Manchester RD.

By the first decade of the twentieth century Liverpool had taken over from Manchester the role of the unhealthiest city in the urban sample, with what remained an extraordinarily high crude death rate in the Liverpool RD of 30.5 deaths per 1,000 inhabitants. This only represented a marginal improvement in absolute terms in comparison with 1871–1880. The differences between the registration districts, however, actually increased as the neighbouring RDs registered substantial mortality improvements. There were strong variations according to age: the younger age-groups (2–45) and the very old (over 65) showed an improvement in death rates in the Liverpool RD, whereas the situation for infants and the age-group 45–65 deteriorated. The particularly prominant causes of death in comparison with other towns in the sample were pneumonia, bronchitis, diarrhoea and dysentery, violence and 'other causes'. In the Liverpool RD digestive diseases continued to take their toll, and the death rate from diarrhoea and dysentery was even worse in the early twentieth century than in the previous period. In the healthier towns, improvements in the death rate affected all age-groups, and the differences between the registration districts became more attenuated.

Despite differences in town planning[33] and the fact that ethnicity did not play a decisive role in the residental structure of nineteenth-century German cities,[34] the pattern of structural change in the largest towns in both countries under observation showed obvious similarities. Increasing social segregation characterized intra-city structures. Residential and commercial areas became more and more separated. As a characteristic of this process the population of the city centre migrated towards the outer borders, and commerce and retailing increasingly dominated the urban core. In many large towns, however, the old inner-city (the *Altstadt*) was not affected by this process (Matzerath, 1985, p. 284). Housing in these areas was cheap, and occupied by inhabitants of low socio-economic status. The houses and flats were of such a low standard that they were frequently called '*unternormale Wohnungen*' (Eberstadt, 1920, pp. 366–73)—sub-normal flats—or, as the English called them, slums. In Hamburg, for example, this situation can be clearly identified, demonstrated by the high population density (inhabitants per room without kitchen) in 1885 in the districts on the Elbe, with particularly high density rates in Steinwärder (1.79), Klein Grasbrook (1.75), Billwärder Ausschlag (1.70), followed by the Altstadt and the Neustadt, Horn and St Pauli, and in the working-class suburbs Barmbeck (1.65) and Winterhude (1.48) (Fig. 28), surpassing the average for the whole town of 1.40 inhabitants per room.[35] Again these conditions found a reflection in the mortality rate (Fig. 29), with a positive coefficient of correlation between the two variables.[36] The interrelationship between housing conditions and health, however, was rather complex, and will be discussed in more detail in a separate chapter (see Chapter 10).

33 See Sutcliffe (1981). See also Chapter 10.

34 Polish migration into the Ruhr area, or the increasing presence of Italian migrants in many German cities by the beginning of the twentieth century, did not lead to a substantial ethnic segregation in the residental structure within the large German towns. Polish in-migrants, for example, often settled outside the towns in the colonies built by the mining companies in close proximity to the mines. See Kleßmann (1978); Stefanski (1984). More general is Herbert (1986).

35 For further indicators see Table 38 and Wischermann (1983).

36 The correlation of the number of inhabitants per room (without kitchen) in 1885 and the crude death rate in 1887, $r = 0.5469$, sig. (two-tailed) = 0.008. It has to be kept in mind in this context that numerous diseases are not associated with population density (digestive diseases, typhoid fever, etc.). This is also the reason why the year 1887 has been selected for the CDR, as Hamburg in 1885 suffered from typhoid fever epidemics (see p. 122). If the density indicator is correlated with the death rate from tuberculosis the correlation is higher, with $r = 0.6564$, sig. (two-tailed) = 0.001. Sources: see Table 28.

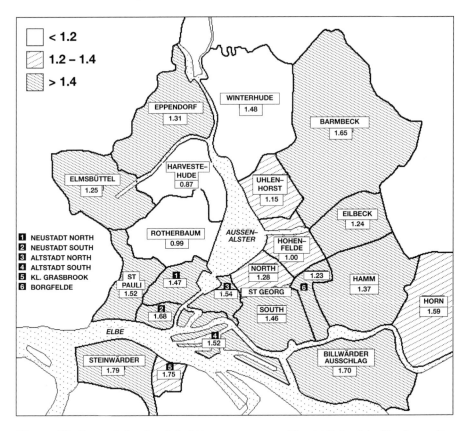

Figure 28: Internal density (inhabitants per room without kitchen) in Hamburg city districts, 1885

Sources: See Table 28.

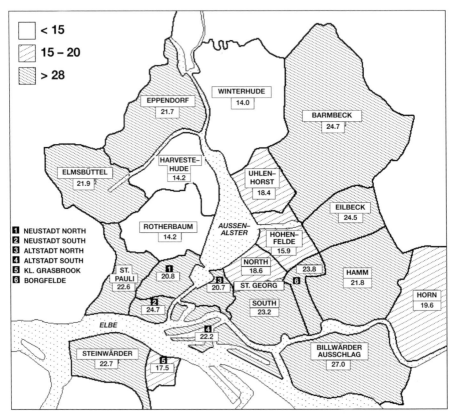

Figure 29: Crude mortality rates in Hamburg city districts (per 1,000 inhabitants), 1887
Sources: See Table 28.

Chapter 7

CONCLUSION TO PART II

An 'urban penalty' can be identified in both countries, yet in Germany it disappeared relatively quickly after peaking in the two decades after the middle of the nineteenth century, corresponding with the breakthrough to large-scale urbanization. After the turn of the century, urban CDRs and SMRs were below the corresponding rates for Prussia. In England and Wales the gap between urban and rural mortality rates was converging from the beginning of the period under investigation, yet the 'urban penalty' was still present at the start of the twentieth century. Comparing the situation in both countries, the following can be stated. In Germany, the mortality rates of the 1870s were significantly higher than in England and Wales, with respect to both urban rates and nationwide, but due to the rapid decline in German urban mortality in the following decades the ten largest towns in both countries registered similar death rates after the turn of the century. By contrast, national figures still reveal better health conditions in England and Wales when compared with Prussia.

In both countries the 'urban penalty' affected almost all age-groups. However, it was predominant in the younger age-groups, particularly concerning infants, as well as among the higher male age-groups. Furthermore, it was evident in relation to almost all important diseases, although the main killers of that period, namely diseases of the respiratory and digestive systems, played a disproportionate role. Mortality rates from digestive diseases, including typhoid fever, made a greater contribution to the spatial variations between the cities than lung diseases. Mortality variations within individual cities, however, surpassed inter-urban differences.

In the disease panorama the major difference between German and English urban mortality was the dominance of the gastro-intestinal disease complex in the former case, with death rates more than twice as high as in the English urban sample. It was the reduction in mortality from this complex which to a large extent was responsible for the rapid disappearance of the 'urban penalty' in Germany. Correspondingly, major improvements can be found in the mortality of younger age-groups, especially amongst infants. This analysis of the course and character of the 'urban penalty' will now be used as a basis for investigating the determinants of the mortality decline, and for evaluating the impact of economic growth, of housing conditions, of the different public health strategies applied in England and Germany to combat disease, as well as of various types of medical supply and intervention on the urban mortality decline.

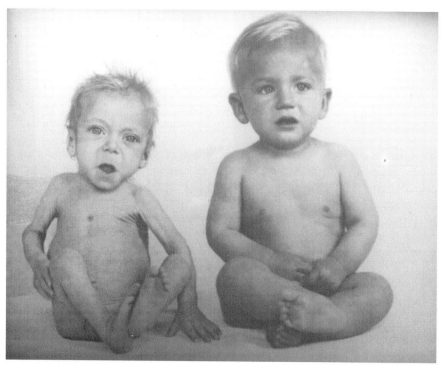

Plate 1: Left: infant, 12 months, nourished with animal milk; right: infant, 10 months, breast-fed c.1904

Source: University of Düsseldorf, Institut für Geschichte der Medizin

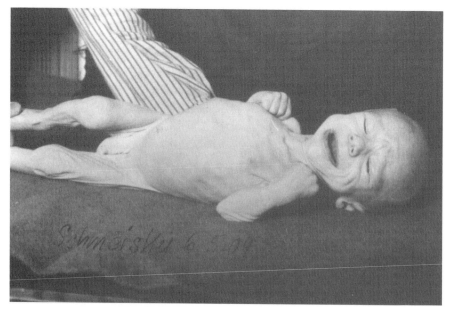

Plate 2: Infant suffering from atrophy, 1904

Source: University of Düsseldorf, Institut für Geschichte der Medizin

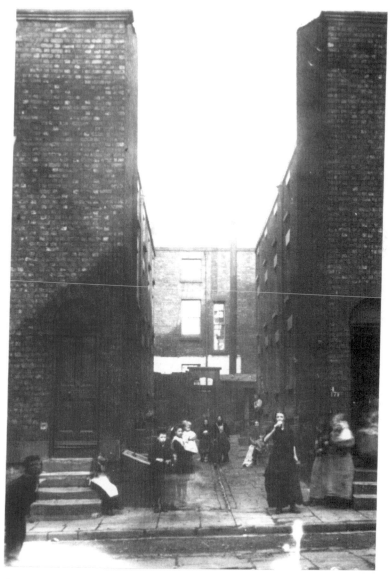

Plate 3: Court No. 7, Llanrwst Street, Liverpool, 1897
Source: Liverpool Record Office, Liverpool Libraries and Information Services; City
Engineers Collection, photograph no. 11

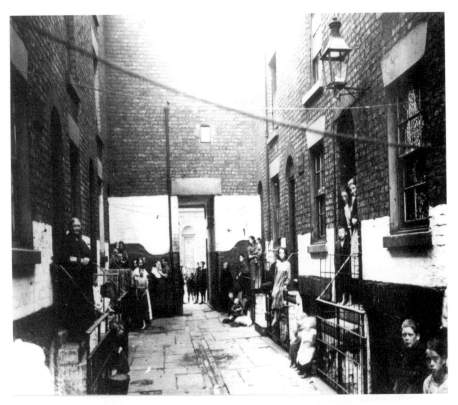

Plate 4: Court No. 2, Silvester Street, Blenheim Street area, Liverpool, 1913
Source: Liverpool Record Office, Liverpool Libraries and Information Services; Photos and Small Prints:
Insanitary Housing, 352 HOU 82/19.

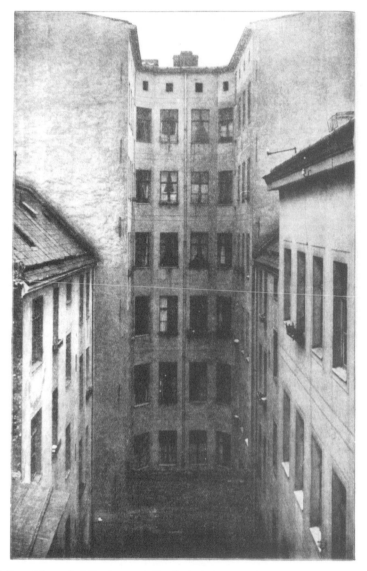

Plate 5: Rental barrack (Mietskaserne), Berlin, built in the 1880s
Source: Eberstadt (1917)

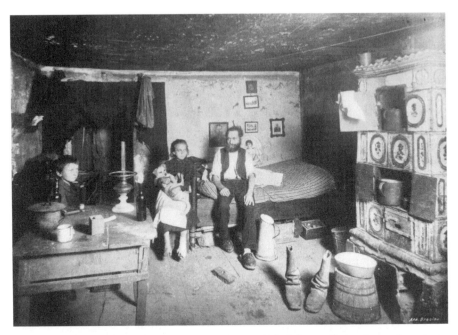

Plate 6: Flat in Breslau, shared by a family of five, 1905: father, suffering from tuberculosis, and son have to share one bed
Source: *Denkschrift zur ersten Wohnungs-Enquete der Orts-Krankenkassen in Breslau* (1906)

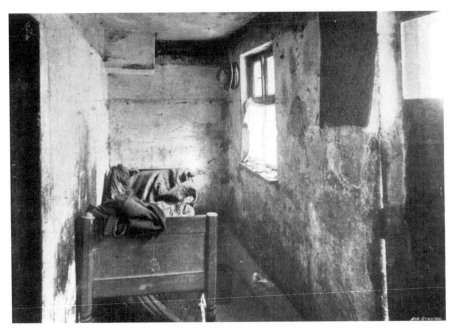

Plate 7: Sleeping room in the same flat in Breslau, 1905
Source: *Denkschrift zur ersten Wohnungs-Enquete der Orts-Krankenkassen in Breslau* (1906)

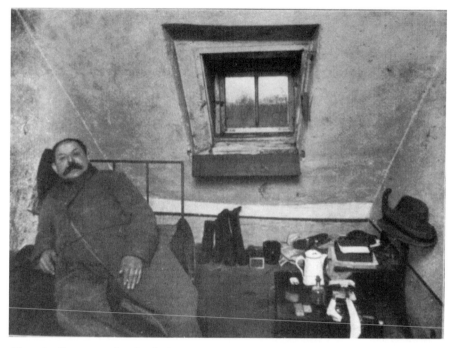

Plate 8: Occupant of a flat in Breslau, 1905, suffering from asthma, rheumatism and stomach trouble

Source: *Denkschrift zur ersten Wohnungs-Enquete der Orts-Krankenkassen in Breslau*, 1906

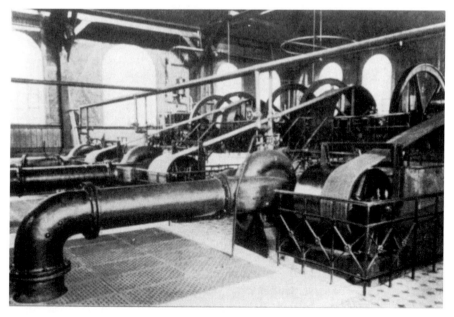

Plate 9: Water pump station, Düsseldorf, c.1904

Source: *Düsseldorf und seine Bauten* (1904)

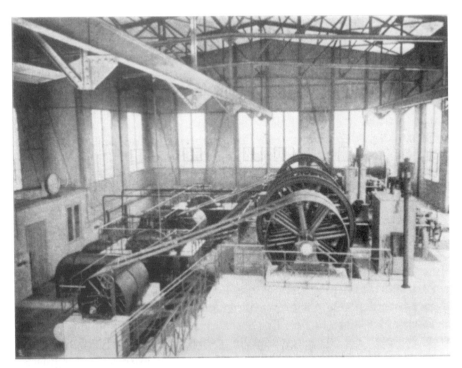

Plate 10: Water pump station, Düsseldorf, c.1904

Source: *Düsseldorf und seine Bauten* (1904)

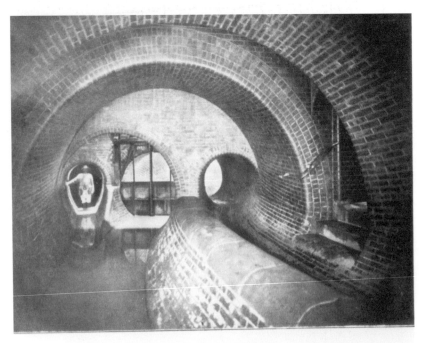

Regenauslasskanal mit Überlaufwehr und Absperrschieber (Königinstrasse).

Plate 11: Part of the sewerage system in Munich, c.1907

Source: *Hygiene und Soziale Fürsorge in München* (1907)

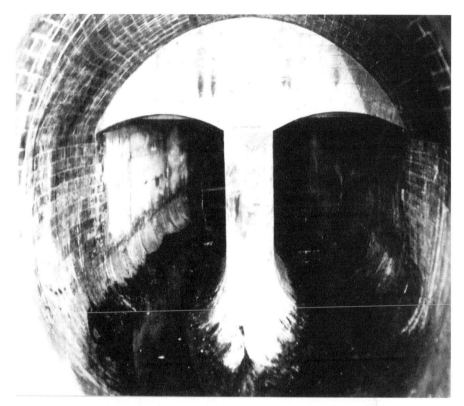

Plate 12: Sewer culvert, Brunswick Street, Liverpool, 1903
Source: Liverpool Record Office, Liverpool Libraries and Information Services; City Engineers Collection, photograph no. 442

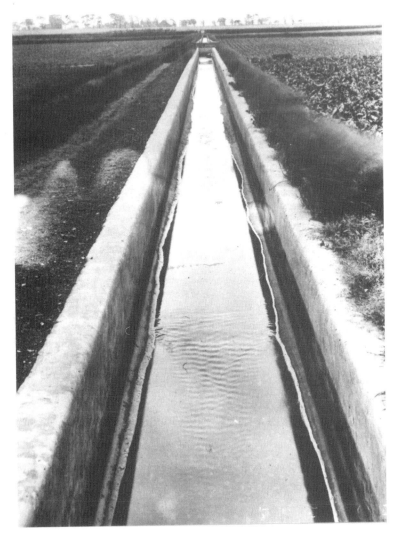

Plate 13: Sewage farm, West Derby, 1897. New carrier
Source: Liverpool Record Office, Liverpool Libraries and Information Services; City Engineers Collection, photograph no. 32

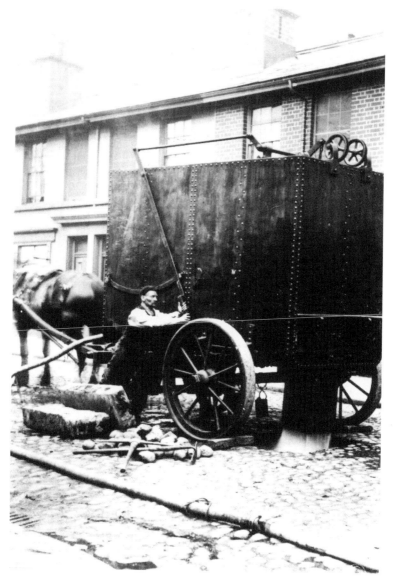

Plate 14: Gully flushing tank, Liverpool, 1897
Source: Liverpool Record Office, Liverpool Libraries and Information Services; City
Engineers Collection, photograph no. 43

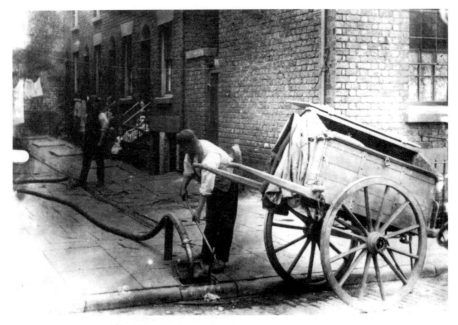

Plate 15: Gully flushing gang, court cleaning, Liverpool, 1897
Source: Liverpool Record Office, Liverpool Libraries and Information Services; City Engineers Collection, photograph no. 48

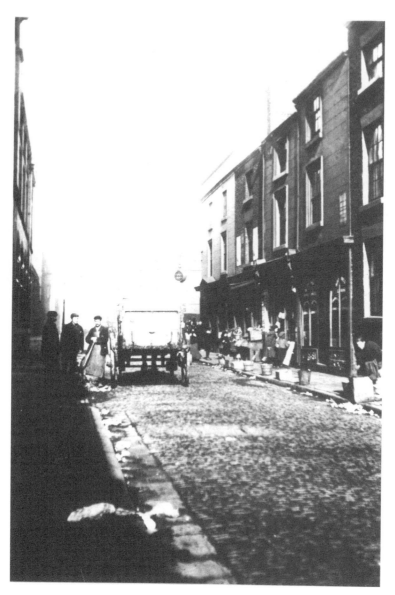

Plate 16: Refuse disposal, Highfield Street, Liverpool, 1902
Source: Liverpool Record Office, Liverpool Libraries and Information Services; City Engineers Collection, photograph no. 248

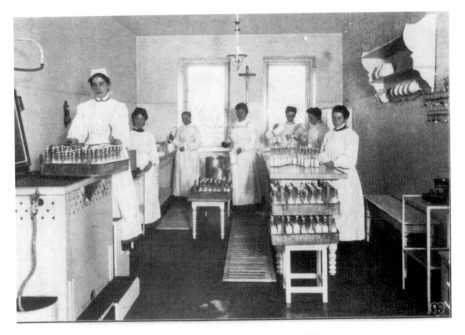

Plate 17: Milk kitchen at a Munich infant welfare centre, c.1907

Source: *Hygiene und Soziale Fürsorge in München* (1907)

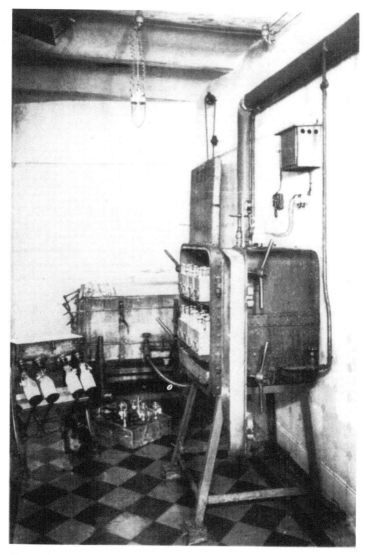

Plate 18: Pasteurization and sterilization of milk, Munich, c.1907
Source: *Hygiene und Soziale Fürsorge in München* (1907)

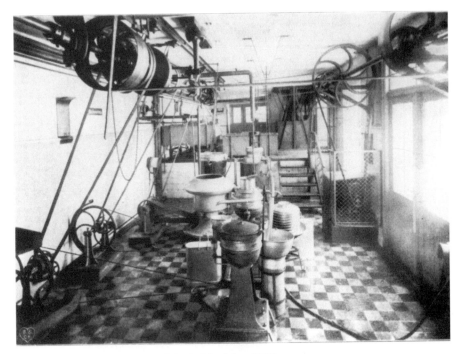

Plate 19: Centrifuge room at a dairy in Munich, c.1907

Source: *Hygiene und Soziale Fürsorge in München* (1907)

III THE DETERMINANTS OF URBAN MORTALITY CHANGE

Chapter 8

INTRODUCTION TO PART III

The most widely accepted explanatory model for analysing nineteenth-century mortality trends remains the 'McKeown-hypothesis', according to which a rise in primary sector output was responsible, not only for an increase in life expectancy, but also for a general improvement of health conditions in Europe. On the other hand, industrialization and urbanization led to a rapid increase in average community size and created specific urban environmental problems, which, of course, required new strategies to fight disease. However, the various age-groups in European society were differentially affected by these developments, and certain diseases, such as plague, which were not directly dependent on the level of living standards, were already in decline or had disappeared. In view of different developments in urban and rural mortality rates, this strongly suggests that other factors apart from the rise in living standards also contributed to the disappearance of the 'urban penalty' in Germany and its decrease in England and Wales.

In order to investigate the reasons for these developments, the analysis will focus on typical urban strategies designed to restrict the incidence of disease, i.e. on the role of different public health measures and types of medical intervention which were introduced during this period. Special emphasis will be placed on water supply and sanitation, overall medical provision and housing conditions. In view of the sharp decline in the 'urban penalty' in Germany, the question arises whether these strategies were applied more rapidly, effectively or on a broader basis than in England. Did the German urban system, therefore, react more appropriately to contemporary health problems than was the case in England? As a start, however, the analysis will turn towards the connection between economic growth and mortality changes, although this study cannot address in detail the broader standard of living debate.

Chapter 9

ECONOMIC GROWTH AND MORTALITY CHANGE

McKeown (1976) estimated that improvements in the quality and quantitity of diet were the prime force behind the European mortality decline in the sense that an under- or malnourished individual presented less resistance to infection. This assumption remains, however, difficult to test in a historical context. McKeown refers to a per capita increase in food supplies, facilitated by structural reform in the primary sector and the introduction of new crops (in particular the potato). His analysis of mortality change is essentially based on developments in five countries: England, Ireland, Sweden, France and Hungary (McKeown, 1976). A direct link between primary sector output and decreasing mortality, however, has not been explored in terms of the German case. Recent research has indicated an improvement in diet during the nineteenth century, from which even the lower classes increasingly benefited in the second half of the century (Teuteberg, 1972; 1979; Dickler, 1975; Abel, 1981; Teuteberg and Wiegelmann, 1986).[1] From the 1870/80s onwards the estimated actual calorific intake increasingly surpassed the recommended amount (Hoffmann, 1965, p. 659). R. Lee, however, has indicated that in the first half of the nineteenth century the McKeown hypothesis is somewhat problematic in the German case, at least at the regional level. For Bavaria there was no clear connection between trends in agricultural output and mortality levels (Lee, 1979; 1980). In this case, nutritional improvements were not directly linked to a decrease in mortality. An increase in per capita food consumption was obviously also dependent on nutritional distribution (social, regional and within the family). This is of special importance in an urban context, where the population was increasingly dependent on money wages in order to purchase the required amounts of food. Furthermore, the neccessary amount and composition of food is dependent on the individual's living and working conditions. A manual working day labourer ideally needs a diet different from that of an office clerk. In order to take this aspect into account, recent research has introduced the term 'nutritional status'. One approach to control for distributional factors and personal requirements is to analyse weight and height of individuals as an indicator for nutritional status.[2] In a recent study W. P. Ward argued that birth weights are a good indicator of maternal nutritional levels (Ward, 1993). He concluded from the data of charitable maternity hospitals in five Western cities (Boston, Dublin, Edinburgh, Montreal, Vienna) that poor women

---

1 For a recent survey in a broader geographical context see Teuteberg (1992). For England see Burnett (1966); Oddy and Miller (1976); Oddy (1982).

2 For attempts to use height as a measure of nutritional status to weight the role of standards of living see Fogel (1986); Floud, et al. (1990). For a recent research review see Harris (1994).

experienced dramatic setbacks in nutrition during the late nineteenth century. All in all, however, information on the actual nutritional status of Europe's population in the nineteenth century is based on cross-sectional and questionable estimates, and comparable material for the selected towns and cities is not available.[3] The next part of this chapter, therefore, will adopt a more classic approach and will focus on economic conditions and growth as a proxy for living standards. This chapter, in particular, will investigate potential links between the prime economic functions of the ten largest towns in England and Germany and their respective mortality levels. It will also provide an analysis of the interrelationship between urban wages and the levels and trends in mortality, including a more detailed assessment of the connections between female labour force participation and infant mortality. Finally, a general comparison between the developments in both England and Germany will be provided.

THE ECONOMIC BASE AND MORTALITY LEVELS

A more direct link between economic growth and demographic development, as provided by an analysis of changes in nutritional status, can be obtained by analysing the primary economic base of the relevant cities and towns. More explicitly, if the standard of living was the major force behind the mortality decline, there should be differences in the mortality development of individual towns dependent on their economic base, at least in the beginning of the period under investigation. After the turn of the century it is likely that these differences between the towns and cities will have disappeared despite remaining regional differences, due to the fact that as a consequence of the growing world market improvements in diet were accessible to the whole urban network of towns, both in England and Germany.

Such an analysis can be undertaken by investigating occupational health, i.e. mortality rates differentiated according to various occupational groups. Social inequality can thereby be assessed. Following the changing interrelationship between health and social class over time also allows a detailed evaluation of the impact of living standards on health. Available data on occupational health, however, are very problematic. In the case of England, for example, they apply only to adult males, and are only available for approximately a hundred different occupations at the national level. German material is differently structured and, again, very heterogeneous, as a consequence of which a comparative approach is not really feasible without losing substantial information. In many cases where information on diseases related to occupation is available there are no data about the population at risk, employed in the specific occupations. What is more, as contemporaries pointed out, occupational classifications used in the official statistics are too crude to represent actual wealth distribution (Prinzing, 1913, p. 31; Silbergleit, 1896, p. 456). To incorporate adequate material on occupational mortality for all the cities in the English and German sample would require an analysis of local data sources, which are invariably

---

3 Contemporary writers had already pointed out that a considerably larger proportion of young males from rural areas were suitable for military service when compared with those from urban areas. See, for example, Teleky (1914), pp. 31–49.

scattered.[4] Furthermore, the number of records to be collated and analysed would far surpass the scope of this study. It would be a task which lies outside the remit of a macro-level approach.

For this reason the following brief discussion of the interrelationship between the economic base of towns and cities and their respective mortality levels will basically rely on established economic classifications (see Appendix 8). Using the German occupational census of 1907 and the methodological approach employed by Blotevogel (1979), Hietala (1987) and Laux (1983; 1989), the sample of the ten largest German towns will be analysed on the basis of primary economic function and occupational structure. A similar classification system, as devised by Greenhow (1858), Welton (1911), and developed by Lawton (1983; 1989), will be applied to the English city sample and combined with the results of the 1911 census.[5] It has to be kept in mind, however, that the census material provides only a static picture of the socio-economic structure in individual cities. Diachronic aspects are excluded, although they might have played a major role where the impact on health is concerned. Laux claims that once the functional character of the towns and cities had been established, it tended to remain relatively stable over time (Laux, 1989). This might be true for the majority of the cities in the sample; it is, however, not true for Düsseldorf, which developed, as already mentioned, from a relatively small residence and garrison town into a modern industrialized town with a significant component of commercial and administrative functions. Furthermore, substantial incorporations of neighbouring municipalities, as for example in Berlin, might have had a profound impact on the economic base of the city. With this limitation in mind, the relationship between occupational structure and urban mortality rates, as well as the link between female participation in formal labour markets and infant mortality will be explored in the following.

A classification of towns according to their economic base remains particularly ambiguous in the case of Germany, because a large proportion of towns had an increasingly multi-functional character (Blotevogel, 1979; Schöller, 1985, p. 283; Laux, 1989). This was reinforced by the persistence of a federal state system in Germany even after political unification in 1871, which meant that most of the towns in the sample retained at least additional governmental functions. In contrast, it is relatively easy to establish a specific economic orientation for most of the English towns in the sample so that an accurate classification can be undertaken more easily (Lawton, 1989). However, bearing in mind the trends towards increasing economic and social segregation within nineteenth-century cities, it will be useful to take advantage of the English registration procedure and analyse the English sample according to urban districts. The differentiation according to registration districts has therefore been kept where possible.

According to these established economic classifications London, Liverpool and its suburb West Derby were dominated by commerce; Bristol by commerce and

---

4 This area is currently being investigated for Sheffield by R. I. Woods and N. Williams, University of Liverpool.

5 See also Banks (1978).

engineering; Birmingham and Aston by hardware, metal and engineering; similarly Sheffield by hardware, tools, steel and metal; the neighbouring registration district of Ecclesall Bierlow by cutlery; Newcastle upon Tyne by commerce, engineering and shipbuilding; and nearby Gateshead by iron, glass, engineering and coalmining. Finally, there was Leeds with woollen textiles, engineering and commerce; Bradford with woollen textiles; Bolton with cotton and engineering; the Manchester area with cotton in Chorlton and Prestwich; and cotton, engineering and commerce in Salford and Manchester. If the results of the 1911 occupational census for the male population are taken as an indicator for the area's economic base the picture becomes more informative.[6] According to the grouped occupations (39 categories), Liverpool's occupational structure was dominated by male workers engaged in the category 'Food, Tobacco, Drink, and Lodging', and in harbour work: 10.5 per cent of all occupied males over 10 years of age were working in the food industry and 9.3 as dock labourers. London and Bristol were dominated by the food business, with 11.1 and 12.4 per cent respectively. In Manchester the predominant category was 'General Engineering and Machine Making', with 11.5 per cent of the male population working within that area. The same was true for Leeds and Newcastle, with 14.6 and 16.7 per cent of the male workforce in this category. Birmingham and Sheffield were dominated by the iron and steel sector ('Iron, Steel, etc. Manufacture; Tools; Dies, etc.; Arms; Misc. Metal Traders'), with 21.9 and 33.8 per cent respectively. In Bradford and Bolton the predominant category was 'Textile Manufactures', with 29.4 and 25.3 per cent.

Relying on these simplistic economic classifications, no direct link can be established for the English sample between the dominant economic base of urban districts and their mortality levels and trends. Districts or towns dominated by commerce, cotton, steel and metal manufacturing can be found anywhere on the scale, ranging from very unhealthy to healthy places in both periods under investigation and with respect to all causes of death, although only tuberculosis and typhoid fever, as repesentatives of the two main disease groups, are represented in Table 24. The question, however, immediately arises whether this is due to the limited utility of such an approach for large urban districts. The largest cities in nineteenth-century England were complex agglomerations with various central functions such that even a more detailed analysis of the economic base might be misleading. It is not surprising, therefore, that differences in the inner-city structures were more decisive in determining mortality levels. As already pointed out in the analysis of spatial variations, the inner centres of the towns, almost as a rule, recorded higher death rates than their surrounding areas. Even in the unhealthy northern towns, where the inner-city districts recorded extremely high death rates, other surrounding local districts had better mortality rates. In 1871–1880, the registration districts of West Derby and Chorlton, suburban parts of the cities of Liverpool and Manchester respectively, were much healthier places than their city centres. The Liverpool RD recorded a crude death rate of 33.6 (per 1,000 inhabitants) compared with 23.4 in West Derby, while the Manchester RD experienced a rate of 31.7 compared with 23.6 in Chorlton (Table 24). In reality,

6 Source: *Published Volumes of the Census of England and Wales* (1911).

despite the ascribed similarity in economic structure, West Derby and Chorlton represented high-status suburbs. Whereas the gap between Manchester and Chorlton became attenuated after the turn of the century, with an even lower death rate from tuberculosis in the Manchester RD (138.6 per 10,000 inhabitants) than the Chorlton RD (151.7), differences in the mortality rates between Liverpool and West Derby became greater, due to the marginal improvement in health conditions in Liverpool.

Despite their ascribed multi-functional character, the occupational census in 1907 reveals that the towns in the German sample were clearly dominated by labourers occupied in industry, mining and construction, followed by trade, transport and food. Civil servants and the self-employed formed the third largest group, though lagging behind somewhat (Table 25). The only exception in the sample is the port-city of Hamburg, where more people were employed in trade (36.7 per cent of the labour force) than in industry (36.1 per cent). As in the English case, mortality levels in German towns also seem to have been quite independent of the economic base. Whether industry, commerce or government administration formed the core activity, this seems to have been an insignificant factor in determining the health conditions in the ten largest towns.[7] For example, the towns with the lowest percentage of the labour force occupied in 'Industry' (Munich, Hamburg and Frankfurt) occupy completely different positions in Table 25, where the towns are ranked according to their CDRs. Again, however, this may be the result of an over-simplistic system of classification. Furthermore, regional mortality patterns, particularly the strong east–west gradient, again appear to have been the main determinant of urban mortality levels and trends in the specific cities under examination.

In relation to tuberculosis, the new industrial towns of western Germany, including Essen, Düsseldorf and Dortmund, recorded relatively low mortality rates.[8] This may, to a certain extent, have been an indirect reflection of the influence of their economic base. These new industrial towns of Rhineland-Westphalia had a relatively low overall proportion of in-migrants (Brückner, 1890, p. 182; Bleicher, 1895, p. 2; Laux, 1989, p. 134),[9] and natural increase was a strong and significant component of population growth (Matzerath, 1984; 1985, p. 310). Düsseldorf, which had a relatively significant level of in-migration—in comparison with other towns of this particular area (Brückner, 1890, p. 182)—nevertheless registered a low percentage of unskilled workers migrating into the city (Köllmann, 1974, pp. 110–12, 120–24). Furthermore, these cities were often embedded in Catholic areas which registered relatively high birth rates (see Table 30), reflecting differences in attitudes and norms regarding sexual behaviour and birth control in comparison with Protestant areas. This large proportion of infants and children

---

7 The correlation of the percentage of labourers in the main occupations and crude death rates gives the following results:

Industry: r = 0.0176, sig. (two-tailed) = 0.962;
Trade: r = -0.3727, sig. (two-tailed) = 0.289;
Civil Servants: r = 0.1921, sig. (two-tailed) = 0.595.

Sources: See Table 25.

8 TB death rates (per 100,000 inhabitants) in 1900–1912 in Essen were 157.5; in Düsseldorf 153.0; in Dortmund 140.4. Source: *Veröffentlichungen des Kaiserlichen Gesundheitsamtes (Beilagen)*.

9 See also Chapter 6.

within the city's total population was also reflected in a relatively high death rate from digestive diseases in most of the periods under discussion in both Cologne and Düsseldorf (in comparison with other towns in the western parts of Germany). All these

Table 24: Economic base and mortality in large English towns, crude death rate (per 1,000 inhabitants), 1871–1880 and 1901–1910, and selected causes of death (per 100,000 inhabitants), 1901–1910

Registration district	Economic base*	Mortality			
		CDR 1871–1880	CDR 1901–1910	TB†	Typhoid
		(per 1,000)		1901–1910 (per 100,000)	
Liverpool	Commerce (food)	33.6	30.5	283.8	13.6
Manchester	Cotton, engineering, commerce (general engineering)	31.7	19.6	138.6	4.6
Salford	Cotton, engineering, commerce (general engineering)	27.7	19.6	173.0	23.8
Sheffield	Hardware, tools, steel, metal (iron, steel, etc. manufacture)	27.4	19.2	122.1	10.8
Prestwich	Cotton	26.8	20.4	240.9	22.7
Leeds	Woollen textiles, engineering, commerce (general engineering)	26.0	17.9	150.7	14.9
Newcastle upon Tyne	Commerce, engineering, shipbuilding (general engineering)	25.9	18.4	162.3	2.6
Birmingham	Hardware, metal, engineering (iron, steel, etc. manufacture)	25.8	22.2	182.9	14.9
Bristol	Commerce, engineering (food)	25.5	14.9	117.8	6.6
Gateshead	coalmining, iron, glass, engineering	24.9	16.9	126.4	7.5
Bolton	Cotton, engineering (textile manufacture)	24.3	16.1	110.8	20.4
Bradford	Woollen textiles (textile manufacture)	23.9	16.1	135.5	12.4
London	Commerce (food)	22.4	15.8	147.7	6.5
Chorlton	Cotton	23.6	16.6	151.7	7.2
West Derby	Commerce	23.4	17.7	142.4	11.5
Ecclesall Bierlow	Cutlery	21.1	14.3	102.3	10.9
Aston	Hardware, metal, engineering	20.7	14.8	115.9	8.4

* Economic base according to the classifications of Greenhow and Welton. In brackets the main occupational category for males over 10 years of age in administrative counties and county boroughs according to the 1911 census.
Mortality rates according to registration districts.
† TB=Pulmonary tuberculosis and phthisis.
Sources: Greenhow (1858); Welton (1911); *Published Volumes of the Census of England and Wales* (1911); *Decennial Supplements to the Annual Reports of the Registrar-General of Births, Deaths, and Marriages in England and Wales* (1871–1880 and 1901–1910).

factors led to a different age-composition of the population, which, in turn, influenced the predominant disease panorama. Returning to age-specific death rates, the potential impact can be demonstrated. In Düsseldorf, for example, low overall death rates from tuberculosis can indeed be attributed to a large degree to these particularities in the age-composition. In the higher age-groups (from 40 years onwards), however, tuberculosis mortality in Düsseldorf was even above the average for the ten largest towns.[10] In this respect, Düsseldorf by no means offered better health conditions than the other towns of the sample. Finally, as in the case of the English cities, mortality from typhoid fever also failed to reveal any significant link with the economic base of individual towns.

Table 25: Economic base, principal occupations (in 1907) and mortality in the ten largest German towns, crude death rate (per 1,000 inhabitants), 1877–1889 and 1900–1913, and selected causes of death (per 100,000 inhabitants), 1900–1913

City/town	Economic base *	Principal Occupations in 1907 (%)†			Mortality			
		Industry‡	Trade‡	CS‡	CDR 1877–1889 (per 1,000)	CDR 1900–1913	TB 1900–1913 (per 100,000)	Typhoid
Munich	Government Commerce	36	24	11	31.7	18.5	269.0	2.8
Breslau	Government Commerce	43	21	9	30.5	21.7	312.6	6.0
Cologne	Commerce	44	25	8	26.5	18.6	191.8	4.6
Nuremberg	Industry	58	19	6	26.4	18.1	248.7	1.5
Berlin	Government Commerce	49	23	7	26.3	15.8	213.5	3.8
Hamburg	Commerce	36	37	6	26.2	15.4	173.6	4.1
Düsseldorf	Industry	50	21	8	24.1	15.7	153.0	3.0
Dresden	Government Industry	45	22	10	24.1	14.9	207.9	4.2
Leipzig	Commerce	50	25	6	22.3	16.0	204.5	3.9
Frankfurt	Commerce	40	27	7	20.0	14.5	208.6	2.4

* Economic classification according to Blotevogel (1979), p. 250; Hietala (1987), p. 97; Laux (1983), pp. 72–73.

†Percentage of the total labour force.

‡ Industry = Industry, mining and construction;
  Trade = Trade, transport and food;
  CS = Civil servants and self-employed.

Sources: *Veröffentlichungen des Kaiserlichen Gesundheitsamtes (Beilagen); Statistik des Deutschen Reichs*, NF **207** (1909/10).

10 From 40 to 60 years—Düsseldorf 29.91 deaths per 10,000 inhabitants in 1907; all towns 28.26. Over 60 years of age—Düsseldorf 34.99; all towns 27.95.

INCOME AND MORTALITY CHANGE

Despite the increasing wealth of the two nations and rising living standards in the second half of the nineteenth century,[11] a large number of the population in both countries were still living in poor and insecure conditions, as rising income was not equally distributed amongst the different classes. In Germany, according to W. Sombart's contemporary analysis of the occupational census of 1895, two-thirds of the population led a proletarian or proletarian-like existence (Sombart, 1903, pp. 531–52). From modern reconstructed time series on nineteenth-century wages it has been estimated that in mid-century Germany two-thirds of the population, and at the end of the century one-half of the population lived in poor conditions (Zapf, 1983, p. 52). Concerning England, Charles Booth concluded in his famous social investigation that in the 1880s and 1890s 30.7 per cent of all the people in London lived on or below the poverty line.[12] His findings were confirmed by Rowntree's pioneering study on poverty in York, first published at the beginning of the twentieth century.[13] The life of the urban working class was inherently unstable; despite working many hours for comparatively little wages, no savings could be amassed. Additionally, both female and male workers were often subject to seasonal unemployment (Treble, 1979, pp. 72–80). It has been estimated that approximately 25 per cent of male workers in late-Victorian Britain could expect interrupted income within the course of a year (Stedman Jones, 1971, pp. 52–66). Within that context continuing unemployment, disease or the death of the main family earner became the biggest threat. Disease and physical exhaustion could reduce the status even of a skilled worker to that of a day labourer. Before sufficient social insurance programmes were launched at the beginning of the twentieth century, incapacity to work, resulting from disability in old age, meant a considerable drop in living standards. If those affected were not taken into their family's or children's home, they had to turn to poor relief and, in Germany, to the benefits of disability and old-age insurance. Yet, even this provided them only with the bare minimum. These risks increased with advancing age, as sharp differences in the standard of living were not related only to social class, but also to stages in the life-cycle (Schomerus, 1979). After years of hard work in unhealthy surroundings the fate of the industrial worker was typically marked by a decline in position and income, and was already apparent around the age of forty (Weber, 1912; Syrup-Gleiwitz, 1914; Rowntree, 1971). Indeed, as demonstrated above in the analysis of age-specific mortality, the risk of dying was especially prominent in an urban environment for males in the higher age-groups (Figs 12 and 13).

---

11 See Feinstein (1990a; 1990b); Gömmel (1979); Orsagh (1969); Zamagni (1989); Zapf (1983).

12 Booth (1889; 1891). Booth carried on with his research in the following years and added these new surveys to a re-issue of his first studies, published 1892–1897 under the title *Life and Labour of the People in London*. For a commented synopsis of his work see *Charles Booth's London* (1969). See also O'Day and Englander (1993).

13 Rowntree (1971). For a comprehensive account on poverty largely based on the investigations of Booth and Rowntree, see Treble (1979).

Table 26: Correlation coefficients of wages for labourers in the building and engineering industries, a rent and price index, 1905, and crude death rates, mortality from selected causes, and infant mortality in the ten largest English towns, 1901–1910

	CDR	TB	Dig	Ty	Dip	Cb	IMR
LBUI	−.3583	.0132	−.3676	−.0875	−.0075	−.2881	−.3269
	P= .309	P= .971	P= .296	P= .810	P= .984	P= .420	P= .356
LENG	−.4744	−.0553	−.4707	−.5862	.0047	−.3052	−.2954
	P= .197	P= .888	P= .201	P= .097	P= .991	P= .425	P= .440
RPI	−.2350	.2809	−.4115	−.7289	−.3655	−.8076	−.2707
	P= .513	P= .432	P= .237	P= .017	P= .299	P= .005	P= .449

LBUI=Wages for labourers in building industries; LENG=Wages for labourers in engineering industries; RPI=Rent and price index; CDR=Crude death rate; TB=Tuberculosis death rate; Dig=Digestive diseases death rate; Ty=Typhoid fever death rate; Dip=Diphtheria death rate; Cb=Childbirth death rate; IMR=Infant mortality rate; P=Two-tailed significance. Sources: 'Cost of Living of the Working Classes' (1908); *Decennial Supplement to the Annual Reports of the Registrar-General of Births, Deaths, and Marriages in England and Wales* (1901–1910).

In order to obtain a closer insight into the interrelationship between income and health,[14] notwithstanding inevitable source problems, use will be made of wages for labourers in the building and engineering industries and of a rent and price index for the sample of English towns in 1905, as well as of the average wage earned for day labour (*ortsüblicher Tagelohn*) paid to female and male workers over 16 years of age in the sample of German towns in 1912 as an indicator of contemporary income levels. It has to be noted that seasonality of work cannot be compensated for in that context.

Expressed as a coefficient of correlation, there is a relatively weak interrelationship between average wages in the building and engineering industries, and crude death rates and infant mortality rates, as well as death rates from various causes, such as tuberculosis, digestive diseases, typhoid fever, diphtheria and childbirth (Table 26). Using a rent and price index as a proxy for costs of living, the coefficients of correlation are similarly weak, except for, surprisingly, deaths from typhoid fever (−0.7289) and at childbirth (−0.8076)—causes of death which are normally rather associated with environmental conditions or medical interventions.

For the German towns, however, there is a relatively strong association between male wages and the crude death rate (−0.7947) as well as with the female tuberculosis death rate (−0.7218) (Table 27), indicating the importance of male earnings for the family. The lack of a correlation between male wages and infant mortality could reflect the difficulties encountered by men on low wages in actually starting a family. This might have been possible, however, with additional female earnings, which would have raised the family's prospective standard of living. Female wages register

14 See also Kunitz and Engerman (1992).

Table 27: Correlation coefficients of average day labour wages for workers over 16 years of age, 1912, and the crude death rate, mortality from selected causes, infant mortality and birth rate in large German towns, 1907 and 1900–1913

	CDR 1907	TB 1907	Dig 1907	Ty 1907	Dip 1907	CDRF 1907	TBF 1907	TyF 1907	Cb	IMR 1900–1913	Br
MW	−.7947	−.6013	−.5395	−.3728	−.1841	−.6652	−.7218	.6803	.1739	−.4559	−.2138
	P=.006	P=.066	P=.108	P=.289	P=.611	P=.051	P=.028	P=.044	P=.631	P=.185	P=.553
FW	−.6473	−.3852	−.7390	−.2157	−.4339	−.4210	−.2094	.3766	−.1477	−.6974	−.4843
	P=.043	P=.272	P=.015	P=.549	P=.210	P=.259	P=.589	P=.318	P=.684	P=.025	P=.156

MW=Male wages; FW=Female wages; CDR=Crude death rate; TB=Tuberculosis death rate; Dig=Digestive diseases death rate; Ty=Typhoid fever death rate; Dip=Diphtheria death rate; CDRF= Crude death rate females; TBF=Tuberculosis death rate females; TyF=Typhoid fever death rate females; Cb=Childbirth death rate; IMR=Infant mortality rate; Br=Birth rate; P=Two-tailed significance.

Sources: *Statistisches Jahrbuch Deutscher Städte,* **19** (1913), p. 8 26; *Veröffentlichungen des Kaiserlichen Gesundheitsamtes (Beilagen)* (1901–1914); Appendix 2.

a negative correlation with digestive diseases primarily affecting infants (–0.7390), and the infant mortality rate (–0.6974). This underlines the complex impact of female labour force participation on the health of infants, which will be the focus of the following chapter. In contrast to the English case, the interrelationship between earnings and death rates from typhoid fever and death at childbirth is rather weak.

However, additional evidence of the interrelationship between the standard of living and people's health can be gained by a more differentiated analysis of city districts. The well-known example of Hamburg reveals a strong correlation between the annual taxable income per capita and the crude death rate (–0.6989), and especially deaths from tuberculosis (–0.7282) (Table 28). City districts with a high per capita income reveal the lowest tuberculosis death rate, and vice versa (Figs 30 and 31). This is supported by a strong correlation between other indicators of contemporary living standards, such as the number of tenements with a bath and the number of households with domestic servants, and the death rate from tuberculosis (–0.7624; –0.7270). Given the overall importance of tuberculosis within the contemporary disease panorama, there was an equally significant correlation between these two variables and the overall crude death rate (–0.6679; –0.6780). A relatively strong correlation between indicators of overcrowding and the tuberculosis death rate, and between population density and typhoid fever, indicates the important impact of housing conditions on health, which will be dealt with in a separate chapter.

The interdependence between income distribution and infant mortality in Hamburg is not quite as strong (–0.5758) as is the case with tuberculosis, primarily because of the absence of a direct connection between wealth and deaths from digestive diseases, which remained the main cause of infant deaths in the late nineteenth century. This indicates that in the case of Hamburg, additional environmental factors played a more prominent role.

Table 28: Health and social class in Hamburg during the 1880s—coefficients of correlation

	CDR	Ty	TB	Ddd	IMR	Inc	Inh	Bath	Derv	Chil	Wom	Dens	Popd	Sinh
CDR	1.0000	.2523	.6685†	-.0165	.5194	-.6989†	-.4985	-.6679†	-.6780†	.6170*	-.6987†	.5469*	.5029	.2851
Ty	.2523	1.0000	.5455*	.2531	-.1662	-.1375	-.3673	-.2411	-.1892	-.2895	-.1106	.1574	.3954	-.2059
Tb	.6685†	.5455*	1.0000	-.1917	.3439	-.7282†	-.4753	-.7624†	-.7270†	.2037	-.5575*	.6564†	.5827*	.3808
Ddd	-.0165	.2531	-.1917	1.0000	-.2186	.1638	-.3070	.1593	.1997	-.1291	.1816	-.3406	.0792	-.4673
IMR	.5194	-.1662	.3439	-.2186	1.0000	-.5758*	-.0440	-.5221	-.6006*	.5747*	-.4783	.4272	.0187	.3983
Inc	-.6989†	-.1375	-.7282†	.1638	-.5758*	1.0000	.4602	.9835†	.9628†	-.5944*	.8427†	-.8360†	-.5626*	-.6541†
Inh	-.4985	-.3673	-.4753	-.3070	-.0440	.4602	1.0000	.4435	.3478	-.1729	.3217	-.1724	-.4236	-.0047
Bath	-.6679†	-.2411	-.7624†	.1593	-.5221	.9835†	.4435	1.0000	.9795†	-.5239	.8482†	-.8730†	-.6092*	-.6670†
Derv	-.6780†	-.1892	-.7270†	.1997	-.6006*	.9628†	.3478	.9795†	1.0000	-.6012*	.8683†	-.9204†	-.6141*	-.7500†
Chil	.6170*	-.2895	.2037	-.1291	.5747*	-.5944*	-.1729	-.5239	-.6012*	1.0000	-.7636†	.4905	.4027	.5793*
Wom	-.6987†	-.1106	-.5575*	.1816	-.4783	.8427†	.3217	.8482†	.8683†	-.7636†	1.0000	-.8256†	-.7020†	-.6813†
Dens	.5469*	.1574	.6564†	-.3406	.4272	-.8360†	-.1724	-.8730†	-.9204†	.4905	-.8256†	1.0000	.6810†	.8481†
Popd	.5029	.3954	.5827*	.0792	.0187	-.5626*	-.4236	-.6092*	-.6141*	.4027	-.7020†	.6810†	1.0000	.4449
Sinh	.2851	-.2059	.3808	-.4673	.3983	-.6541†	-.0047	-.6670†	-.7500†	.5793*	-.6813†	.8481†	.4449	1.0000

N of cases: 22   Two-tailed signif: *-.01 †-.001

CDR=Crude death rate (1887); Ty=Typhoid fever death rate (1885–1888); TB=Tuberculosis death rate (1887); Ddd=Diarrhoea and dysentery death rate (1894); IMR=Infant mortality rate (1894–1900); Inc=Annual taxable income per capita (Marks) (1886); Inh=Inhabitants per tenement (1885); Bath=Number of tenements with baths (1885); Derv=Number of households with domestic servants (1885); Chil=Number of children under age 15 (1885); Wom=Women in the labour force (1900); Dens=Number of inhabitants per room (without kitchen); Popd=Population per hectare (1885); Sinh=Share of inhabitants to the total population in per cent (1885).

Sources: Reincke (1890), pp. 16, 17, 19; *Die Gesundheitsverhältnisse Hamburgs* (1901), pp. 221, 291; *Statistik des Hamburgischen Staates*, **14** (1887), p. 14; **15** (1894), p. 57; **17** (1895), p. 8; Wischermann (1983), pp. 443, 445, 460, 463, 469, 475, 476.

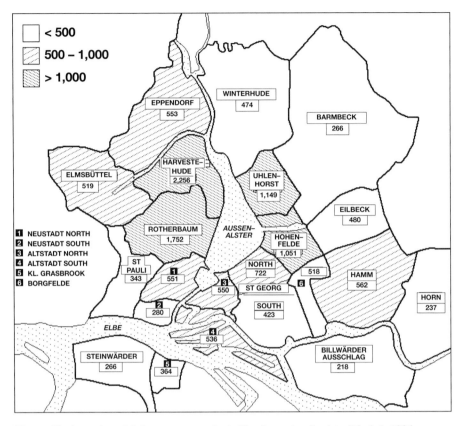

Figure 30: Annual taxable income per capita in Hamburg city districts (Marks), 1886
Sources: See Table 28.

Similarily, on a larger aggregate level, there was quite a strong interrelationship between social class and infant mortality, although this does not explain all the differentials. Using Prussian statistics, Reinhard Spree has shown the immense differences in infant mortality according to parental occupation, with the lowest figures reported in relation to civil servants and extraordinary high rates amongst domestic servants, where the percentage of illegitimate infants was also high (Spree, 1981a, p. 59; 1995). Spree has demonstrated that decreasing infant mortality in Prussia in the late nineteenth century affected the various social classes differently so that class-specific variations increased substantially. As the major differences, however, did not occur between 'capital' and 'labour', he suggests that additional factors must have been operating. A similar widening of infant mortality rates according to the father's social class has been suggested for England and Wales during the nineteenth and early twentieth centuries (Titmuss, 1943, pp. 44–45; Watterson, 1988; Woods et al., 1993, p. 46). Using the census of 1911, class-specific rates of infant mortality have been produced for the period 1895–1911, demonstrating a clear inverse association in infant mortality rates from the highest to the lowest classes.[15] The levels declined for every class at different rates so that social inequality increased. In this case, however, the broad occupational categories do not allow a judgement to be made on whether the increasing differentials might be the result of growing inequalities in income distribution. The benefits of rising living standards were far from being equally spread over the various social classes. Moreover, in 1895–1897 agricultural labourers registered lower infant mortality rates (110 per 1,000 births) than the professional class (121). After the turn of the century the ratio changed: in 1910 the professional class registered an infant mortality rate of 59 per 1,000 births, agricultural labourers 87. Obviously, at the end of the nineteenth century rural living conditions outweighed the higher incomes available in an urban environment, stressing again the role of environmental factors. N. Williams has pointed out recently that urban class differentials became accentuated in areas with poor environmental conditions (Williams, 1992). Other influential factors can be found in socio-cultural areas. For example, in the United States around 1900, occupational differences

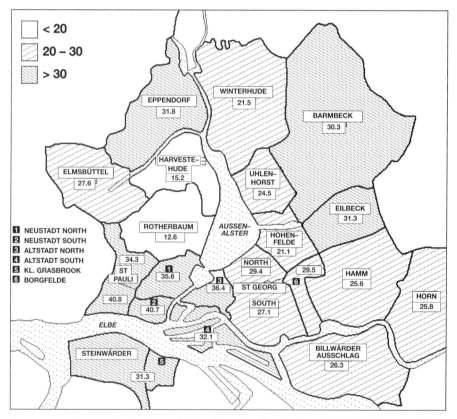

Figure 31: Tuberculosis death rates in Hamburg city districts (per 10,000 inhabitants), 1887
Sources: See Table 28.

15 For a recent survey see Haines (1991).

were far less pronounced when compared with differentials by ethnic group (Preston and Haines, 1991). Irish and German families, for example, with high infant mortality in a nineteenth-century European context, still registered their traditionally high infant mortality rates. In conclusion, it can be stated that the standard of living had a substantial impact on health, although additional factors were also at work. These included culturally-determined behaviour and environmental conditions.

FEMALE LABOUR FORCE PARTICIPATION

A further indicator frequently used to analyse the possible interrelationship between living standards and health conditions is the proportion of women in the labour force, or conversely the proportion of women 'mainly engaged in household duties'. Many contemporaries attributed high infant mortality rates primarily to the participation of women in the labour force, particularly in industrial work. High female labour force participation was associated with an absence of breast-feeding, and a general neglect of child care (Jones, 1894, pp. 54–56; Dyhouse, 1978, pp. 251–53). Contemporary studies examining the reasons why women did not breast-feed pointed out that many women were physically incapable of breast-feeding as a result of hard work and poor living conditions. Investigations in a Munich children's hospital, for example, claimed that in 58 per cent of all cases the reason for not breast-feeding was a physical one (Escherich, 1887, p. 257). Whatever the actual reasons were, medical personnel regularly blamed the mothers for not breast-feeding, pointing out that breast-feeding was relatively cost-free, so that the mothers actually did not need to go to work. Consequently, health authorities proposed excluding women from the formal economy for the benefit of their children. This was a clear misjudgement of the situation, as mothers often sold their milk in order to provide a little extra income. Furthermore, it was a complete misjudgement of the female economy and women's work. This section will explore the nature and structure of women's work in both countries and will analyse its impact on health, in particular where mother and child were concerned.

Table 29 indicates that in England and Wales the number of women not actively participating in the formal labour force was constantly increasing from mid-century onwards, both nationwide and in the largest towns.[16] In 1911 the percentage of females officially registered as being engaged solely in household work varied between 57.1 in London and over seventy in Sheffield and Newcastle (including Gateshead). Nationwide the average was 63.2 per cent. Agriculture remained the largest source of female employment.[17] Despite industrialization, women in an urban environment remained concentrated in a few occupations, which frequently revealed affinities to

16 Although data on women above the age of 10–20 over time may well reflect improved legislation on child employment and increased schooling, this effect is supposed to be counterbalanced by a reduction of the age limit for inclusion in the census from 20 to 10 from 1891 onwards.

17 For an introduction to the subject see Higgs (1987); Hudson and Lee (1990); John (1986); Lewis (1984; 1986); Roberts (1988); Tilly and Scott (1978).

Table 29: Wives and others mainly engaged in households (%), mortality in combined registration districts, female crude death rate (per 1,000 inhabitants), selected female causes of death (per 10,000 inhabitants) and IMR, 1901–1910

City/town	f >20 1851	f > 20 1871	f >10 1891	f >10 1911	CDR(f) /1,000	TB(f)* /100,000	IMR /100	Childbirth† /10,000
London	50.7	54.1	55.7	57.1	14.4	106.0	15.5	1.59
Bristol	47.0	50.0	53.0	59.0	14.0	103.6	14.3	1.85
Birmingham	57.8	58.9	56.6	59.3	16.4	125.9	19.5	2.22
Liverpool	58.6	63.4	64.4	66.7	17.7	122.1	18.6	2.18
Bolton	54.3	48.9	49.3	55.3	15.2	89.8	17.3	2.55
Manchester	51.3‡	51.9‡	54.7	59.3	17.3	134.7	19.4	2.25
Salford	–	–	57.0	60.3	18.1	132.4	20.1	2.14
Bradford	53.3	49.6	48.0	53.9	14.9	107.0	16.7	2.41
Leeds	57.5	61.7	58.8	60.9	16.2	109.1	18.2	2.35
Sheffield	67.8	71.4	68.0	70.9	15.9	69.3	20.6	2.70
Gateshead	72.6	77.4	76.1	76.3	16.3	113.4	18.5	3.28
Newcastle	62.3	65.9	68.1	71.7	16.9	132.6	17.8	2.36
England/Wales	54.1	56.1	60.8	63.2	14.4	96.9	15.0	2.11

Wives and others mainly engaged in household duties and widows, daughters and scholars over 20 years of age, 1851; wives and others mainly engaged in household duties over 20 years of age, 1871; unoccupied females over 10 years of age (excluding retired, pensioners, own means), 1891; unoccupied females (students, scholars, others) at ages 10 years and upwards, 1911.

1851, 1871 principal towns = cities and boroughs having defined municipal limits, except for Manchester (city) and Salford (borough) 1851, 1871 = parliamentary limits; London = registration division.

1891 urban sanitary districts, London = registration division.

1911 principal towns: Bristol, Liverpool, Manchester, Newcastle, Birmingham, Bradford, Leeds, Sheffield = county boroughs (city); Birkenhead, Bolton, Salford, Gateshead = county borough; Aston Manor = municipal borough; London = administrative county.

Mortality rates for London; Bristol; Birmingham=Birmingham and Aston; Liverpool= Liverpool, Birkenhead, Toxteth Park and West Derby; Bolton; Manchester= Manchester, Prestwich and Chorlton; Salford; Bradford; Leeds; Sheffield=Sheffield and Ecclesall Bierlow; Gateshead; Newcastle.

* TB=Pulmonary tuberculosis and phthisis.

†Childbirth=childbirth and puerperal fever.

‡ Manchester and Salford.

Sources: *Published Volumes of the Census of England and Wales* (1851, 1871, 1891, 1911); *Decennial Supplement to the Annual Reports of the Registrar-General of Births, Deaths, and Marriages in England and Wales* (1901–1910).

housework. In Britain in 1911 35 per cent were employed as domestic servants, 19.5 per cent as textile workers and 15.6 per cent as garment workers (Hudson and Lee, 1990, p. 21). The 1911 census gives further details for the English sample of towns (grouped occupations; 32 categories). In most of the towns the predominant occupation for females over the age of ten was domestic indoor service. The exceptions were Birmingham with a predominance of women employed in the metal industries, Leeds with women working as tailors, and Bolton and Bradford with the textile industries.[18]

Pressure from the organized labour movement for a 'family wage' as well as state intervention led to married women being increasingly excluded from the formal economy (Hudson and Lee, 1990, pp. 23–26). Indeed, according to the census, the vast majority of the women in employment (over the age of ten) were unmarried (see also Tilly and Scott, 1978). In Leeds, for example, of all the women in the labour force 55,235 were unmarried, 11,112 married and 5,228 widowed. This corresponds to 77.17, 15.52 and 7.30 per cent respectively. The situation in the other largest towns of the sample ranged from 8.69 per cent of women employed in Newcastle and 11.67 employed in Liverpool being married to 19.04 in Bradford and 20.29 in Birmingham.[19] On a national average the number of women who worked in the formal econ-

18 Predominant female occupation and the percentage (of all women in the labour force over the age of ten) employed in it in the ten largest English towns (county boroughs), 1911:

Predominant occupation		Percentage
Bristol	Domestic indoor service	20.69
Liverpool	Domestic indoor service	21.87
London	Domestic indoor service	28.01
Manchester	Domestic indoor service	12.88
Newcastle	Domestic indoor service	28.28
Sheffield	Domestic indoor service	24.39
Birmingham	Metals, machines, implements, and conveyances (including electrical apparatus)	26.58
Bolton	Textile manufactures	64.18
Bradford	Textile manufactures	60.26
Leeds	Tailoresses	22.10

Source: *Published Volumes of the Census of England and Wales* (1911).

19 Marital status of women over ten years of age in employment in the ten largest English towns (county boroughs), 1911:

	Unmarried	Married	Widowed
Birmingham	70.62	20.29	9.09
Bradford	74.37	19.04	6.59
Manchester	74.39	16.16	9.46
Leeds	77.17	15.52	7.30
Bolton	79.50	14.73	5.77
London	75.75	13.91	10.35
Sheffield	77.15	13.47	9.39
Bristol	78.96	13.32	7.72
Liverpool	76.60	11.67	11.73
Newcastle	82.26	8.69	9.05

Source: *Published Volumes of the Census of England and Wales* (1911).

omy was about ten per cent in the early decades of the twentieth century. In terms of age-specific participation rates, the number of married women in official employment decreased from their early twenties onwards; once married women had left the official labour market, they tended not to rejoin it (Lewis, 1984, p. 150).

The actual number of women in employment, however, might have been higher because of persistent underregistration of women's work (Higgs, 1987; Roberts, 1988, pp. 17–20; Tilly and Scott, 1978, p. 125). Furthermore, census returns do not include the whole range of seasonal and casual part-time work. For the early twentieth century, for example, Ayers and Lambertz's oral interviews revealed a substantial hidden female economy in Liverpool (Ayers and Lambertz, 1986; Ayers, 1990). Women increased inadequate family income by chopping and selling kindling, taking in laundry, sewing, keeping small shops in front rooms and cellars. Prostitution as well has to be mentioned in this context. And finally, a large number of women worked full-time at home for no wage at all.

Similarly in Germany most women's work was labour-intensive, low-skilled, irregular and low-paid. Women folded cartons, sewed, plaited wicker, knotted fishnets and rolled tobacco (Franzoi, 1984, p. 258). In Imperial Germany almost 50 per cent of the female labour force was employed in the clothing industry, another third worked in foods and tobacco ('Frauenerwerbsarbeit', 1912; Franzoi, 1984, p. 258). According to the 1907 occupational census the majority of the women in the labour force in the German sample of towns were working in industry, domestic service (including domestic servants living outside the household and hired labour with changing employers) and trade.[20] Industry dominated in Nuremberg (43.8 per cent), Berlin (39.1), Leipzig (38.3), Dresden (34.0) and Breslau (31.5), whereas domestic indoor service was the predominant occupation in Frankfurt (30.3 per cent plus 5.8

20 Predominant female occupation and the percentage (of all women in the labour force) employed in it in the ten largest German towns, 1907:

	AG	ID	TR	CS	WO	DS(HL)	DS
Berlin	0.1	39.1	18.1	3.9	16.6	8.2	13.9
Breslau	0.9	31.5	14.5	5.1	22.5	6.2	19.0
Cologne	1.1	23.4	18.2	5.7	22.2	4.9	21.2
Dresden	0.6	34.0	16.8	4.4	21.5	6.0	16.7
Düsseldorf	1.7	21.6	18.4	5.2	22.1	6.2	24.6
Frankfurt	1.6	22.9	16.5	5.3	17.6	5.8	30.3
Hamburg	0.2	22.6	20.3	5.5	20.9	8.5	22.0
Leipzig	0.6	38.3	18.4	3.6	18.0	4.5	16.6
Munich	0.5	22.4	24.0	5.7	20.2	8.1	19.0
Nuremberg	1.9	43.8	17.4	2.3	15.5	3.0	15.6

AG=Agriculture; ID=Industry, mining and construction; TR=Trade, transport and food; CS=Civil servants and self-employed; WO=Without occupation (excluding household members); DS(HL)=Domestic servants living outside the household and hired labour with changing employers; DS=Domestic servants living in the household.
Source: *Statistik des Deutschen Reichs*, NF **207**, **2** (1910).

Table 30: Wives and others mainly engaged in households/without profession (%) and mortality in German towns and selected causes of death, 1900–1913

City/town	f >14 in households	Mortality 1900–1913					
		CDR	Tuberculosis	Typhoid	Childbirth	IMR	Birth rate
		f	f	f			
	(1907)	(per 1,000)		(per 100,000 inhabitants)		(per 100 births)	(per 1,000 inhabitants)
		1907	1907	1907		1900–1913	
Munich	54.49	16.6*	216.0*	2.1*	5.68	20.6	28.12
Nuremberg	54.57	18.1§	248.7§	1.5§	4.15	21.9	32.55
Breslau	57.73	19.0	274.2	0.7	5.03	22.6	29.49
Berlin	58.28	14.7	186.7	3.4	8.69	18.1	23.37
Dresden	61.04	13.7*	150.8*	2.7*	7.58	16.3	26.19
Frankfurt	61.39	13.9	200.3	1.7	2.53	14.0	26.12
Leipzig	61.91	12.3‡	156.4‡	2.0‡	7.82	19.8	27.60
Hamburg	65.64	12.8†	141.6†	2.4†	8.95	15.8	25.13
Cologne	66.78	17.2	170.9	2.7	6.90	20.3	33.45
Düsseldorf	68.89	14.6	157.5	1.6	3.04	16.9	32.58

* 1910 death rates for both sexes.
† 1910.
‡ 1912.
§ 1900–1913 death rates for both sexes.
Sources: *Statistik des Deutschen Reichs*, NF **207**, **2** (1910); *Veröffentlichungen des Kaiserlichen Gesundheitsamtes (Beilagen)* (1901–1914); Appendix 2.

living outside the household and hired labour with changing employers), Düsseldorf (24.6 and 6.2), Hamburg (22.0 and 8.5), Cologne (21.1 and 4.9) and Munich (19.0 and 8.1). Between 15 and 22 per cent of women were without registered occupation (excluding those registered as household members), indicating a substantial hidden female economy. Married women, including widows and separated women, constituted 21 per cent of Germany's female labour force in 1907, although they represented approximately 50 per cent of homeworkers, i.e. before the Home Work Act of 1911 they worked in an unregulated, little protected and low-paid area of production (Franzoi, 1984, p. 258; Hudson and Lee, 1990, pp. 29–30). In the sample of German towns, the total number of females over the age of 14 staying at home ranged from over 50 per cent in the south-eastern and eastern towns (54.5 per cent in Munich, 54.6 per cent in Nuremberg, 57.7 per cent in Breslau) to considerably higher rates in the western towns, with 66.8 per cent in Cologne and 68.9 per cent in Düsseldorf (Table 30). Again, as in the English case, estimates of female work have to be treated with great care. The extent and range of the hidden female economy is hard to analyse quantitatively. Especially in the cities the domestic industry of wives and daughters was often deliberately concealed in order to avoid paying taxes (Franzoi, 1984, p. 259).

The effects of female labour force participation on the health of mother and child, however, remain controversial. Statistical evidence has to be restricted to the impact of the formal female economy. In this respect we have a fairly weak, but positive correlation between the percentage of women not in paid work and the female crude death rate in the ten largest English towns for the period after the turn of the century.[21] This was, to a large degree, a result of risks at childbirth, reflected in the higher correlation of this indicator with infant mortality rates and especially with deaths from childbirth and puerperal fever. In general, however, these correlations are not as strong as might have been expected. This implies that the connections between female work and demographic trends were more complex. In Liverpool, for example, where official employment was concentrated in the food trade, physical dock and warehouse work as well as the male-dominated clerical service, census material registered a higher number of women staying at home (not taking into account the unofficial female economy) accompanied by high infant mortality rates. As mentioned earlier, improved hygiene conditions tended to reduce mortality differences between breast-fed and artificially-nourished infants. Against this background the working mother's wage, which brought a better standard of living for the family, may have become a more important factor in the survival chances of infants (Dyhouse, 1978, pp. 254–57). In this sense, a mother's working wage could influence hygiene conditions via an increased calorific intake or with respect to food quality. Contemporary statistical observers were certainly puzzled by the negative relationship between female earnings and the infant mortality rate (*Forty-Second Annual Report*, 1913, p. 56; Woods et al., 1989, p. 115). It also suggests, however, that along with economic factors, the role of the environment has to be taken into account, or as A. Wohl puts it, cities with a good general environment could afford to have a high proportion of women in the labour force (Wohl, 1983).

German data (Table 30) also show a positive correlation between the percentage of females not participating in the labour force and the female crude death rate. However, there is a negative correlation between the number of females staying at home, infant mortality and the birth rate. This indicates that in Germany, women shortly before or after delivery were, to a greater degree than in England, still

---

21 The correlation of women not participating in the labour force and mortality rates gives the following results:

for the English towns:

CDR (fem)	: r = 0.3863, sig. (two-tailed) = 0.215;
TB (fem)	: r = –0.0002, sig. (two-tailed) = 1.000;
IMR	: r = 0.3962, sig. (two-tailed) = 0.202;
Childbirth	: r = 0.5924, sig. (two-tailed) = 0.042.

for the German towns:

CDR (fem)	: r = 0.4340, sig. (two-tailed) = 0.210;
TB (fem)	: r = 0.6177, sig. (two-tailed) = 0.057;
IMR	: r = –0.1106, sig. (two-tailed) = 0.761;
Childbirth	: r = –0.3131, sig. (two-tailed) = 0.378;
Birth rate	: r = –0.3570, sig. (two-tailed) = 0.311.

Source: See Tables 29 and 30.

participating in the official labour market.[22] In England various 'Factory Acts' (start-ing with the 1802 Health and Morals of Apprentices Act) provided at least some reg-ulations concerning the protection of the individual's health at work, although their actual accomplishment in practice was often unsatisfactory. By contrast, Germany remained without regulations for a considerably longer period (Hirt, 1873, pp. 1–28). The *Reichsgewerbeordnung* of 1878 prohibited factory work for women in the first three weeks after delivery (Teleky, 1950, p. 105), but demands from the medical pro-fession for legislative regulations preventing women from factory work in the last two months of pregnancy and the first two months after delivery were not fulfilled (Selter, 1902, p. 390; Schneck, 1975). The impact of this liability for labour service on health is supported by the relatively good positive correlation between this vari-able and the female tuberculosis death rate, whereas there is basically no correlation in the sample of English towns. The coefficient of correlation with reference to infant mortality, however, is very low. Whereas higher female wages for day labour appear to have reduced infant mortality in towns, the lack of correlation between female labour force participation and infant mortality, particularly in the German case, could be the result of regional differences, which possibly disguised potential interrela-tionships. With reference to the two demographic patterns of eastern and western regions of Germany with higher death rates and especially high infant mortality in the east and south-east, attributed to the absence of breast-feeding, it is remarkable that the towns of the sample belonging to this area (Breslau, Munich and Nuremberg) registered a high proportion of female labour force participation. Whereas in the highly industrialized western areas of Germany, differences in infant mortality rates between breast-fed and artificially-fed infants increasingly vanished, they remained evident in the less industrialized eastern areas. In these regions high female labour force participation could not counterbalance low living standards so that the absence of breast-feeding had a stronger negative impact on the survival chances of infants than in the better-off, more industrialized western areas. For families at the lowest end of the income distribution scale, additional income gains outweighed the impact of reduced breast-feeding (see also Brown, forthcoming). Industrialization, there-fore, reinforced contemporary regional differences (Lee, 1979, p. 156).

ECONOMIC GROWTH AND HEALTH

Having established strong, but not exclusive, links between living standards and health, we now in conclusion follow the developments of industrialization and urban health change on a broader scale. The comparative analysis of urban mortality change from the 1870s to 1910 confirms a clear interrelationship between economic growth and mortality change. The national absolute death rates in Germany were still substantially higher than in England at the end of the period under investigation. This corresponds with the economic situation in both countries. On the eve of the First

---

22 Low income, however, may have promoted the extension of the hidden female economy despite increasing legislation and protective measures.

World War Germany was, in terms of gross national product, still a poorer country than England (Pollard, 1987, p. 189).[23] Germany's per capita income has been estimated at about £44 as opposed to Britain's £55. Real wages were still about 10 to 20 per cent lower than in England (Saul, 1980, p. 10; Zamagni, 1989, pp. 114–18; Zapf, 1983, pp. 57–58).[24] At the beginning of the twentieth century actual working-class money wages in Germany were substantially lower, despite the fact that longer hours were worked. In addition, the general level of prices was distinctly higher in Germany as compared with England (Zamagni, 1989, p. 119). A contemporary report on the living conditions in both countries concluded that the ratio of expenditure on food, fuel and rent per capita in Germany and England was 119 to 100, the hourly rates of money wages 75 to 100 ('Cost of Living in German Towns', 1908, pp. li–lii). As the relationship between life expectancy and income is non-linear, i.e. the same extra income will extend life more effectively nearer the margin of malnutrition (Fogel, 1986), and Germany was a relatively poor country in comparison with England, a similar rise in the standard of living in both countries towards the end of the nineteenth century would have lifted more people over the essential minimum income barrier and consequently saved more lives in Germany than in England. As a result, the accelerated industrialization of Germany in the late nineteenth century apparently produced a faster relative rise in the standard of living, with both quantitative as well as qualitative improvements in diet, which brought about an even more rapid improvement in German health conditions. In terms of world industrial production, England lost its leading role to the USA from the 1880s onwards; by 1900 Germany had caught up with England and registered almost the same level of production (Kuczynski, 1965, p. 154; Kindleberger, 1975). The growth rate of real wages in Germany surpassed that in England, especially from the 1880s onwards (Gömmel, 1979, p. 18). Between 1871 and 1913 the average growth rate of real wages (1.3 per cent per annum) was significantly higher than in England (0.9 per cent per annum) (Orsagh, 1969, p. 483). Real wages, together with numerous other variables, are a significant indicator of socio-economic conditions, and the parallels between their development and trends in mortality cannot be overlooked in this context. German mortality rates from the 1870s onwards declined rapidly from a very high level, whereas the improvements in England were more equally distributed over the nineteenth and early twentieth centuries.

The results of this analysis correspond with some general demo-economic models for modern Third World countries, which stress the necessity of a big push in economic development in order to obtain lasting changes, whereas small gains in income tend to produce a decline in mortality and hence a stronger population

---

23 A direct comparative analysis of the state and development of the economies in the two countries has been provided by Saul (1980). See also Landes (1969).

24 Standard of living is a complex concept that includes substantially more variables than wages and prices. Already contemporary comparisons emphasized in this context that German workers benefited to a higher extent from social insurance schemes than their English counterparts. See Ashley (1904), pp. 16–18.

growth that pushes the population back to its original income level.[25] The steadier increase in gains in nineteenth- and early twentieth-century England may have produced a steadier decline in mortality, the accelerated industrialization in Germany a correspondingly accelerated decline. In the period 1888–1912, rising real wages reduced mortality in German towns with over 15,000 inhabitants in almost all cases (Brown, forthcoming). The towns in both countries seem to have benefited more from this rise in the standard of living than the countryside, which remained more static and followed the pattern of urban development more slowly. This would also explain the higher mortality rates in the less industrialized eastern parts of Germany, as throughout the nineteenth century there are signs of an accentuation in regional economic divergence, which could neither be overcome by the *Zollverein* (custom union) nor by improvements in transport (Lee, 1988, p. 355). For example, the eastern provinces of Prussia registered very high infant mortality with maximum rates in Silesia between 24 and 27 per 100 births after the middle of the century, as opposed to lower figures in the west, where IMR fluctuated in the Rhineland, for example, between 13 and 20 (Prinzing, 1899, p. 587). In Eastern Prussia the growth of Junker estates based on grain monoculture led to a peasant class which needed to exploit the labour of its female members in order to subsist. This resulted not only in high adult female mortality, but also in high infant mortality, caused by the inability of many mothers to breast-feed. In Western Prussia, on the other hand, land reforms in the early nineteenth century led to a wider distribution of peasant land ownership, greater crop variations and more livestock, which, in turn, brought about better health conditions (Lee, 1984a, pp. 168–72). Similarly, in the course of industrialization, living standards in the new industrial towns of western Germany experienced considerable growth. Wages both for females and for males were highest in this area.[26] Düsseldorf played an outstanding role in that context. In 1907 day labourer wages were higher than in all other towns of the Rhineland. Together with Leipzig they were higher than in all other towns over 100,000 inhabitants, surpassing even those in the world cities of Berlin, Hamburg and Frankfurt.[27] Furthermore, annual day labourer wages for male adults in Düsseldorf rose from 720 to 1,050 Marks between 1893 and 1910. At 31.4 per cent this growth rate surpassed the average of 26.6 for all towns over 200,000 inhabitants substantially.[28]

In southern Germany the impoverishment of the vast majority of the population, originally caused by the Thirty Years War, continued for generations. Regions which suffered most from the Napoleonic Wars of 1796–1809 registered high infant mortality rates. Battles, troop movements, harvest failure, the requisition of cattle, as well as war contributions led to severe pauperization (Prinzing, 1899, p. 598). In addition, these agricultural regions were hit severely by the spread of potato-rot. Yet, even in periods of bad harvest and hunger crisis, corn was exported to neighbouring foreign

25 For an overview see Preston (1975).
26 Source: *Statistisches Jahrbuch Deutscher Städte*, **19** (1913), p. 826.
27 Source: *Statistische Monatsberichte der Stadt Düsseldorf* (1907), p. x.
28 Source: *Statistische Monatsberichte der Stadt Düsseldorf* (1910), p. xi.

countries (Vögele, 1989, p. 37). Finally, a peasantry poor in purchasing power made the survival of small-scale traders in the towns difficult. All this and particularly the lack of cattle led to notorious infant feeding practices using a thick and sweetened meal-pap. Dummies were often filled with mashed rusk and sugar. Even poppy-seed extracts and opium were added as a sedative. As a result of this poor situation, Arthur Imhof claims that the local population developed a fatalistic mentality, based on a deeply rooted 'system of wastage of human life' (Imhof, 1981b). Particularly in Catholic areas, the death of an infant was accepted with indifference, or relief, as now there was an 'angel in heaven' who could pray for the family (Maier, 1871, p. 195). As a consequence, not the survival of the infant, but its baptism was the most important objective. The infant was often taken to the church within a few hours or days after birth, even in the winter and even when the church was more than an hour distant (Maier, 1871, p. 194). Spatial correlation between areas devastated by war and regions of high infant mortality rates is seldom convincing, and, as W.R. Lee has pointed out, the role of religion may have served as a means of justifying rather than as a cause of human behaviour (Lee, 1984b, p. 236). With reference to Prussia, Lee stresses that peasant life in all areas was harsh, but that the critical difference lay in the nature of structural change in the east, which affected the key variable, the nature of women's work outside the house, in a more negative way as far as the purely domestic role of peasant women was concerned than in the west (Lee, 1984b, p. 248). Certainly, for the south it remains dubious whether there was such a deeply rooted attitude in view of the fact that economic growth and industrialization from the late 1860s, the expansion of the railway network, and numerous good harvests, led to a decline in infant mortality. Indeed, this decrease started even earlier than in the northern parts of Germany (Prinzing, 1899, p. 599). In other south German agricultural areas, however, the situation may even have deteriorated. With ever-falling grain prices resulting from the rising world-market, Germany was transformed from a grain-exporting to a grain-importing country, which destabilized the economic base of traditional grain-producing areas, such as the regions on the northern border of Lake Konstanz (Vögele, 1989). Deprived of its traditional role as the granary for north-eastern Switzerland, the region failed to develop new income resources, and consequently experienced a fall in the standard of living, which was accompanied by high mortality rates. Conversely, other areas, dependent upon the purchase of grain, i.e. the towns, may have benefited from cheaper corn prices (Dickler, 1975).

CONCLUSION

In conclusion, a strong link between national economic development and improvements in health conditions can be established. The cities and towns as the focus of industrialization at first suffered most under the radically changing living conditions which accompanied urbanization and the development of an industrial economy. Yet, in the longer term, urban areas profited most from rising living standards. The interrelationship between economic growth and mortality change, however, was quite complex. Although a direct link between the primary economic base of the relevant towns in the two national samples and mortality levels could not be elaborated within the framework of a comparative macro-analysis, there were clear links between income, wages and health that had varying effects on different age-groups. The complexity of the subject becomes even more obvious when the effect of female labour force participation on health is analysed. At some stages of economic development, which found their expression and reflection in regional variations, additional family income improved the survival chances of infants, while in others it increased the risks for mother and child. Finally, the results of this analysis indicate that additional factors were at work determining the level and development of urban health conditions in the two countries under examination.

Chapter 10

HOUSING CONDITIONS AND MORTALITY CHANGE

The physical conditions of housing were generally poor during the period under investigation, both in urban and rural areas. Yet, population density in the country-side was more advantageous. In 1901, for example, there were on average 4.6 persons per inhabited building in rural districts of England and Wales, whereas in urban districts the corresponding rate was 5.4 (Table 31), making rural housing conditions that bit more tolerable (Pooley, 1992, p. 77). In contrast, rapid population growth and the increasing concentration of people in towns during the urbanization period led to major problems as far as urban housing conditions were concerned. The housing market could not keep pace with the growth of urban agglomerations. Population increase and housing construction cycles were not congruent (Tilly and Wellenreuther, 1985). Pressure on the housing market was aggravated by the need to live close to the place of employment and by continual population displacements caused by street construction, commercial development and railway building (Wohl, 1971, pp. 17–21). The functional change of many nineteenth-century towns with their increasing social segregation also brought about the rise of immensely over-crowded inner-city residential areas with particularly bad living conditions. This rapid growth of nineteenth-century towns led to horrific housing conditions, described in detail by prominent contemporary middle-class observers (e.g. Kay, Engels, Chadwick), and which have been the subject of both contemporary investigations and a number of modern historical analyses.[1] The following section will therefore be restricted to a synthesis of key aspects of this development process in both England and Germany, and then focus on the potential impact of housing on nineteenth century urban health conditions. First of all, however, some basic methodological considerations have to be taken into account.

In view of the devastating conditions in nineteenth-century Europe, recent research has criticized McKeown's narrow link between diet and tuberculosis and has high-lighted the strong correlation between overcrowding and tuberculosis. Several studies claim that poor housing conditions were primarily responsible for high urban

---

1 For further details in relation to Germany see Eberstadt (1909; 1920); Flügge (1916); Niethammer (1976); Teuteberg (1985); Gransche and Rothenbacher (1988); Zimmermann (1991). For an impressive micro-study see Wischermann (1983). For England see Burnett (1978); Daunton (1983); Dyos and Wolff (1973); Gauldie (1974); Rodger (1989); Wohl (1977). For a recent survey of national housing policy in both countries see the contributions of Pooley on England and Wales and Teuteberg and Wischermann for Germany in Pooley (1992). For selected European and American cities see Daunton (1990). Dealing with housing conditions within the broader context of town planning see Sutcliffe (1981).

Table 31: Housing density in selected English towns, 1851–1911, crude death rate (per 1,000 inhabitants), and mortality from pulmonary tuberculosis and phthisis (per 100,000 inhabitants), 1901–1910

Registration district	Average number of persons per inhabited building						CDR	TB*
	1851	1871	1881	1891	1901†	1911†		
London	7.7	7.8	7.9	7.6	7.9	7.9	15.8	147.7
Bristol	7.2	7.1	6.7	6.7	5.6	5.3	14.9	117.8
Clifton/Barton	6.0	6.2	6.2	6.0	–	–	–	–
Birmingham	5.1	5.0	5.1	5.0	4.8	4.8	22.2	182.9
Aston	5.0	5.0	5.1	5.0	4.8	4.7	14.8	115.9
Birkenhead	–	6.3	6.2	5.6	5.6	5.4	15.2	113.7
Liverpool	7.3	7.0	6.6	6.2	5.6	5.6	20.0	164.6
Toxteth Park	–	–	5.7	5.5	–	–	19.3	136.0
West Derby	6.1	5.9	5.7	5.5	–	–	17.7	142,4
Bolton	5.7	5.1	5.1	4.9	4.7	4.5	16.1	110.8
Chorlton	5.4	5.1	5.1	5.0	–	–	16.6	151.7
Salford	5.6	5.2	5.2	5.1	5.0	5.0	19.6	173.0
Manchester	6.2	5.3	5.1	5.0	5.0	4.9	18.8	176.9
Prestwich	–	–	5.3	5.3	–	–	20.4	240.9
Bradford	5.3	4.8	4.8	4.6	4.4	4.1	16.1	135.5
Leeds	4.8	4.7	4.8	4.8	4.5	4.4	17.9	150.7
Ecc. Bierlow	5.0	5.0	5.0	4.8	–	–	14.3	102.3
Sheffield	5.0	4.9	5.0	4.9	4.8	4.7	19.2	122.1
Gateshead	6.4	6.7	6.5	7.0	8.0	7.3	16.9	126.4
Newcastle	8.3	7.7	7.2	7.2	8.2	8.1	18.4	162.3
England/Wales	5.5	5.3	5.4	5.3	5.2	5.1	15.4	116.1
urban districts	–	–	–	–	5.4	5.2	–	–
rural districts	–	–	–	–	4.6	4.5	–	–

London=registration division.

*TB=Pulmonary tuberculosis and phthisis.

† Principal towns: Bristol, Liverpool, Manchester, Newcastle, Birmingham, Bradford, Leeds, Sheffield=county boroughs (city); Birkenhead, Bolton, Salford, Gateshead=county borough; Aston Manor=municipal borough.

Mortality rates for London; Bristol; Birmingham; Aston; Liverpool=Liverpool, Toxteth Park and West Derby; Bolton; Manchester=Manchester, Prestwich and Chorlton; Salford; Bradford; Leeds; Sheffield=Sheffield and Ecclesall Bierlow; Gateshead; Newcastle.

Sources: *Published Volumes of the Census of England and Wales* (1851, 1871, 1891, 1911); *Decennial Supplement to the Annual Reports of the Registrar-General of Births, Deaths, and Marriages in England and Wales* (1901–1910).

mortality rates (Cronjé, 1984, p. 101; Kearns, 1988a, p. 232; Szreter, 1988, p. 13; McFarlane, 1989; Hardy, 1993), as the important primary factor lies in the close and regular proximity to people who expectorate tubercle bacilli, especially in an open case of the disease. Consequently, it has been argued that the decline of mortality from tuberculosis and other respiratory diseases might be attributed to an improvement in housing rather than nutritional status. Such a close relationship between housing conditions and the tuberculosis death rate was, in fact, postulated by some nineteenth-century observers. Contemporary investigations into the impact of housing conditions on health focused on the prevailing insanitary conditions, and, from the 1880s onwards, increasingly on overcrowding and tuberculosis. The results of these studies showed that specific streets and districts of individual towns were more exposed to the disease than others, and that these areas were usually characterized by bad housing conditions and overcrowding. This led to the conclusion that tuberculosis was the housing-disease par excellence (Flügge, 1916, p. 44). Certainly the Hamburg data have demonstrated a positive correlation between the number of inhabitants per room as an indicator of housing conditions and the death rate from tuberculosis (see Chapter 6, 'Mortality Patterns inside the City'). The problem remains, however, whether this interrelationship represents a causal link, with tuberculosis mortality as a direct result of poor housing conditions. Tuberculosis, as a chronic disease, caused death on average 6.5 years after the start of the disease (Flügge, 1916, p. 48). In view of high contemporary inner-city migration rates there might be no connection between the dwelling where death occurred and the location where the disease originated.[2] Or, to put it more emphatically, the dwelling where death occurred might not have been the cause of the disease, but the result, as the onset of tuberculosis brought about the economic decline of the family. When the wage-earner of the family caught tuberculosis and the disease broke out, this was often eventually accompanied by the loss of employment. It was definitely the final stages of the disease that ultimately made it impossible for individuals to continue to work. The consequent reduction in the family's income frequently necessitated a move into cheaper and, no doubt, unhealthier accommodation. In this context social security systems in the case of disease, like the Friendly Societies in England or the National Health Insurance scheme in Germany, may have played an important role by granting at least minimal additional financial support (see Chapter 12). Finally, the sex-specific distribution of deaths from tuberculosis outlined in the previous chapters, indicating a strong predominance of deaths from tuberculosis amongst adult males, again pinpoints that additional factors such as working conditions may have played a part in influencing the relative level and trends in tuberculosis mortality.

2 According to early housing statistics of large German towns, mobility was substantial. In the 1880s, for example, 26.6 per cent of all the houses in Leipzig, 29.1 in Dresden, 35.0 in Berlin, and 35.2 in Breslau were occupied by the same lodgers for less than one year. Over 40 per cent in Leipzig and Dresden, and over 50 per cent in Breslau and Berlin were occupied for less than two years. See Neefe (1886).

Unfortunately, the source material concerning housing conditions is often insuffi-
ciently differentiated and unsystematic, so that a comprehensive analysis of working-
class housing is almost impossible (Niethammer, 1976, pp. 63–68). A comparative
approach for both countries encounters even more limitations, due to the predominance of different types of working-class housing (see pp. 140–43). A quantitative
comparison can only be undertaken on the basis of housing figures, i.e. the number of
persons per inhabited building (*Behausungsziffer*). In this respect the figures for Germany appear to be much worse than for England, with buildings housing two to
fifteen times the number accommodated in English dwellings. Historians have concluded from these statistics that overcrowding was much more severe and housing
conditions were dramatically worse in Germany than in England (Niethammer, 1976,
pp. 90–91). Such a conclusion, however, seems to be problematic and even misleading, as these figures reflect important differences in housing construction. The English back-to-back houses inevitably had lower population density in comparison with
the German multi-storeyed 'rental barracks' (*Mietskasernen*). The extent to which the
average number of persons per inhabited building is only a crude indicator of the
actual housing density becomes obvious when it is compared with data relating to the
number of persons per tenement. In Dresden in 1875, for instance, the average number of persons per inhabited building was 32, whereas the number of persons per tenement was only 4.6 (see Table 32). A more informative comparison of housing

Table 32: Housing density in selected German towns, 1875 and 1900, crude death rates (per
1,000 inhabitants) and mortality from tuberculosis (per 100,000 inhabitants), 1877 and 1900

Town	Average number of persons per inhabited		Mortality		Average number of Persons per inhabited		Mortality	
	building 1875	Tenement 1875	CDR 1877	TB	building 1900	Tenement 1900	CDR 1900	TB
Berlin	57.9*	4.4	29.8	355.0	77.0*	3.9	18.9	235.3
Breslau	45.0*	4.3	29.5	298.4	53.3*	4.0	26.1	339.1
Cologne	-	-	25.7	462.7	15.8	4.3	23.2	239.7
Dresden	32.0	4.6	24.6	379.4	28.7	4.1	18.9	244.2
Düsseldorf	-	-	22.0	330.8	20.0	-	19.4	200.8
Essen	-	-	24.8	359.1	18.7	4.9	24.4	216.3
Frankfurt	16.5	4.7	19.5	379.2	18.7	4.7	17.4	256.1
Hamburg	26.0*	4.7	26.5	348.8	35.6*	4.4	17.6	204.0
Leipzig	38.0*	5.1	23.6	341.7	27.8	4.5	19.5	227.5
Munich	-	-	34.0	387.9	36.6*	3.8	25.0	322.9
Nuremberg	-	-	26.3	542.7	19.5	-	23.8	295.7

* Persons on estate.

Sources: Eberstadt (1909), p. 129; Lindemann (1901), p. 285; *Statistisches Jahrbuch Deutscher
Städte*, **11** (1903), pp. 72–83; *Veröffentlichungen des Kaiserlichen Gesundheitsamtes (Beilagen)*
(1878 and 1901).

conditions in England and Germany, therefore, can only be obtained by examining the actual number of persons per flat or dwelling, but such an analysis is unfortunately impossible, as the data are not available for the English sample from the census publications. Even this would not take the actual size of the flats into consideration. Furthermore, improvements in the ratio over time might actually not be the result of enforced building activities, but simply the effect of reduced family size that resulted from declining birth rates. As a consequence of these limitations a comparison of housing conditions between the two countries has to rely basically on qualitative information, and on broad statistical measures. This, however, should not obstruct the realization of the objectives of this study too severely. The intention is not to explain differences between the health risks of the two populations in a direct comparison on the basis of various indicators, but rather to analyse the structural mechanisms behind urban mortality change in the period under examination. Therefore, after a brief account of housing differences in England and Germany, the potential links between urban housing conditions and health, especially with respect to crude death rates and tuberculosis mortality, will be explored. The analysis will focus on whether substantial improvements in housing conditions were achieved in the period under investigation, and whether or to what extent this affected the decline in urban death rates. Finally, some more speculative considerations about health within the house will conclude this chapter.

HOUSING IN ENGLAND AND GERMANY

Housing in England and Germany was, and is, based on two very different traditions. At the beginning of the twentieth century the British Board of Trade summarized the essential differences in working-class housing between the two countries as follows: 'The German working classes are housed almost exclusively in large tenement buildings, frequently constructed round a central courtyard, each building containing a number of separate dwellings … On the other hand, the English working man for the most part, if we except a few towns chiefly in the north of England, rents a small separate house. In the case of Germany, tenements of two rooms and three rooms are the most frequent for working-class households; in England, tenements of four and five rooms are the predominant types. At the same time the rooms of the German tenement are as a rule distinctly both larger and loftier than the English' ('Cost of Living in German Towns', 1908, p. xl).

The reasons for these differences in housing systems are complex. The roots may go back to medieval times when many towns and cities on the continent were fortified with walls which restricted the available space and encouraged the construction of high buildings. By contrast, in England the walls of most towns, except in the northern areas still subject to Scottish incursions, were removed or ignored as early as the fifteenth century (Sutcliffe, 1974, pp. 6–11). When population growth accelerated, both countries had already established divergent housing traditions. This process was reinforced during industrialization, largely as a result of different relationships in the ownership of land and buildings. In England the ownership of land and houses was often separate. Instead of selling their ground (freehold system) many landowners preferred to lease it for the purpose of house-building for periods up to 99 years, the so-called leasehold system (Eberstadt, 1920, pp. 596–97). In Germany the owner of the land also owned the houses built on it. The acquisition of building land in order to construct working-class housing was often undertaken by large, highly-capitalized companies, often associated with some of the big investment banks (Sutcliffe, 1981, pp. 14–15). The high costs of land and capital for building favoured the construction of multi-storeyed housing, which in its extreme form took the shape of *Mietskasernen* (rental barracks), large tenements arranged around one or more courtyards. Berlin took the lead in multi-storeyed housing. From the middle of the nineteenth century it spread to other large towns, whereas such housing could not be found to the same extent in small and medium-sized towns. Rental barracks were especially prominent in the east, and gained ground increasingly in the west, with the exception of some areas in north-western Germany, in particular in and around Bremen. This development corresponded with a clear east–west gradient in housing density, with the western parts registering a lower 'person per house' ratio (*Behausungsziffer*) than eastern Germany (Flügge, 1916, pp. 4 and 9). This is reflected in the sample of towns, with especially high rates in Berlin and Breslau (Table 32). The towns famous for their rental barracks, however, did not register the highest housing density in terms of the average number of persons per tenement. In 1875 Berlin and Breslau actually had the lowest rates judging from the sparse data available for the sample. By 1900 the trend for multi-storeyed housing had considerably increased in most of the towns in the sample, i.e. the number of persons per inhabited building increased, whereas the average number of persons per tenement had decreased in most places (except for Frankfurt, where it remained stable at 4.7). Major elements of town planning, as for example zoning building regulations, in which Germany led the world, were established relatively late so that they had hardly any importance for city development before the First World War (Teuteberg and Wiegelmann, 1992, p. 242). One significant exception was the physical development plan for Berlin (the 'Hobrecht-Plan'—carried out by James Hobrecht, an official in the police building department), published in 1862 (Hartog, 1962, p. 32). In practice, however, it produced high land values and aided the spread of rental barracks, even in the suburbs (Sutcliffe, 1974, p. 9; 1981, pp. 20–21). As a result of these developments 90 per cent of all dwellings in the large towns of Germany were based on a rental scheme (Tyszka, 1914, p. 178).

With increasing urbanization land prices rose, and these higher costs were passed on to the lodgers. Therefore, in general, housing was more expensive in Germany than in England, where strong building societies cushioned similar tendencies (Leuthold, 1886, p. 9; Eberstadt, 1920, p. 600; Sutcliffe, 1981, p. 14).[3] At the national

---

3 In England, the rents of working-class dwellings usually included taxation based on the rentable value of the dwelling, whereas in Germany local taxation was not included in the rent. If net rents in England, excluding taxation, stood at 100, the equivalent figure for Germany would have been 123. See 'Cost of Living in German Towns' (1908), p. xl.

level the ratio of wage to net rent was 1.0 in England and Wales and 0.7 in Germany (Daunton, 1990, p. 9). From 1880 to 1900 rents rose about 20 per cent nationally, but in London by only about 12 per cent. After the turn of the century rents even decreased in London, Liverpool, Nottingham, Plymouth and Edinburgh or remained stable as in Manchester, Glasgow, Birmingham, Bradford and Leeds (Eberstadt, 1920, p. 600). Whereas in England the building cycle determined the demand for capital, in Germany less capital was available, and the ability to mobilize funds influenced building (Daunton, 1990, p. 11). In Germany at least 80 per cent of the working class was dependent on the speculative rental housing market. Confronted with increasing demand in the rapidly growing cities, rents rose significantly. In Berlin, for example, the rental levels per capita tripled between 1855 and 1895 (Reich, 1912, p. 127). This development particularly affected small flats (one room), so that the poor had to pay more not only in relative but also in absolute terms (Niethammer, 1976, p. 81). Moreover, it was this class that registered a particularly high migration rate within the city. In Berlin in 1876, 45.9 per cent of all flats with a rent of up to 100 *Taler* recorded a change of lodgers, in comparison with 24 per cent for flats of over 1,000 *Taler* (Reich, 1912, p. 9).

In England, working-class housing was dominated by smaller self-contained terraced houses, with a generally lower ratio of persons per inhabited building in the English registration districts and towns of the sample (Table 31). High-density terraced housing with a common back wall (back-to-back houses) was essentially an urban, industrial type which was in regular use in Birmingham, Bradford, Leeds, Liverpool, Manchester, Sheffield and other towns, especially in the Midlands, the West Riding and South Lancashire ('Cost of Living of the Working Classes', 1908; Burnett, 1978, p. 74). The highest concentration of houses was achieved by eliminating streets so that various rows of terraced houses formed a court, which was only accessible by narrow passages or tunnels. One end of the court was usually closed either by houses or by the privies and ashpits. Flats were relatively rare, and accounted for only 3.4 per cent of the total stock of dwellings in England and Wales according to the 1911 census. They were, however, concentrated in the London and Tyneside areas. Consequently, Newcastle upon Tyne (8.1), Gateshead (7.3) and London (7.9) registered the highest average number of persons per inhabited building. Although the flat was not common in English industrial towns, this did not mean there was no high-density working-class housing. Three-storey, three-room type back-to-back houses, concentrated in Birmingham, Sheffield and other towns, produced a high population density ('Cost of Living of the Working Classes', 1908; Burnett, 1978, p. 74; Sutcliffe, 1974, p. 13). In Liverpool, for example, mass casual employment of unskilled labourers in the neighbourhood of the docks and restricted growth possibilities led to gross densities as high as 700 persons per acre by the middle of the nineteenth century (Taylor, 1974, pp. 43–45). This was the highest density in the whole of England, and made the city infamous for its high share of court and cellar dwelling.

Various early legislative measures, like the Nuisances Removal Acts 1855 and 1860, Sanitary Acts 1866 and 1874, the Public Health Act 1875, and the Housing of the

Working Classes Acts from 1885 onwards were supposed to provide means to abolish these conditions. According to these acts, local authorities could inspect their districts. Inspectors of Nuisances, however, were too few in number, often living in poor conditions themselves, and, what is more, dependent on the vestry often consisting of the house-owners and landlords of these districts, who had no interest in investing additional money (Ruprecht, 1884, pp. 68, 83; Aschrott, 1886, pp. 103–06; Leuthold, 1886, p. 20; Tyszka, 1914, p. 179). Finally, the practice of municipal extension planning in England was almost non-existent before the First World War. One major exception to this lack of municipal interference was slum clearance. On the whole, however, early local and national legislation on slum clearance (Artisans' and Labourers' Dwellings Improvement Acts 1875, 1879 and 1882) was ineffective, and, what is more, often failed to provide new housing (Aschrott, 1886, p. 114; Sutcliffe, 1981, p. 47).

Despite these differences, housing conditions in both countries under consideration were generally characterized by overcrowding and by a lack of light and fresh air. In London, according to the Royal Commission to inquire into the housing of the Working Classes, 60,000 families were living in one-room flats in the mid- 1880s (Aschrott, 1886, p. 97). In early twentieth-century Berlin, there were 251,550 one-room flats housing 768,837 people (Flügge, 1916, p. 6). In some inner districts of London more than 50 per cent of all the tenements were overcrowed according to the 1891 census (Pooley, 1992, pp. 76–77). Overcrowding was worsened by the huge number of *Schlafgänger* or bed-lodgers. In Berlin in 1880 more than 15 per cent of all households had between one and 34 bed-lodgers (Fuchs, 1911, p. 884). In some cases the beds were rented out during the day, when the main user was at work (Flügge, 1916, p. 6). There were especially bad conditions in the dark, damp and airless cellar-flats, mostly without windows, and directly underneath the roof. They were hot in the summer, cold and filled with smoke from the ovens or heaters in the winter. Living and sleeping rooms were used as kitchens, or as workplaces, especially in the textile industries where mainly female home-workers were employed in the so-called 'sweating system'. In Berlin around the turn of the century, for example, home work was carried out in 20,000 dwellings by 9,919 males and 11,749 females (Fuchs, 1911, 879). In general, contemporary reformers considered English urban housing conditions to be superior to those of Germany due to the predominant small houses, but all in all, housing conditions provided a range of health-damaging factors and, once acute or chronic infectious diseases broke out, they found ideal conditions for transmission.

HOUSING AND HEALTH CONDITIONS

Poor housing conditions, overcrowding and frequent inner-city migration characterized the situation of most towns in both England and Germany, with especially bad conditions in city centres. The developments in the largest towns confirm the extent and impact of increasing social segregation. In English towns, registration districts covering the inner-city area usually had a higher population density, and recorded a worse crude death rate and a higher tuberculosis mortality than the surrounding districts. At the beginning of the twentieth century the registration district of Liverpool, for example, still had a high mortality rate of 30.5 deaths per 1,000 inhabitants, with more than 284 people dying from tuberculosis per 100,000 inhabitants. For German towns, the well-known example of Hamburg reveals similar results. The inner-city area of the Altstadt registered almost double the population density of corresponding working-class districts on the city's borders (Fig. 32), accompanied by high death rates from tuberculosis (Fig. 31). For Berlin, reports exist which indicate clusters of disease in specific houses. In 1873, for example, 150 out of 153 persons suffering from typhus in the 61st sanitary district (*Medizinalbezirk*) could be found in one particular house, the Müllerstraße 31. Of the total of 575 poor sick in the 18th sanitary district, 30.8 per cent (177 cases) were traced to one house in the district. All registered cases of cholera, 46 per cent of all the dysentery cases, and 80 per cent of all the diphtheria cases in the district occurred in this house. A complex of houses with the same owner in the Johanniterstraße 215, housing more than 1,000 inhabitants, reported 53 per cent of all the sick in the 13th sanitary district (Leuthold, 1886, p. 10). First results of an analysis of the patients in the Düsseldorf hospitals in the 1880s reveal similar tendencies.[4] The domicile of many patients can be traced back to a small number of houses in poor areas. Yet, it remains unclear to what extent these high mortality rates were actually caused by housing conditions. Comparing the sample of towns in the 1870s, the connection between housing density—expressed by the average number of persons per inhabited building—and mortality was rather weak.[5] Moreover, in both countries the relationship remained weak around the turn of the century (Tables 31 and 32), even between the crude death rate, tuberculosis mortality and the proportion of cellar-flats in relation to all inhabited dwellings, judging by the data available for the German sample.[6] Similar results can be achieved with respect to

---

4 J. Vögele, W. Woelk and B. Schürmann, 'The Patients of the Düsseldorf Hospitals in the Late 1880s' (current research project).

5 Correlating housing density (average number of persons per inhabited building, England 1871), the crude death rate and mortality from tuberculosis (1871–1880) gives the following results:

CDR: $r = 0.0731$, sig. (two-tailed) $= 0.773$;

TB: $r = 0.1442$, sig. (two-tailed) $= 0.568$.

Sources: See Table 31 and *Decennial Supplement to the Annual Reports of the Registrar-General of Births, Deaths, and Marriages in England and Wales*, 1871–1880. German data are so rare for this decade that they do not permit a correlation analysis.

6 Correlating housing density (average number of persons per inhabited building, England 1911; Germany 1900), the crude death rate and mortality from tuberculosis gives the following results:

CDR for the English towns: $r = -0.1035$, sig. (two-tailed) $= 0.725$;

CDR for the German towns: $r = -0.0254$, sig. (two-tailed) $= 0.941$;

TB for the English towns: $r = 0.1164$, sig. (two-tailed) $= 0.692$;

TB for the German towns: $r = 0.2387$, sig. (two-tailed) $= 0.480$.

Using the rates for the average number of persons per tenement for the German sample of the same period similarly does not suggest that the incidence of tuberculosis increased with higher housing density. Similar results were obtained by correlating mortality and the percentage of cellar-flats from all inhabitated dwellings in German towns:

CDR: $r = -0.0440$, sig. (two-tailed) $= 0.904$;

TB: $r = 0.0431$, sig. (two-tailed) $= 0.906$.

Sources: See Tables 31 and 32.

overcrowding and deaths from various diseases.[7] Even within an individual city, mortality was surprisingly weakly correlated with population and housing density. In Manchester, housing density accounted for only 17 per cent of the variance in crude mortality rates during the period 1871–1875 (Pooley and Pooley, 1984, pp. 171–72). Furthermore, despite increasing legislation, major qualitative changes in housing conditions during the second half of the nineteenth century remain dubious (Brockington,

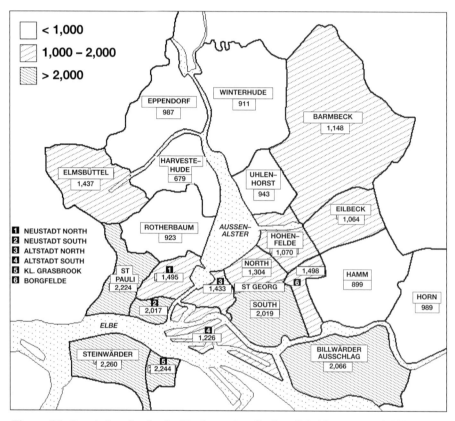

Figure 32: Population density in Hamburg city districts (inhabitants per 10,000 square metres), 1885

Sources: See Table 28.

7 In the census of England and Wales 'the percentage of population occupying overcrowded tenements of not more than four rooms (more than two persons per room)' was used as an indicator for overcrowding in individual cities; no corresponding data exist for Germany. Correlating overcrowding (1901), the crude death rate and mortality from tuberculosis (1901–1910) in the ten largest English towns gives the following results:
CDR: $r = -0.0591$, sig. (two-tailed) = 0.871;
TB: $r = 0.1910$, sig. (two-tailed) = 0.597.
Sources: 'Cost of Living of the Working Classes' (1908), pp. 592–93; *Decennial Supplement to the Annual Reports of the Registrar-General of Births, Deaths, and Marriages in England and Wales* (1901–1910).

1966, pp. 92–93). There were advances in structural standards and the use of sounder material may have improved insulation from cold, damp and noise (Burnett, 1978, p. 158), but it is, however, questionable to what extent the working classes benefited from these developments. Municipal housing was only provided to a limited extent from the last decade of the nineteenth century onwards, and public intervention failed to ameliorate the adverse housing conditions of most working-class households (Niethammer, 1979; von Saldern, 1979). Programmes to improve working-class housing, such as the garden city movement, only operated on a small scale, and were available for just a priviliged few (Flügge, 1916, pp. 27–28; Burnett, 1978, pp. 173–83; Pooley, 1992, p. 79). In quantitative terms the situation improved only slightly. The private market was able to provide new housing for the more affluent working class, but it contributed little to the low-rent housing stock the masses relied on (Pooley, 1992, pp. 76–77). In Hamburg, for example, only the number of expensive dwellings increased in the 1870s and early 1880s, whereas the number of cheap dwellings (with a rent of up to 150 Marks) even decreased, despite the absence of a corresponding rise in income (according to the income tax statistics) (Koch, 1886, p. 45). In the English sample Newcastle RD, Liverpool RD and Manchester RD registered the strongest improvements until the 1890s. From the twentieth century onwards, housing density rates refer to municipal boroughs instead of registration districts. Between 1901 and 1911 most of the boroughs registered small improvements, whereas the figures for London (registration division) remained stable. Slight improvements in the persons-per-building ratio in the sample of English and German towns may therefore be less attributable to larger-scale house building than to reduced family size.[8] Appalling slums remained. In Leeds, for example, in the Quarry Hill area, where 10,500 people lived in 2,200 houses, the death rate was nearly twice that of the borough as a whole in 1893–1895 (Morgan, 1980, p. 68). The more pronounced improvements recorded for the English sample (Table 31) seem to be the result of boundary changes rather than actual improvements. In some places, for instance in London, housing conditions remained stable or even deteriorated. Yet in Germany, even towns such as Frankfurt am Main saw an improvement in the tuberculosis death rate, while, by contrast, towns with improved housing density (such as Breslau) showed a deterioration in mortality from tuberculosis. It was only the twentieth century which brought substantially improved housing conditions for the working class. Reduced overcrowding was the result both of an improving housing market and of smaller family size as a consequence of declining fertility rates.

INSIDE THE HOUSE

Nineteenth-century urban housing was additionally characterized by increasing social differences within the house. Rapid population growth led to a substantial shortage of accommodation facilities. Low-status in-migrants not only moved into

---

8 In Prussia, for example, the average size of family households declined in urban areas from 4.65 in 1875 to 4.38 in 1910, whereas in rural areas it even increased slightly from 4.98 to 5.01. *Preußische Statistik*, **39** (1877) and **234** (1913).

the cheapest and worst city districts, but also occupied the corresponding rooms or flats within the buildings in these areas. In 1844 Engels found in Liverpool 'a full fifth of the population, more than 45,000 human beings, living in narrow, dark, damp and badly ventilated cellar dwellings of which there are 7,862 in the city' (Engels, 1892). E. W. Hope, Medical Officer of Health in Liverpool from 1894 to 1924, described the city's court and cellar dwellings as 'disease factories'. In Berlin in 1880 more than 100,000 people lived in cellar dwellings (Fuchs, 1911, p. 878). In Germany, multi-storeyed housing and particularly the infamous rental barracks were considered to be especially unhealthy,[9] as it was difficult for the town-dweller to obtain easy access to fresh air or to get enough physical exercise outside the house (Flügge, 1916, p. 123).[10] After several visits to a working-class district of London, Alfred Grotjahn, a leading German social hygienist,[11] was surprised at the good health of the people. This he attributed to English housing which enabled the children to go outside often and easily. 'And it is definitely not by chance', he concluded, 'that in the large Scottish towns, which are built in a German way as high rental barracks [*Mietskasernen*], there were many children with rickets' (Grotjahn, 1915, p. 260; my translation), just like in Germany. Whether this was solely the fault of housing conditions cannot be further considered here. In any case, Germany's multi-storeyed housing reflected also social inequalities within the house itself. According to James Hobrecht, rents in a rental barrack in the late 1860s could range from 50 Thaler in the cellar-flats, under the roof and in the back house, to 500 Thaler on the first floor, the *belle étage* (Hobrecht, 1868, p. 15). As a result, the poorest in many places lived in cellar-flats (*Kellerwohnungen*), often dark and humid, or on the highest floor directly underneath the roof. On one and the same floor, flats or rooms with windows facing the street offered more air and light than those facing the dark backyard, which was surrounded by other houses. The effects on health are difficult to prove statistically in this context, as source material is limited and haphazard, and there is no information about the demographic structure of the population (such as age- and sex-distribution, and family size) within the house. Moreover, the locational position of an individual within the house also changed within the life-cycle. Poor in-migrants from other towns or rural areas first moved into the cellar-flats or found accommodation directly underneath the roof. With increasing income they tended to move towards the middle floors of the house, or from backyard flats to the front of the building. Despite the fact that differences in the age-structure and the sex-composition of the dwellers cannot be controlled for, there are, however, indications that mortality was dependent on the position within the house. In Berlin in 1885/86 the crude death rate was highest in the cellar-flats (21.1 per 1,000 occupants) and underneath the roof (21.4), whereas the middle floors showed lower rates (ground floor:

---

9 For an impressive description see Treue (1969).
10 For a visual impression see the collection of photographs of the Berlin Wohnungs-Enquête between 1903 and 1920 in Asmus (1982).
11 For a recent synthesis see Kaspari (1989).

20.4; first floor: 18.4; second floor: 18.8; third floor: 19.0) (Prinzing, 1906, p. 448).[12] By the 1890s the cellar-flats had lost their disadvantage to some extent, whereas the most extreme death rates were still recorded on the highest floor: in 1890/91 the crude death rate in Berlin houses was 21.3 in the cellar, 20.7 on the ground floor, 22.1 on the first floor, 21.4 on the second, 20.3 on the third, and 22.8 on the fourth (Fuchs, 1911, p. 890). A differentiation according to selected causes of death is possible for Berlin in the period 1900–1902, but unfortunately there is no information concerning the population at risk. Prinzing calculated the distribution of different causes of death within the house per 100 deaths. A low percentage of deaths from phthisis (5.2 per 100 deaths) and diarrhoea and dysentery was registered in the cellar-flats (5.4) (Prinzing, 1906, pp. 448–49). However, this might be attributed to the young average age of the lodgers, who were probably unmarried, so that there were only a small number of infants and children living in these places. More evident was the higher proportion of deaths from diarrhoea or dysentery on the top floor (22.6). Just underneath the roof, lodgers and their infants were directly exposed to climatic influences. Such unhealthy conditions, combined with a low economic status, may have been responsible for the higher level of mortality from these diseases. Despite these conditions and growing criticism of multi-storeyed housing, the rental barrack system was defended by stressing the educational momentum provided by it. James Hobrecht argued that the mixture of various social classes within one building would inevitably lead to social peace, and elements of the good education of the richer inhabitants, especially with respect to personal and domestic hygiene, would transfer to the poorer inhabitants of the house (Hobrecht, 1868, p. 15). In practice, the contrary was the case, with a clear division between the various inhabitants. Ignorance and arrogance on the one side were confronted with envy and hatred on the other (Beier, 1982, p. 267).

CONCLUSION

In conclusion, industrialization and urbanization led to appalling housing conditions. Without doubt, these were largely responsible for the widespread diffusion of disease and death in the city. Overcrowding and poor quality housing may well be a major cause of the 'urban penalty' in both countries. Improvements in urban health conditions and especially the decline in infant mortality and deaths from tuberculosis, however, can hardly be attributed to changes in housing conditions. Qualitative improvements in housing during the period under investigation were few and far

---

12 Similar differences in the CDRs were recorded for Berlin in the 1870s:

	1875/76
Cellar	35.6
Ground floor	29.4
First floor	28.6
Second floor	29.2
Third floor	32.9
Fourth floor	36.5

Source: Fuchs (1911), p. 890.

between, and not available to the vast majority of the urban population. In quantitative terms, the private housing market could not keep pace with the population increase. It contributed little to the low-rent housing stock that was most needed. Private programmes to improve working-class housing operated on a small scale. Similarly, municipal housing remained rather limited in the period under observation.

Chapter 11

IMPROVING THE ENVIRONMENT:
THE IMPACT OF SANITARY REFORMS
ON THE PEOPLE'S HEALTH

The sanitary movement focused on infrastuctural measures that were intended to improve the hygienic conditions of the urban environment. Particular importance was placed on the provision of an improved drinking water supply, a more efficient removal of excrement and waste disposal. Street cleaning, the establishment of slaughter houses, disinfection plants, food inspection, the provision of healthy nutrition (in this connection, great emphasis was placed on the establishment of milk disinfection stations [*Kindermilchstationen*]) and, after considerable delay, municipal housing provision and even the reduction of noise in the city were all included in this concept (Weyl, 1904, p. 1). Illness and disease were no longer regarded as natural and therefore a matter of destiny, but rather as something that could be positively influenced or prevented by improving environmental conditions. This led to discussions amongst doctors, politicians and local authorities that stressed the need to improve urban living conditions, particularly by providing an adequate sanitary infrastructure. Specific measures were carried out in an increasingly systematic manner during the last decades of the nineteenth and the early twentieth century. At the turn of the century public health measures had become a significant and growing component of municipal budgets in the large towns of both countries. Munich, for example, spent 16.3 per cent of its 1894 budget on public health issues (Singer, 1895, p. 19).

Although a wide range of public health measures were adopted, the following section will focus on two key aspects of the sanitary infrastructure during the late nineteenth and early twentieth centuries, namely the provision of a central water supply and the construction of sewerage systems, as well as municipal milk supplies. These two areas of public intervention received special attention from contemporaries and, consequently, constituted the most widespread measures in terms of urban public health strategies. Considering further the substantial role of digestive diseases within the urban cause of death panorama and the predominance of infant mortality, these two areas of public health intervention should have registered the strongest and most far-reaching impact on urban health conditions. Other components of sanitary reform (like, for example, food inspection) were taken up on a relatively small scale during the period under consideration and therefore could have had only a limited potential to influence the health conditions of urban populations on a large scale. Nevertheless, they may have supported the reduction in the high urban death rates.

THE EXPANSION OF CENTRAL WATER SUPPLY AND SEWERAGE SYSTEMS IN ENGLAND AND GERMANY

A major intervention in the living environment during the second half of the nineteenth century was the installation and expansion of central water supply and sewerage systems. Again England was the pioneer in this field and soon became more advanced than other countries. Legislative and administrative proceedings have been described in detail.[1] After a preliminary period of national public health legislation and organization in the 1840s—the Royal Commission on the Health of Towns (1843) and the Public Health Act of 1845 (Uffelmann, 1874; Frazer, 1950; Brockington, 1966)—such sanitary reforms were increasingly implemented from mid-century onwards, following Edwin Chadwick's report on the *Sanitary Conditions of the Labouring Population* (Chadwick, 1842). Apart from London, the northern industrial and commercial towns, namely Manchester and Liverpool, were at the forefront in terms of administrative measures and the actual establishment of new public health facilities. In Manchester a voluntary board of health had already been formed in 1795 as a consequence of various typhus fever epidemics. Yet opposition to and neglect of its programme rendered the board ineffectual (Rosen, 1958, pp. 158, 201). Successful intervention only started with the 1844 Police Regulation Act. The first comprehensive health legislation passed in England, however, was the Liverpool Sanitary Act of 1846, which made the town council responsible for drainage, sewerage and street cleaning. It allowed the appointment of a Borough Engineer, an Inspector of Nuisances, and the first ever Medical Officer of Health (Midwinter, 1969, p. 84). The well-known William Duncan of Liverpool was appointed Medical Officer of Health in 1847 (Brockington, 1966, pp. 26, 40). In the same year, the Liverpool Corporation Waterworks Act empowered the city to purchase existing undertakings, so that Liverpool had control of its major health utilities well before the comprehensive Public Health Act of 1875 was passed. Parliament successively gave greater responsibility and powers to local authorities, and municipal enterprises experienced a substantial expansion in the last decades of the nineteenth century (Falkus, 1977, p. 145).

After a period of predominantly private ownership—by 1846 only 10 out of about 190 local authorities possessed their own waterworks—a modern ownership structure was established during 1861–1881. During this period the proportion of towns supplied municipally increased from 40.8 to 80.2 per cent (Stern, 1954, p. 999; Hassan, 1985, pp. 533–35), and in 1907, 81 per cent of the net output of water undertakings in England and Wales came from municipal concerns (Falkus, 1977, p. 136). After the often disastrous effects of municipalization in the early stages, in the long run these municipal waterworks worked more efficiently in terms of actual water

---

1 For a comprehensive overview of the development of public health from early civilizations to nineteenth- and twentieth-century development in Europe and the United States see Rosen (1958). With special emphasis on the administrative concerns of the developments in Britain see Brand (1965); Brockington (1965; 1966); Frazer (1950); Wohl (1983). For information about E. Chadwick see Lewis (1952); Finer (1952).

supply. By 1882 average consumption was 50 per cent higher in towns supplied municipally. In terms of financial returns, private water supply companies achieved only an insignificantly higher return than municipal enterprises (Hassan, 1985, p. 540). However, private enterprise was increasingly on the decline in terms of water supply. The Public Health Act of 1875 obliged urban authorities to ensure a satisfactory supply of water, and the municipalities were authorized to construct, purchase, lease or hire waterworks subject to the consent of the Local Government Board (Falkus, 1977, p. 145). As a consequence, the last decades of the nineteenth century brought about great progress in sanitary administration and the actual construction of sanitary works. Indeed these years were the high point of the public health movement in England.

In Germany sanitary reform spread only hesitantly at first. Whereas Manchester and Liverpool, for example, had already spent more than £1 million on the construction of waterworks by the end of the 1850s, expenditure in Hamburg only amounted to £170,000 (Strang, 1859). Without a legislative framework, the initiative for central water supply and sewerage in Germany was completely in the hands of the traditionally self-governing and powerful local communities.[2] Private enterprise was sparse. In 1907 only 4.5 per cent of all waterworks were in the hands of private companies (Mombert, 1908, p. 10). As the provision of central water supply was rather expensive in terms of capital investment particularly in relation to construction, municipalities reacted very carefully at first. Only a few towns in the 1840s (Hamburg, 1849, financed by the state) and 1850s (Berlin, 1852; Würzburg, 1854; Glauchau, 1856; Homburg, 1858; Altona, 1859) had witnessed the establishment of a central water supply (Grahn, 1904a; Steuer, 1912). Increasingly, other towns followed this development in the succeeding decades, with major building activity being undertaken particularly in the 1870s and 1880s. By 1900 all the larger towns (with a population exceeding 25,000 inhabitants) had a central water supply, whereas only 47 per cent of the smaller towns (2,000–25,000 inhabitants) had such facilities (Table 33). There were wide regional differences; 67 per cent of the smaller towns in Prussia and 35 per cent in the other German states still had no central water supply by the turn of the century (Grahn, 1904a, p. 309). The expansion of sewerage systems followed the construction of waterworks after an interval (see Appendix 9); the main period of construction occurred around the end of the nineteenth and beginning of the twentieth century (Fig. 33).

In the case of the large towns, Germany was quickly catching up with English developments of municipal enterprise. In England the municipal franchise was based on ratable values, a system which resulted in a small electorate. In 1861 only 3 per cent of the population of Birmingham could vote for the town council; the figure for

2 For a detailed description of municipal self-government and administrative powers in Germany from one of the leading contemporary British experts on Germany, see Dawson (1914). He summarizes the differences between England and Germany as follows '... while the German town, grown to man's estate, exercises the freedom and independence of manhood, the English town is still protected and chaperoned by its ever present and often fussy nurse, the "Board above"' (p. 36). See also Krabbe (1979).

Leeds was 13 per cent. The franchise and property regulations relating to individuals able to sit on town councils led to local authorities that were dominated by property interests that advocated the maintenance of low rates. A survey of one-fifth of the sanitary districts in 1886 revealed that those administering public health acts at the local level were mainly shopkeepers (30.8 per cent of the local sanitary officials), followed by manufacturers (17.5 per cent), gentlemen (11.8 per cent), merchants (8.6 per cent), farmers (7.7 per cent) and builders (7.6 per cent) (Wohl, 1983, p. 167). Many of these middle-income rate-payers became alarmed by plans for expensive local sanitary investments and, being an influential pressure group, they were often successful in blocking reform (Midwinter, 1969, pp. 69, 111; Smith, 1979, p. 216; Wohl, 1983, p. 101; Thompson, 1984, pp. 141–42). It has been argued that this led to an under-investment in urban social overhead provision, that was only overcome in the last third of the nineteenth century (Williamson, 1987; 1990).

In Germany, due to the three-class electoral system (in most of Prussia and some other parts of the Reich) or other sharp restrictions of the franchise (the distinction between residents and citizens in Hamburg, Bavaria and Wurtemberg), political power at the municipal level was concentrated in the hands of a minority of residents. Major control functions were put in the hands of a largely entrepreneurial upper bourgeoisie. The town councils in the cities of the Rhineland, for example, were increasingly dominated by representatives of the large industries (Lenger, 1990, pp. 120–21), who most probably received the most significant net economic benefits from sanitary reform. On the one hand, as entrepreneurs, they profited directly from the increasing revenue surplus of public utilities, such as central water supply and sewerage provision. On the other hand, as employers, they benefited from the increased health of their factory workers (Smith, 1979, p. 216; Wohl, 1983, chs 4 and 7; Hassan, 1985; Brown, 1989, p. 8). This group also dominated the wide range of municipal boards, the duties of which ranged from preparing forthcoming town council meetings to the direction of the local gas- and waterworks (Lenger, 1990, p. 133). This, combined with the widespread employment of professional administrators and, by British standards, a highly trained corps of bureaucrats (*Leistungsverwaltung*) (Dawson, 1914; Krabbe, 1985), ensured a more ready accomplishment and acceptance of reform measures (Sutcliffe, 1981, p. 26). On the eve of the First World War the city of Cologne, for example, employed 3,000 civil servants, the city of Düsseldorf 2,000 (Lenger, 1990, p. 131). These professional administrators initiated ambitious programmes of municipal reform and enterprise with the help of police powers that gave municipal government abundant opportunities to intervene in private property rights and to regulate municipal building measures.[3] It should not be neglected in that context that there were often strong social and family links between the administrative and economic elites in the cities which alleviated the pursuit of their interests (Lenger, 1990, p. 167). Both groups were also strongly represented in the *Niederrheinische Verein für öffentliche Gesundheitspflege*, an association set up in 1869 for the promotion of public health in the lower Rhenish cities (Ladd, 1990, pp. 38–41). In addition, the higher

---

3 For the English situation see Kearns (1988b).

population density of German towns that resulted from the characteristic pattern of multi-storeyed housing, reduced the required capital investment. Also on the technical side, progress was more easily facilitated in Germany by the direct use of British know-how and engineering skills. Numerous constructions in Germany were carried out by employing British sanitary engineers (e.g. William Lindley in Hamburg and Frankfurt am Main and as adviser in Düsseldorf, Krefeld and Chemnitz; Joseph Gorden in Frankfurt am Main) and by applying techniques developed in Britain (Hartog, 1962, p. 24).[4] Yet despite this, German towns could not apply ready-made, fully

Table 33: Increase in number of German towns with central water supply (absolute figures and percentage [in brackets])

Towns	Up to 1870		1870–1880		1880–1890		1890–1900		Up to 1900		No. of towns
Up to 25,000 inhabitants	20	(1)	94	(6)	201	(14)	381	(26)	696	(47)	1,490
Over 25,000 inhabitants	23	(15)	58	(39)	35	(23)	34	(23)	150	(100)	150
Total	43	(3)	152	(9)	236	(15)	415	(25)	846	(52)	1,640

Source: Grahn (1904a), p. 309.

Table 34: Expansion of the health-related infrastructure in the ten largest German towns, 1888–1912

Town	Length of water supply (m)		Properties served		Domestic water consumption/capita per day (litres)		Length of sewerage system (m)	
	1888	1912	1888	1912	1888	1912	1888	1912
Berlin	661,246	1,176,719	20,403	30,726	51.0	80.7	567,967	1,108,100
Breslau	157,873	423,035*	6,242	11,128	51.3	60.7	231,263	343,600
Cologne	137,796	460,028	11,620	29,184	158.3†	150.6†	56,600	438,500
Dresden	165,134	529,730	7,544	17,244	70.4	110.9†	149,133	455,800
Düsseldorf	107,975	481,290	6,072	19,731	69.5	114.9	32,000	349,000
Frankfurt	188,626	848,582*	7,788	26,334	97.3	163.5†	191,600	400,000
Leipzig	140,457	506,624	4,256	18,468	92.5†	70.9†	9,4280	435,300
Hamburg	394,095	771,027*	16,397	25,970	208.2†	133.8	287,731	527,000
Munich	184,912	549,906*	5,366	17,251*	8.9	158.6	109,392	327,200
Nuremberg	103,044	285,638	4,550	14,578	34.2	65.3	93,418	242,400

* Includes areas outside the town.
† Complete water consumption per capita and day.
Sources: *Statistisches Jahrbuch Deutscher Städte*, **1** (1890) onwards.

4 Reformers in Germany were more in favour of groundwater theories where the rise and transmission of cholera and typhoid fever were concerned, and therefore put theoretically more emphasis on sewerage systems; in England the drinking-water theory was more predominant. See Knorr (1958).

developed construction techniques in the development of central water supply and sewerage systems. Sanitary engineering was still in its initial stages and there was no consensus with respect to construction methods and operational procedures.

Technical standards determined the efficiency and quality of the infrastructural measures. All the ten largest German towns, for instance, had a centralized sewerage system, mainly using the so-called '*Mischsystem*' (mixed system). On the one hand, as the provision of centralized water supply was a relatively new development, the availability of natural resources was often a critical factor. The use of ground or surface water was dependent on the local geographical and topographical situation. On the other hand, sanitary engineering was still in a phase of experimentation and a variety of different systems were tested or applied. The municipalities were therefore confronted with a multitude of various systems. Mechanical, biological and chemical processes were available for the purification of the waste water (Fig. 34).[5] Berlin and Breslau used irrigation or sewage farms (*Rieselfelder*), with waste water pumped onto special fields. Only Munich and Nuremberg had no water purification at all (see Appendix 9). In addition to technological difficulties, urban authorities were constantly in fear of committing budgetary resources to relatively untried and unproved experiments (Wohl, 1983, p. 169), as many of the earlier sewerage systems had not brought about the expected solution to river pollution (Hamlin, 1988, p. 67).

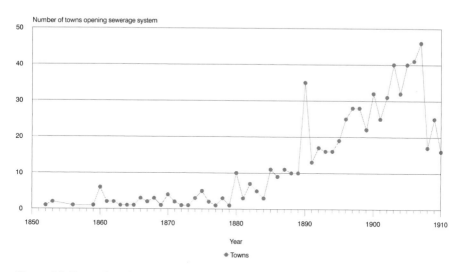

Figure 33: Expansion of sewerage systems in German towns
Sources: Salomon (1907, 1911).

5 For the various techniques see Imhoff (1979); Stanbridge (1976).

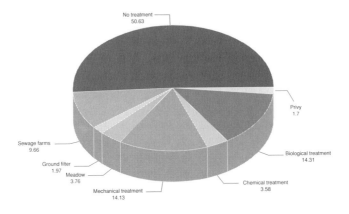

Figure 34: Sewage treatment in German towns, 1907

Sources: Salomon (1907, 1911).

For these reasons, in terms of technical standards and the number of houses joined to central sanitary facilities, the real phase of expansion of centralized water supply and sewerage in both countries was not before the 1870s. In Berlin for example, the construction of a central water supply had already been initiated in 1853, but by 1873 only 54 per cent of the properties, and 50 per cent of the housing, were connected. And it was not until the end of the nineteenth century that domestic water supply became almost universal in German towns (Table 33 and Fig. 35). Similarly, in St Helen's the number of inhabitants centrally supplied with water rose from 56,000 in 1880 to 98,000 in 1908 (an increase of almost 100 per cent); in Sheffield the whole town was only effectively supplied by 1906 (Smith, 1979, p. 228). In London it was only in the 1890s that half of the population had access to a constant central water supply (Luckin, 1984, p. 112). In Germany a special problem arose as a result of the characteristic multi-storeyed housing. In the early phases of developing a central water supply, the water pressure was often only strong enough to reach the lower floors of houses, leaving the inhabitants on the higher floors without flowing water. Therefore, especially in the German case, the number of houses connected to a central water supply is only a rough and crude indicator of the actual overall supply to the urban population. On the whole, the expansion of water supply was undertaken with a different timing and different intensity, so that a diverse variety of houses and households in each town were served by these facilities. Although average water consumption generally increased in the German towns between the late 1880s and 1913 (Fig. 36), there remained substantial variation in the actual amount of water available (Table 34). Even as late as 1912, domestic water consumption per capita and day in the ten largest German towns varied between 60.7 litres in Breslau and 158.6 litres in Munich. The supply of flowing water was often restricted in quantity or to specific hours or days, and in Bristol in the 1830s the Puritan Corporation even closed all the conduits on Sundays, making it a punishable offence to draw water on that day (Wright, 1963, p. 149). Hot summers could interrupt the constant supply of water until late in the nineteenth century.

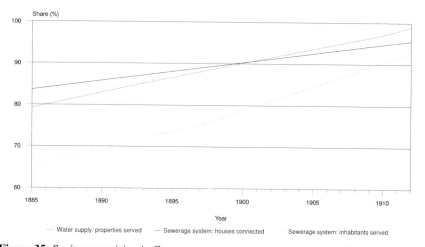

Figure 35: Sanitary provision in German towns—average access to central water supply and sewerage systems

Source: *Statistishes Jahrbuch Deutscher Städte*, **1** (1890) onwards.

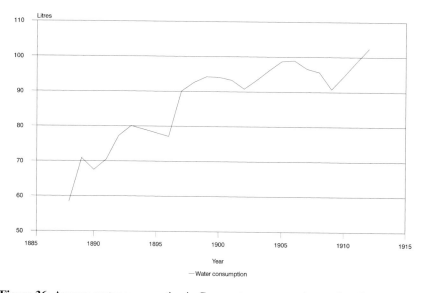

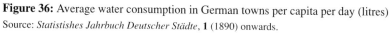

Figure 36: Average water consumption in German towns per capita per day (litres)

Source: *Statistishes Jahrbuch Deutscher Städte*, **1** (1890) onwards.

Similar developments can be registered with respect to drainage and sewerage systems. Again Liverpool and Manchester were leading the way (Wohl, 1983, pp. 97–102; Sheard, 1993, pp. 158–63), although Manchester did not adopt a water-borne sewerage system, but decided instead to install a dry conservancy pail system. Other towns followed, some with considerable delay. In Sheffield in 1873 only four per cent of all houses were served by water-closets; the conversion of privies only really began after 1894, yet in the 1890s some 40,000 houses still had privies (Williams, 1989, p. 147). In Leeds in 1871 there were 30,335 privy-middens, with 277 pail closets, and only 6,348 water-closets (Stanbridge, 1976, vol. 1, pp. 35). In Birmingham during the same year only six per cent of the population had access to water-closets. About 20,000 inhabitants were being served by 7,065 water-closets and about 325,000 by 19,551 privy-middens (Stanbridge, 1976, vol. 1, p. 35). Bolton in 1889 had 1,252 water-closets, 8,632 privy-middens and 6,000 pail closets (Stanbridge, 1976, vol. 1, p. 36). According to an 1894 survey, Bradford still had 30,000 privies, Manchester, Preston and Sheffield over 20,000 each, Birmingham, Bolton, Leeds and Salford between 10,000 and 20,000; Manchester still had nearly 70,000 pail closets, Birmingham 33,000 and Gateshead more than 10,000 (Stanbridge, 1976, vol. 1, p. 36). In Bradford, even by 1900, less than 25 per cent of the houses had the use of water-closets (Thompson, 1984, p. 140). In 1902 Manchester had 80,000 pail closets and 46,000 water-closets (Stanbridge, 1976, vol. 1, p. 36). Quality was also a problem: of 1,747 houses inspected in 1885 by the Jewish Sanitary Committee for the East End of London, 90 per cent had water-closets which were broken or 'could not flush' (Smith, 1979, p. 222). The situation in rural areas was even more worrying. The change from the conservancy system to the water-carriage system did not really start before the passing of the Rural Water Supplies and Sewerage Act of 1944 and is still not completed. In 1975 it was reported that in England and Wales there were still about 900,000 ratepayers not on main drainage (Stanbridge, 1976, vol. 1, p. 28).

As the expansion of infrastructural sanitary measures was often a slow process, a town or city frequently required several years before it was sufficiently supplied and the majority of the population had access to such facilities. It is therefore important to examine the spatial diffusion pattern of central water supply and sewerage systems in individual cities. As mentioned earlier, the poor often lived in the inner-city centre. As this area was often congruent with the old nucleus of the town, which, in many cases, was situated on the traditional trade-routes, the rivers, it was these districts which could have been served most easily from a technical point of view. Yet the connection to central water supply and sewerage systems was often first undertaken in the wealthier districts (Oldendorff, 1904, pp. 350–51; Falkus, 1977, p. 142; Stanbridge, 1976, vol. 1, p. 28). In the *First Report of the Commissioners for Inquiring into the State of Large Towns and Populous Districts* (published in 1844) there was also concern about water access for the poorer classes. A regularly occurring statement for the individual towns is that 'the poor are badly supplied'. For Bolton it is reported that the 'poorest people beg water', for Liverpool that 'many of the poor beg or steal it' (*First Report*, 1844). It took quite a long time and in some towns well into the twentieth century before the poor had access to piped water and drainage. Figure 35 supports this point with respect to access to the sewerage system. Considering that the working class in Germany lived in multi-storeyed houses and the wealthier groups of the population inhabited smaller houses, the fact that the number of houses connected to the sewerage system surpassed the number of inhabitants actually served until the early twentieth century supports this view for the ten largest

German towns. Similarly, in England, and especially in the industrial towns of the Midlands and north, only houses in the upper-class districts had water-closets (Stanbridge, 1976, vol. 1, p. 35). In Liverpool the introduction of water-closets was spatially biased towards the wealthier districts, with the conversion of privies to water-closets coming last in the courts (Sheard, 1993, pp. 175–81).

CHOLERA AS THE 'BIG SANITARY REFORMER'
OR
THE MOTIVES FOR SANITARY REFORM

The reasons and motives for establishing sanitary facilities were many and varied from town to town, as well as, of course, between the two countries under compari-son. Explanations range from very practical factors—a central water supply was considered to be an essential aid against fire—to questions of power between munic-ipal and state authorities.[6] One common argument, frequently put forward either in combination with others or as a key factor, was that the cholera epidemics, which affected both countries from the 1830s onwards, provided the impetus for sanitary reforms (Gottstein, 1901, p. 244; Fischer, 1933, vol. 2, p. 502; Rath, 1969, p. 76; Wohl, 1983, p. 173; Labisch, 1988, p. 1079). Cholera in this context is seen by mod-ern historians as 'the reformer's best friend' or the 'big sanitary reformer'. In a more general way, it has been argued that the most extensive sanitary reform was under-taken in the unhealthiest places, whereas in cities where health problems were per-ceived to be less acute the stimulus to action was lacking (Hennock, 1973, pp. 112–13). However, there are some serious objections to the hypothesis that cholera or generally bad health conditions initiated sanitary reform or acted as a driving force behind the expansion of public health measures in the period under consideration.

First of all, many contemporaries, for example Engels and Chadwick, tended to explain the urban crisis with respect to housing and employment conditions. Cholera was not their primary focus of attention. Pauperism was regarded as the main threat. With widespread Malthusian fears of overpopulation, cholera was even regarded as a necessary check, keeping population growth within the limits of available nutri-tional supply. In this view cholera functioned as 'the police of nature'. It is not sur-prising, therefore, that urban health conditions in Germany did not play a special role within the public health movement, which from the 1840s onwards replaced the old system of the medical police. Medical research into cholera did not focus on urban living conditions (Bleker, 1983, p. 126). The unhealthiness of towns was taken as an obvious fact that did not require any further confirmation as a result of epidemio-logical research. In the rare cases of scientific investigations into urban health con-ditions to any great extent, early medical-statistical scholars in Germany, like Oesterlen, used statistical material relating to conditions in English industrial towns (Oesterlen, 1874). At mid-century, when urban death rates were highest in Germany, contemporary medical literature showed only a marginal interest in urban living

---

6 For a discussion of various factors see Hamlin (1988); Krabbe (1985), pp. 26–27.

conditions. Towards the end of the century, however, when death rates improved and the towns registered better health conditions than rural areas, many authors in the medical profession tended to dramatize urban health conditions (Bleker, 1983, pp. 123–32). Although there was a growing statistical literature about urban health conditions, it was obviously not analysed. Indeed, contemporary hostility against the towns and their perceived unsanitary conditions even increased. This indicates that an analysis of urban health conditions from medical history sources is not only incomplete (Bleker, 1983, p. 133), but that contemporary medical opinion may be completely misleading. The absence of any clear link between the extensive cholera literature and sanitary reform in contemporary German reports places in severe doubt the general view that cholera functioned as the initial driving force for sanitary reform. More importantly, it implies that the sanitary movement in Germany was an imported reform from England, which simply occurred at the right time when historical urban health risks were most acute.

Additional support for this hypothesis is provided by the fact that the systematic expansion of these facilities in Germany only started after a delay of 30 to 40 years following the outbreak of the first cholera epidemics. Even in England a number of decades passed between the first outbreaks of cholera and the systematic take up of sanitary measures. Local reports reveal that the threat of cholera was not connected with sanitary reforms. Public health issues were frequently raised by engineers or members of the local sanitary boards, and not by the medical officers of health (Hamlin, 1988, p. 68). In fact, the first General Board of Health (1848–1854) in England had no specific medical representative (although it co-opted Southwood Smith on the occasion of the 1849 cholera epidemic). Cholera came and went, and an epidemic was easily forgotten, no matter how many victims had been taken. Moreover, there was no conclusive theory concerning the causes of many diseases, and a much stronger conflict in Germany than in England between supporters of the drinking-water and ground-water causation theories. Consequently there were acrimonious disputes concerning the utility and effects of different sanitary techniques (see for example Varrentrapp, 1868). In many towns the construction of expensive sanitary facilities had been begun despite the absence of any significant risk of cholera or a clear theory concerning the origin and transmission of many diseases. In Frankfurt am Main, for example, six million Marks had been spent by 1877, although the town was never affected by cholera epidemics (*Frankfurt am Main*, 1881, p. 34). In England, sewage works were often constructed or enlarged in response to injunctions obtained by a private party to stop river pollution, so that the individual towns were forced to act not because of public health acts but because of common English law (Hamlin, 1988, pp. 60–61).

Whereas the direct link between disease and sanitary reform seems to have been of minor importance, it becomes crucial if economic considerations are interposed between the two terms. The pioneers of sanitary reform—Chadwick, Farr and Pettenkofer—estimated on the basis of human capital economics that the projected savings in human life resulting from improved sanitary facilities far exceeded the cost of sanitation investment. Increasingly, contemporaries calculated in a cost/benefit analysis the value of productive workers or human life, yet this approach seldom permeated public debate (Williamson, 1987, p. 30). In more practical terms, it was realized that sanitary reform was crucial for the functioning of modern industrial towns. Traditional forms of state intervention relying on quarantine and isolation (*cordon sanitaire*) were completely counter-productive in the context of a modern economy based on the free exchange of goods and services.[7] The famous Munich hygienist Max von Pettenkofer, the main advocate of miasmatic-localistic theories and holder of the first chair of hygiene in Germany, emphasized that an interruption of trade in order to avoid the spread of cholera would be a bigger misfortune than cholera itself, and that many people would prefer an epidemic to an extended restriction of their livelihood.[8] Considering the increasing emphasis on the need to maintain the daily functioning of economic life, it is therefore not surprising that sanitary reforms were first carried out in the new industrial and commercial towns, irrespective of their actual health conditions. In England, both factors coincided: the new industrial and commercial towns were invariably very unhealthy. Liverpool and Manchester, for example, had excessively high death rates (see Chapter 6), and both towns became frontrunners with respect to sanitary reforms. However, the new industrial towns in the western part of Germany registered relatively good health conditions in terms of low mortality and, what may be even more important when analysing the motives for initiating sanitary reforms, they perceived themselves as healthy towns, even healthier than they actually were. For example, from a comparison of the crude death rate in Düsseldorf (21.3 per 1,000 inhabitants) and the Rhineland in general (22.0) with Prussia (22.6) and Germany (22.7) at the end of the nineteenth century, it was concluded in a local report that Düsseldorf was a very healthy town (Brandt, 1902, p. 139). Düsseldorf indeed was amongst the healthiest of the ten largest towns. Yet, as was demonstrated by a more differentiated analysis in earlier chapters of this study, this was attributable to a large extent to differences in the age-structure of the population at risk. The contemporary judgement in this case betrays clear elements of local patriotism. However, the industrial towns of Rhineland-Westphalia were among the frontrunners in the German public health movement, both in terms of organization (Labisch, 1988) and in the actual provision of sanitary measures (see Appendix 9). In addition, miasmatic-localistic theories, which were still taken seriously in certain circles, made isolation and quarantine superfluous, even in times of severe epidemics. It was not by chance that the officials of the old Hanse town of Hamburg were inclined to rely on such theories relating to the origin of cholera during the famous epidemic of 1892 in order to maintain the trade that was so essential for the town's prosperity (Evans, 1987; see also pp. 170–72).

7 See Labisch (1986; 1992), pp. 124–32.
8 For further information about Pettenkofer's life and theories see Hume (1927); von Voit (1902); Winslow (1943), pp. 311–36; Breyer (1980).

There were, however, even more direct links between economics and sanitary reform. Sanitary engineering quickly became an important branch of the economy with its own strong financial interests (see for example Koch, 1911; Steuer, 1912). Furthermore, communal enterprises became a substantial income source for the municipalities. The pricing policy of the communities was also aimed at making a profit (Mombert, 1908, p. 3), and, in German towns with more than 25,000 inhabitants, for example, until the 1930s between 15 and 20 per cent of the municipal budget was covered by income from municipal enterprises (including gas, water and electricity works) (Ambrosius, 1987, p. 141). In short, 'water' became big business, and individual communities viewed municipal water supply as a major income source, which became even more significant after the main investments had been undertaken and whole towns were connected to the central supply system (Table 35).

Table 35: Revenue-surplus of waterworks in German towns (Marks)

| Town | 1889–90 | | 1903–1904 |
	Surplus	Costs for new constructions or extension works	Surplus
Berlin	4,920,745	2,514,144	5,421,635
Hamburg	1,395,691	286,699	2,035,641
Munich	553,362	83,100	1,555,815
Breslau	786,131	89,374	1,208,435
Leipzig	291,340	570,000	1,461,175
Cologne	767,872	261,282	1,293,344
Dresden	777,394	34,147	1,156,933
Frankfurt	1,065,299	618,019	2,011,787
Düsseldorf	352,980	–	701,457
Nuremberg	329,607	56,624	507,191

Revenues without revenue-surplus tranfers from the preceeding year and transfers from funds, loans or other municipal sources; expenditures excluding transfers to community funds, interest rates, redemptions and amortizations, as well as without costs for new constructions or extension works.

1903–1904 no information about costs for new constructions or extension works.

Source: *Statistisches Jahrbuch Deutscher Städte*, **2** (1892); **14** (1907).

Municipal enterprises in the big towns were large-scale undertakings. The Metropolitan Water Board in London, for example, was capitalized in 1903 at nearly £47 million. The total annual expenditure by Manchester Corporation (including loans, repayment and interest) was about £363,000 on water; in Birmingham, capital investment in water supply was about £8 million in 1906; even smaller towns like Leeds or Bradford had invested well over £1 million in water supply (Falkus, 1977, p. 137). Many waterworks were among the top fifty industrial concerns in England, and the total capitalization of these fifty concerns was about the same as that of the capital raised by the municipalities for their water, gas, electricity and tramways (Falkus, 1977, p. 137). Moreover, there was an increased need for an appropriate quantity and quality of water for industry, which in some places, such as in the mining-dominated towns in the industrial area of the Rhineland and Westphalia, even led to subsidence of the ground-water level so that many wells ran dry (Zadek, 1909, pp. 38–39). How desperate the cry for water was can be gauged from Liverpool, with its notorious water shortage in the early stages of water supply, where a local newspaper printed the apparently serious idea of shooting cannons at the clouds (Sheard, 1993, p. 127). Especially in the case of English textile towns, local industry needed a specific quality of water, 'soft water', which could no longer be obtained from the polluted rivers, so that a central water supply from outside the town became absolutely essential (Hamlin, 1988, pp. 72–73). In some cases, this soft water had to be transported over long distances through lead service pipes. Occasional cases of lead-poisoning were seen as an acceptable risk, as iron pipes were considered to colour 'soft water' (Silverthorne, 1884, pp. 31–32). Other towns sought to attract new industries by the provision of sufficient amounts of water (Krabbe, 1985, p. 27), even using surface water for this purpose, although this was often polluted and made effective purification and filtration even more difficult (Gärtner, 1904, p. 759; Zadek, 1909, p. 35). Finally, the reputation of spa towns relied entirely on the provision of good quality water.

In England the development of municipal sewerage systems was also begun with promises of profit, but there was an increasing number of towns where sewage treatment plants failed to live up to contemporary expectations, both in terms of effluent quality and operating costs (Hamlin, 1988, p. 67). From this experience German municipal authorities regarded sewerage systems as less profitable than central water supply (Krabbe, 1983, p. 379). Consequently their expansion followed after a delay of some decades, despite the persistence of miasmatic-localistic theories relating to the origin and transmission of many diseases. With the expansion of central water supply, however, the amount of water within the city often created problems, which made systematic drainage absolutely necessary. In Düsseldorf, for example, after the installation of the municipal waterworks in 1870, the lower-lying city districts were increasingly exposed to flooding (Geusen, 1908, p. 31). And, after all, in many places the cost involved in these subsidized municipal undertakings were relatively limited. In Munich, for example, the costs of the sewerage system stood at 54,183 Marks in 1885 and 433,686 Marks in 1906 (Busse, 1908, p. 70), and financial considerations did not justify a postponement of their construction for so many years. In the case of the city of Leipzig, for instance, the additional expenditure for the sewerage system rose from 229,687 Marks in 1898 to 408,531 Marks in 1907, but these sums were no more than the city's additional expenditure for the administration of its municipal gardens (Weigel, 1909, p. 108).

These examples suggest that economic factors and entrepreneurial interests were the crucial and decisive element behind sanitary reform rather than the medical or hygienic reasons given in the official version of events. Arthur Silverthorne had already noted in 1884 that 'the hygienic view is invariably put forward to support schemes which aim at obtaining supplies of magnitude from distant watersheds in preference to extending and improving original sources; but it may be depended upon that the real and less apparent object is to obtain soft waters suited to the manufacturing interests' (Silverthorne, 1884, p. 31).

THE IMPACT OF CENTRAL WATER SUPPLY AND SEWERAGE SYSTEMS ON URBAN HEALTH

Although the concern about health conditions was after all in many cases not the primary impetus for sanitary reforms, their positive effects on health were considered to be obvious, and taken as a good opportunity to justify the massive expenditure on infrastructural extensions. A classic test for assessing the impact of adequate water supply and sanitation on health was and still is the level and trend of the death rate from typhoid fever. By comparing indicators of sanitary reform for one specific town, mostly the opening dates of the local waterworks and the completion of the sewerage system or the number of houses connected to the central water supply or sewerage system, and the course of typhoid fever mortality, contemporaries concluded from the apparent coincidence between increased supply and the reduced incidence of typhoid fever that there was a causal link between the two developments. Modern studies approach the subject in a similar way, but with more sophisticated methods (e.g. Sydenstricker, 1933, p. 182; Goubert, 1975; Luckin, 1986). The results, however, are primarily determined by the precise methodology applied in each specific case. Typhoid fever mortality was definitely decreasing during the period that corresponded with the expansion of municipal water supply and sewerage systems. Yet, whether there was a causal link between these two developments has still to be elaborated and tested. Studies at the level of city districts including a broader range of indicators are normally more cautious concerning the impact of sanitary reform (e.g. Pooley and Pooley, 1984, on Manchester; Sheard, 1993, on Liverpool; Woods, 1984a, on Birmingham), especially if they also take other determinants of the mortality decline into account and incorporate them into the analysis. Instead, they argue that only changes in social conditions could lead to a long-term decline in mortality. Similarly, a number of macro-level studies including correlations and regressions for a number of Amercian cities suggest a rather weak interrelationship between sanitary reform and water- and food-borne diseases (Condran and Crimmins-Gardner, 1978; Condran and Crimmins, 1980; Higgs, 1979; Higgs and Booth, 1979). In a recent analysis, J. Brown suggests from the application of regression analysis for a sample of German towns in the late period of sanitary reform (1886–1912) an important impact of sanitary improvements on the reduction of typhoid fever mortality (Brown, forthcoming). As spatial and chronological aspects remain largely neglected in his study, this hypothesis still needs to be tested using a systematic comparative approach.

In order to reach some general conclusions concerning the impact of sanitary reform on urban health, the following analysis will employ a comparative macro-level approach utilizing more detailed references to intra-urban conditions in selected cases. Attention is focused on the interrelationship between phases of expansion of the centralized water supply and sewerage systems in the urban communities under analysis on the one hand and trends in disease-specific mortality on the other. Particular attention will be paid to typhoid fever, diseases of the digestive system, and—as the age-group most at risk of dying from the latter—infant mortality as an additional control variable. An emphasis on infant mortality and diseases of the digestive system is of special importance in relation to the German sample, as a decline in the proportion of women breast-feeding in German towns meant that the quality of water used to prepare artificial food became a decisive factor in determining the incidence of deaths from digestive diseases. An analysis of the annual trend of relevant causes of death during the 'sanitary revolution' in various towns with a different temporal and technical approach to their sanitation facilities will provide an insight into the specific interrelationship between sanitary reform and contemporary mortality trends. An additional perspective can be obtained by analysing the death rate trends at the national level and for all towns with a population exceeding 15,000 inhabitants, especially in the early phase of sanitary reform when the number of urban communities supplied with these facilities was not substantial enough to be represented in these figures. Was the trend in death rates influenced by the opening of new waterworks, by the number of houses served, by the specific source of water supply (ground water or surface water), or by the implementation of a filter plant?

When comparing individual towns with respect to these questions, it has to be kept in mind that they also formed a kind of interactive network (via trade, migration, etc.). The impact of this network on health and disease was dependent on the degree of intercommunication between individual cities. In view of major inter-urban migration flows and increasing exchange of goods in the course of industrialization, the network can be assumed to have been highly active. Infectious diseases and epidemics could spread along these routes. If individual towns were situated on the same river, water pollution caused by the towns upstream could cause the situation to deteriorate for the towns downstream. Improvements in the infrastructure of individual cities could have interrupted this chain and served to provide a quarantine for cities adequately supplied with public health facilities. If the number of such cities had become substantial, this also could have had a positive side-effect on those towns with an insufficient public health infrastructure as their degree of exposure was reduced. Hence, as soon as a large proportion of towns were provided with an adequate water supply and sewerage systems, with resultant positive effects on mortality from typhoid fever and from gastro-intestinal infectious diseases, this was likely to have contributed to the decline of these diseases even in towns without such facilities. If nine out of ten towns had successfully eradicated typhoid fever as a result of sanitary reform, this would have reduced the risk of the typhoid fever agent being spread by human contact or via polluted rivers. It is therefore of special importance to take a close look at the early stages of sanitary reform, when only a small number of towns were provided with sanitary facilities and when the urban network effect was marginal.

To approach the question of the potential interrelationship between sanitary reform and urban health from another angle, the analysis will also study a series of typhoid fever epidemics that occurred in the Hanse town of Hamburg in the 1880s. Although not as severe in their demographic consequences as typhoid fever epidemics in the ear-lier decades of the nineteenth century, excellent source material for Hamburg allows an analysis of the spread of the epidemics throughout the city and its various districts, and permits an epidemiological approach within a broader socio-economic framework.

The potential impact of sanitary reform on health becomes obvious if one ascribes the decline of mortality from gastro-intestinal disorders in urban areas completely to the positive effects of the sanitary revolution. In Germany the impact of such mea-sures on the mortality decline had a larger possible impact than that assumed by McKeown for England and Wales. In the ten largest German towns, overall mortal-ity declined from 26.77 to 15.73 per 1,000 inhabitants between 1877 and 1907, but the mortality rate from the digestive disease complex (including typhoid fever and dysentery) fell from 6.74 to 2.35 per 1,000 inhabitants during the same period. If the mortality decline is taken to equal 100, the fall in mortality from gastro-intestinal dis-eases accounted for 39.8 per cent of the overall decline in mortality (digestive dis-eases 34.5 per cent, typhoid fever 4.0 per cent, dysentery 1.3 per cent) (see Table 11). In relation to all German towns with a population of more than 15,000, this calcula-tion can only be applied to acute diseases of the digestive system and typhoid fever (see Chapter 7). The average crude mortality rate of these towns fell from 26.99 per 1,000 inhabitants in 1877 to 14.02 in 1913. The cause-specific mortality rate from acute diseases of the digestive system (typhoid fever included) declined from 2.97 per 1,000 inhabitants to 1.25. That is, the relative contribution of acute gastro-intesti-nal infectious diseases to the overall mortality decline was 13.23 per cent. In relation to the ten largest German towns, the reduction in acute diseases of the digestive sys-tem contributed between 2.65 per cent (Cologne) and 30.28 per cent (Berlin) to the overall mortality decline in this period. The higher the mortality rates from such dis-eases initially were in a specific town, of course, the greater the possible potential effects of the sanitary revolution were likely to be.

If this kind of calculation is applied to England and Wales for the period under obser-vation, the impact of such measures in English towns on the mortality decline was less than the assumed contribution of one-fifth estimated by McKeown for the country as a whole (McKeown, 1976). In the ten largest towns overall mortality declined from 24.0 to 16.8 per 1,000 inhabitants between 1871–1880 and 1901–1910, but the mor-tality rate from the digestive disease complex fell from 2.6 to 2.2 per 1,000 inhabitants.[9] The fall in gastro-intestinal disease mortality, therefore, accounted for only 5.6 per cent of the overall decline in mortality, which is much less than in the German case.

Due to the immense importance of the digestive disease complex in Germany and its significant contribution to the decline in urban mortality, the German case will be used as the focus of the analysis and will be discussed in greater detail, with the Eng-lish data employed for comparative purposes rather than as an independent investi-gation. However, the analysis will start with an examination of the course of typhoid fever mortality in English towns in order to set the framework.

9 Diarrhoea and dysentery, enteric fever and simple continued fever, 1901–1910 and diseases of the digestive system, 1891–1900 (with a death rate of 2.13 per 1,000 inhabitants). See Chapter 3, Table 11 and Appendix 3.

Annual death rates from typhoid fever (enteric and simple continued fever) were recorded in the Annual Reports of the Registrar-General from 1869 onwards.[10] From this year on, mortality declined both in the urban centres and in the case of England and Wales as a whole (Fig. 37). In the early 1870s various towns, amongst them Leeds, Manchester and especially Liverpool, were struck by epidemic occurrences of typhoid fever, far exceeding the national aggregate mortality rates. Thereafter, epidemics disappeared and the mortality rates for the ten largest English towns tended to converge with the national figures. Despite this, the majority of the ten largest towns continued to register death rates well above the national average, although there were some with lower rates (London, Bristol, Birmingham and, from 1900 onwards, Sheffield). It is, however, problematic to infer direct links between the extent of the fall in mortality from typhoid fever and the impact of sanitary reform. Due to national legislation, water supply in England was not as exclusively a phenomenon of the largest towns as it was in the case of Germany during this period (Smith, 1978, p. 187; see also the previous sections).

For Germany in the 1860s and early 1870s, disease-specific death rates from typhoid fever are only available for a handful of the selected towns (see p.152), but the available data suggest that the level of urban typhoid fever mortality was quite similar in England and Germany during this period. From 1877 onwards we can compare the annual rates for both countries (Figs 37 and 38). In England, the decline in typhoid fever seems to have occurred slightly earlier than in German towns of over 15,000 inhabitants, which might have been a consequence of the earlier commencement of sanitary reforms. Some of the ten largest German towns, such as Berlin, Hamburg and Munich, were struck by years with high typhoid fever mortality even as late as the 1870s and 1880s. The rates for most of the ten largest German towns, however, were soon declining to a lower level than the rates for the corresponding English towns. Was this due to the fast and effective installation of sanitary facilities in the large German towns? Indeed by the 1890s, the typhoid fever mortality rate in almost all of the ten largest towns was constantly below the average of all towns with a population of more than 15,000 inhabitants; and their average rate was below the Prussian average until around the turn of the century (Dornedden, 1939, p. 228); thereafter mortality rates converged at a similarly low level. Moreover, in the last third of the nineteenth century, typhoid fever mortality was inversely proportional to town size (Table 36). In 1881, for example, the typhoid fever death rate was 3.2 per 10,000 inhabitants in large towns, 5.1 in medium-sized towns, and 6.5 in small towns.

Table 36: Mortality from typhoid fever in Prussian communities (per 10,000 inhabitants)

Year	Small rural communities	Small towns	Medium towns	Large towns
1876	6.2	8.1	6.4	6.0
1881	5.4	6.5	5.1	3.2
1891	1.9	2.4	2.3	1.4

Source: Kruse (1897), p. 139.

Source: *Statistisches Jahrbuch Deutscher Städte*, **2** (1892); **14** (1907).

The only exception was typhoid fever mortality in small rural communities, which recorded an average death rate from typhoid fever. Bearing in mind the fact that sanitary infrastructural improvements were first applied in the largest towns, the relatively low death rates from typhoid fever in these towns seem to support the hypothesis that the sanitary revolution had positive effects on urban health conditions. The convergence of the rates after the turn of the century might reflect both the increasing diffusion of municipal reforms and the urban network effect.

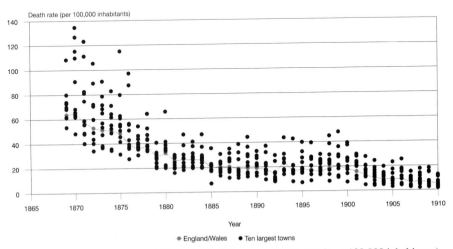

Figure 37: Mortality from typhoid fever in English towns, (1869–1910 per 100,000 inhabitants)
Typoid fever = enteric fever and simple continued fever.

Sources: *Annual Reports of the Registrar-General of Births, Deaths, and Marriages in England and Wales* (1856–1910).

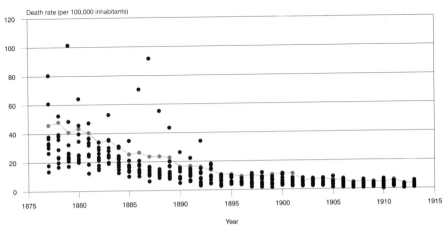

Figure 38: Mortality from typhoid fever in German towns, (1877–1913 per 100,000 inhabitants)
Source: *Veröffentlichungen des Kaiserlichen Gesundheitsamtes (Beilagen) (1878–1914).*

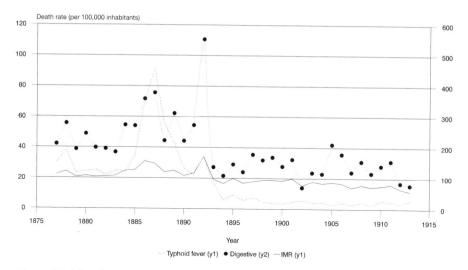

Figure 39: Mortality from typhoid fever, digestive diseases (per 100,000 inhabitants), and infant mortality (per 100 births) in Hamburg, 1877–1913
Sources: *Veröffentlichungen des Kaiserlichen Gesundheitsamtes (Beilagen)* (1878–1914).

Yet, there is also evidence that points in the opposite direction. Although the timing and extent of the expansion of the health-related infrastructure, as well as its technical standards, were very different in the largest German towns, mortality from typhoid fever in urban areas generally (all towns with over 15,000 inhabitants) had shifted almost uniformly onto the same level by the 1890s (Fig. 38). And, what is more, the decline in typhoid fever mortality had already commenced in numerous towns at an earlier stage, when sanitary reforms remained rudimentary (see pp. 152–54). In Berlin, for example, typhoid fever mortality fell from 96 per 100,000 inhabitants in the period 1854–1860, to 83 in the years 1861–1870 and to 62 in the period 1871–1880; in Frankfurt am Main from 54 (1861–1870) to 44 (1871–1880); in Hamburg from 100 (1851–1860) to 75 (1861–1870) and to 44 (1871–1880); and in Munich from 138 (1863–1870) to 115 (1871–1880) (Prinzing, 1930/31, p. 486).

Further light can be cast on this issue by focusing on the towns which registered higher typhoid fever death rates than the average for all towns over 15,000 inhabitants. In this case Munich and Hamburg are particularly interesting, with mortality figures well above the average for several years. Munich, however, was well known for its high mortality rate from diseases of the digestive system during the whole of the nineteenth century (*München*, 1902, pp. 18–32), while the high peaks of mortality in Hamburg refer to typhoid fever epidemics in the second half of the 1880s, which demonstrated the persistent dangers of using a non-filtrated central water supply. The resulting exposure to water-borne infection meant that the likelihood of an epidemic was high, whereas the inhabitants neighbouring town of Altona, which had a filter plant installed, was not affected by the epidemics at all, despite its geographical proximity. In any case, it seems remarkable that both typhoid mortality and morbidity in Hamburg declined to a significantly lower level immediately after the installation of a filter plant in 1893 (Fig. 39 and Table 37).

Table 37: Morbidity and mortality from typhoid fever in Hamburg, 1884–1895 (per 1,000 inhabitants)

Year	No. of sick persons	Morbidity	No. of deaths	Mortality
1884	1,053	2.35	108	0.24
1885	2,172	4.65	160	0.34
1886	3,890	8.09	333	0.69
1887	6,543	13.26	446	0.90
1888	3,199	6.23	275	0.54
1889	3,172	5.89	222	0.41
1890	1,539	2.73	147	0.26
1891	1,197	2.06	128	0.22
1892	1,941	3.30	203	0.35
1893	1,094	1.84	106	0.18
1894	462	0.76	37	0.06
1895	597	0.96	57	0.09

Source: Reincke (1896), p. 412.

The protection provided by a fully-filtered water supply against the recurrence of epidemics becomes more obvious if a closer look is taken at the typhoid fever epidemics in Hamburg.[11] Since 1849 drinking water had been taken from the river Elbe and led through subterranean channels into sedimentation basins and from there into the town itself. As a consequence of a rapid increase in water consumption the sedimentation period was increasingly shortened, which is said to have led to there being hardly any difference between the quality of the drinking water and the non-purified water from the river Elbe. Without a filter plant, a central water supply system was the ideal mechanism for the spreading and diffusion of certain pathogenic agents and inevitably led to the outbreak of epidemics. An increasing population, rising market density and an unfortunate shifting of the locations where the water was taken from the Elbe to the area where sewage was actually pumped into the river increased the risk significantly (Simmonds, 1886). After the middle of the 1880s, several typhoid fever epidemics broke out. In contrast to earlier epidemics, they spread over the whole town at the same time and affected all social classes (Curschmann, 1888; Reincke, 1896, p. 417). So two different transmitters of pathogens were taken into consideration: air and water. In the context of the dominant

11 See also Evans (1987), especially concerning the cholera epidemic in Hamburg of 1892, but also referring to the development of central water supply and mortality from typhoid fever.

theories about the aetiology of disease, contemporary doctors, physicians and epi-
demiologists preferred the latter explanation. It was controversial, however, whether
ground or drinking water played the decisive part in the spread of disease. For quite a
long time the local government in Hamburg stuck to the ground-water theory of Max
von Pettenkofer. According to this theory pernicious miasma rising from the ground
was responsible for the spread of various diseases, especially cholera and typhoid
fever. A sewerage system provided a means of regulating the local ground-water level
and so allowed officials to control the spread of diseases. This theory, of course,
agreed with the mercantile spirit of the 'Hansestadt Hamburg', for it not only seemed
to make the construction of an expensive filter plant unnecessary, but also avoided
trade-damaging measures, such as quarantine. As a consequence, no such improvements to the city's central water supply were undertaken, and Hamburg became the
victim of a water-borne epidemic caused by inadequate sanitary facilities.

Like all water-borne epidemics, typhoid fever spread quickly from the river Elbe
throughout the whole town into the more distant city districts, affecting all social
classes, although it was most severe in the city districts close to the rivers Elbe and
Alster (Curschmann, 1888; Reincke, 1896 p. 417) (Fig. 40). There was a clear overlap
between the areas affected by typhoid fever and the distributional network of the
central water supply, for the epidemics stopped on the border of the neighbouring town
of Altona (Reinsch, 1894; Wallichs, 1891; Reincke, 1899), which had its own filtered
central water supply. The epidemic failed to appear either in the barracks of the 76th
Infantry Regiment in Grindel or in neighbouring Wandsbeck, neither of which was
connected to the central water supply of Hamburg. As a result, the mechanism by
which the typhoid epidemic was spread throughout the city was affected more by its
geographical configuration than its social and sex-specific composition. Typhoid fever
mortality rates were higher in the inner-city and also in upper-class districts situated by
the river (Rotherbaum, Harvestehude, Hohenfelde and Uhlenhorst) than in the working-class settlements on the periphery of Hamburg (Barmbeck and Winterhude) (Fig.
40). Similarly, in the two districts Steinwärder and Barmbeck, which had the same low
level of income per capita of 266 Marks (Table 38), the former, which was situated
directly on the river Elbe, registered a typhoid fever mortality rate almost twice as high
as that of the latter. In the city districts situated directly on the river Elbe (Altstadt,
Neustadt, St Pauli, St Georg), men were more severely affected by the epidemic than
women; in the other city districts, however, the opposite was the case. In the inner-city,
dock workers took their drinking water directly from the Elbe and were encouraged to
do so even during these epidemics, so that a high proportion of them were infected. In
the better-off districts, however, it was predominantly females in domestic service who
were exposed to a high risk of infection (Reincke, 1890, pp. 13–19).

This spatial distribution was also visible in terms of typhoid fever morbidity and case
fatality rates (Figs 41 and 42; Table 38). Here as well, the districts close to the river were
more seriously affected by the epidemics than the more distant areas. Social inequality
in respect to disease still remained high, but was caused mainly by other diseases, as can
be seen from the strong relationship between social status and the crude death rate
(Table 39), and can be attributed to a large extent to tuberculosis (see Chapter 9).

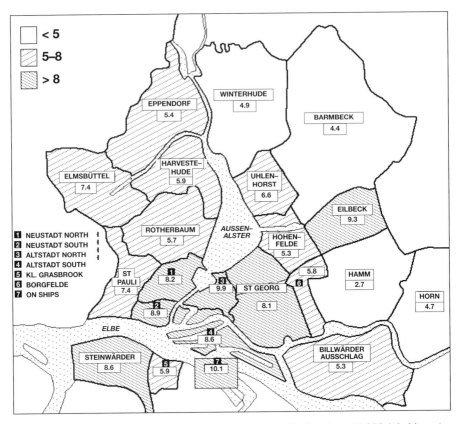

Figure 40: Typhoid fever death rates in Hamburg city districts (per 10,000 inhabitants), 1885–1887
Source: Reincke (1890), pp. 17, 19; *Statistisches Handbuch für der Hamburgischen Staat* (1891), p. 19; *Statistik des Hamburgischen Staates* (1894), p. 57

Even in the wake of these epidemics, confidence in Pettenkofer's theory remained unchanged, few conclusions were drawn, and so Hamburg became the only large German town to fall victim to the great cholera epidemic of 1893. This revealed a similar diffusion pattern to that of typhoid fever, but with 8,616 deaths it had a far greater number of victims (Evans, 1987). Subsequently a filter plant was constructed in record time by workers working day and night (Meyer, 1894), and immediately after its opening on 28 June 1893 typhoid fever mortality and morbidity declined to a lower level (Reincke, 1896, p. 412), whereas mortality actually increased amongst people living on ships (Reincke, 1896, p. 410). Smaller typhoid fever epidemics in the following years were attributed to infected food, and consequently showed a specific social and spatial distribution (Wilckens, 1898).

The Hamburg case reveals that central water supply *per se* has no effect on health conditions. In the proper sense of the word it just implied that water was taken from a specific source and distributed throughout the town. Although a single water source

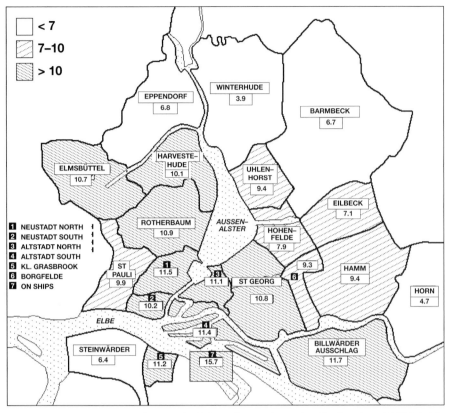

Figure 41: Morbidity rates from typhoid fever in Hamburg city districts (per 1,000 inhabitants), 1885–1887

Source: Reincke (1890), pp. 17, 19; *Statistisches Handbuch für der Hamburgischen Staat* (1891), p. 19; *Statistik des Hamburgischen Staates* (1894), p. 57

facilitates quality control, in the absence of knowledge about the true origin and spread of disease this advantage remained hypothetical. Whereas supporters of miasmatic-localistic theories denied the need to control drinking-water resources, the increasingly scientific analysis of water encouraged growing opposition to this theory. With the rise of bacteriology, scientists focused their investigations on a number of unidentified and obscure germs. As scientists were still unable to identify pathogens, it was assumed that the critical value was 1,000 unidentified germs per one cubic centimetre water, i.e. if the number of germs surpassed this limit it was very likely that there were pathogens amongst them (Grahn, 1904c, p. 975).[12] In the course of time the limit was reduced first to 300, then 100 and finally to 30–40. Even after the identification of the typhoid fever agent, however, it remained difficult to prove its presence in water. This, together with the belief in the power of the self-purification of flowing water, did not help to encourage the construction of artificial sand filtration, adequate

12 See also Hamlin (1991).

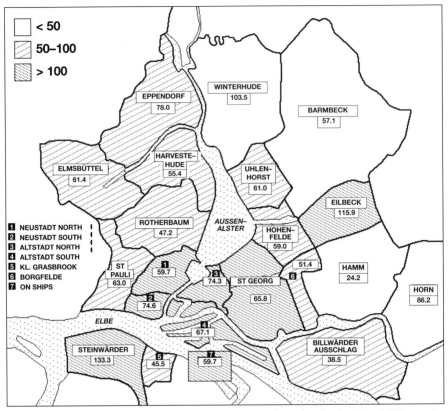

Figure 42: Case fatality rates from typhoid fever in Hamburg city districts (per 1,000 cases), 1885–1887

Source: Reincke (1890), pp. 17, 19; *Statistisches Handbuch für der Hamburgischen Staat* (1891), p. 19; *Statistik des Hamburgischen Staates* (1894), p. 57

Table 38: Social inequality and typhoid fever in Hamburg, 1885–1888 (per 1,000 inhabitants)

City district	Mortality	Typhoid fever Morbidity	Case fatality	Crude death rate (1887)	Income/ head (Marks) (1886)	Inhabitants/ tenement (1885)	Tenements with bath (1885) per hundred	Domestic servants (1885)*	children <15 yrs (1885)†	Women in employment (1900)‡
Altstadt North	9.94	11.14	74.31	20.7	550	4.5	2.8	9.0	27.5	29.3
Altstadt South	8.59	11.39	67.11	22.2	536	4.8	3.6	12.8	28.1	25.4
Neustadt North	8.21	11.54	59.68	20.8	551	4.6	5.0	11.2	28.5	30.3
Neustadt South	8.86	10.18	74.61	24.7	280	4.4	0.6	5.1	31.9	25.2
St Georg	8.06	10.80	65.75	–	–	–	–	–	–	–
North	–	–	–	18.6	722	4.6	9.9	19.8	27.4	32.4
South	–	–	–	23.2	423	4.7	3.4	9.4	35.4	19.7
St Pauli	7.39	9.94	62.96	22.6	343	4.7	1.6	10.1	32.4	–
North	–	–	–	–	–	–	–	–	–	24.8
South	–	–	–	–	–	–	–	–	–	24.5
Rotherbaum	5.74	10.92	47.18	14.2	1752	5.0	31.8	41.4	23.6	39.3
Harvestehude	5.85	10.13	55.36	14.2.	2256	5.4	44.8	49.2	26.2	52.3
Elmsbüttel	7.44	10.65	61.40	21.9	519	4.6	8.5	16.2	36.0	25.0
Eppendorf	5.44	6.78	78.01	21.7	553	4.9	10.9	17.8	32.9	29.5
Winterhude	4.90	3.92	103.45	14.0	474	5.3	4.3	9.3	30.9	34.1
Uhlenhorst	6.64	9.44	61.01	18.4	1149	5.2	19.4	24.4	36.6	26.8
Barmbeck	4.37	6.66	57.14	24.7	266	5.2	3.1	7.8	35.2	23.9
Hohenfelde	5.31	7.90	58.97	15.9	1051	4.3	21.5	34.5	28.4	39.4
Eilbeck	9.31	7.10	115.94	24.5	480	4.4	5.7	14.5	33.4	28.8
Borgfelde	5.81	9.27	51.35	23.8	518	4.2	7.2	14.5	36.6	28.6
Hamm	2.74	9.41	24.24	21.8	562	4.8	8.5	14.7	38.4	25.3
Horn	4.74	4.65	86.21	19.6	237	4.6	2.1	6.0	35.4	24.0
Billwärder A.	5.26	11.72	38.46	27.0	218	4.5	0.4	2.2	42.5	14.7
Steinwärder	8.57	6.43	133.33	22.7	266	4.7	0.1	4.1	38.1	16.8
Kl. Grasbrook	5.89	11.18	45.45	17.5	364	4.8	0.8	6.5	35.6	16.8
On ships	10.10	15.66	59.70	–	–	–	–	–	–	–

* Per cent of households with domestic servants.
† Per cent of the population.
‡ Per cent of all persons in employment.

Sources: Reincke (1890). pp. 16, 17, 19; *Statistik des Hamburgischen Staates* (1894), p. 57; (1895), p. 8; Wischermann (1983), pp. 445, 463, 469, 475, 476.

Table 39: Social inequality and typhoid fever in Hamburg, 1885–1888—correlation coefficients

| | Mortality | Typhoid fever Morbidity | Case fatality | Crude death rate (1887) | Income/ head (Marks) (1886) | Inhabitants /tenement (1885) | Tenements with bath (1885) per hundred | Domestic servants (1885)* | children <15 (1885)† | Women in employment (1900)‡ |
	TM	TM1	TC	CDR	I	IT	TB	DS	CH	WE
TM	1.0000	.3371	.4827§	.2597	-.1317	-.3587	-.2337	-.1908	-.2862	-.0913
TM1	.3371	1.0000	-.6207**	.1347	.2225	-.1998	.1361	.1479	-.1621	-.0295
TC	.4827§	-.6207**	1.0000	.0484	-.2623	-.0443	-.2731	-.2684	-.0245	-.0902
CDR	.2597	.1347	.0484	1.0000	-.6989**	v.4985§	-.6679**	-.6780**	.6170**	-.6960**
I	-.1317	.2225	-.2623	-.6989**	1.0000	.4602§	.9835**	.9628**	-.5944**	.8418**
IT	-.3587	-.1998	-.0443	-.4985§	.4602§	1.0000	.4435§	.3478	-.1729	.3209
TB	-.2337	.1361	-.2731	-.6679**	.9835**	.4435§	1.0000	.9795**	-.5239§	.8479**
DS	-.1908	.1479	-.2684	-.6780**	.9628**	.3478	.9795**	1.0000	-.6012**	.8673**
CH	-.2862	-.1621	-.0245	.6170**	-.5944**	-.1729	-.5239§	-.6012**	1.0000	-.7680**
WE	-.0913	-.0295	-.0902	-.6960**	.8418**	.3209	.8479**	.8673**	-.7680**	1.0000

* Percentage of households with domestic servants.

† Per cent of population.

‡ Per cent of all persons in employment.

§=Signif. LE .05.

**=Signif. LE .01 (two-tailed).

TM=Typhoid fever mortality; TM1=Typhoid fever morbidity; TC=Typhoid fever case fatality; CDR=Crude death rate (1887); I=Income/head (Marks) (1886); IT=Inhabitants/tenement (1885); TB=Tenements with bath (1885) per hundred; DS=Domestic servants (1885); WE=Women in employment (1900).

Sources: Reincke (1890), pp. 16, 17, 19; *Statistik des Hamburgischen Staates* (1894), p. 57; **17** (1895), p. 8; Wischermann, (1983), pp. 445, 463, 469, 475, 476.

sewage disposal and river conservation. Similarly, a conversion from a traditional dry conservancy system to the installation of water-closets could negate all theoretical advantages if there was not enough water available to flush them properly. In Liverpool, notoriously short of water until the 1890s, a spatial analysis of the distribution of sewers compared with mortality rates from typhoid fever and diarrhoea in the various districts, did not yield any clear results (Sheard, 1993, pp. 69–90). Also for a healthier place like Birmingham, a strong correlation between a range of sanitary variables, such as the location quotient of water-closets, and mortality from selected diseases (typhoid fever, scarlet fever, measles) could not be established for the 1880s; the highest association (0.771) could be found between measles and the percentage of back-to-back houses (Woods, 1984a). Without recognizing that all these components contribute to an integrated circulatory water system, which is only as good as its weakest point, lasting improvements in health conditions were not guaranteed and set-backs had to be taken into account. Appropriate sanitary reform required at least sufficent quantities of water, good quality water (through the installation of a filter plant) and an adequate sewerage system. By contrast, a poorly balanced programme of water services could even increase health problems. Rivers became increasingly polluted from untreated water-borne waste disgorged from overloaded sewers (Hassan, 1985, p. 543; Stern, 1954, pp. 999–1000). In 1849 the London sewers delivered over nine million cubic feet of sludge into the Thames. According to *The Spectator*, the companies were paid collectively £340,000 per annum '...for a more or less concentrated solution of native guano' (quoted from Wright, 1963, p. 151). The spread of piped water amongst the comfortably off elements of society led to a deterioration in the environment of the poor (Smith, 1979, p. 219), and enlarged the risk of cholera outbreaks, diarrhoea and typhoid fever (Luckin, 1986, pp. 69–138). In the case of an epidemic, an inadequate central water supply would imply that it was serving only to distribute the disease over the whole area that was connected.

In addition to the case of Hamburg there are various examples where the spread of typhoid fever or cholera epidemics followed the course of the central water supply system. This was the case in relation to the typhoid fever epidemics in Zürich in 1884, in Plymouth in Pennsylvania, USA in 1885, Halle 1871, as well as in Caterham and Redhill in 1879 (Hueppe, 1887, pp. 7–8). Better known are similar cholera outbreaks in Genoa in 1884 and especially in London in 1854. The famous epidemiologist John Snow, a medical practitioner in London, could prove that only areas supplied by the Vauxhall Water Company suffered severely from cholera (Snow, 1855). Still around the turn of the century there were indeed numerous outbreaks of typhoid fever epidemics, for example in Bochum (1900) and in Gelsenkirchen (1901) (Grahn, 1904b). In some towns, typhoid fever death rates even increased after the introduction of the sewerage system. There was a 5 per cent increase in Chelmsford, a 6 per cent rise in Penzance, and even a 23 per cent increase in Worthing (Dreyfuss, 1899, p. 162). Even as late as 1888 there was quite a strong positive correlation in the largest German towns between water consumption (litres per capita) and the death rate from typhoid fever, highlighting the inadequacy of the central water supply, which even increased the risks of infection and epidemics. Only after the turn of the century did this correlation become weak and negative.[13]

In Germany even in the early twentieth century, supporters of miasmatic-localistic theories of disease dissemination still found an audience for their opposition to bacteriological evidence. In the autumn of 1901 a typhoid fever epidemic broke out in the area of Gelsenkirchen.[14] In his report about the causes of the epidemic, the discoverer of the tubercle bacillus Robert Koch assumed that because of water shortage additional quantities of water were taken directly from the river Ruhr and added to the filtrated water. Nine-tenths of the water was actually delivered for industrial purposes, for more than a hundred local coal mines and contracts had been agreed between the waterworks and industry, which under no circumstances could be broken. So, the guilty men were the directors of the Gelsenkirchen waterworks. A trial was announced, and after two-and-a-half years the case went to court in the neighbouring town of Essen in July 1904.[15] The waterworks' directors were accused of being responsible for the outbreak of the epidemic. Robert Koch himself and a number of supporters appeared as referees and reported their views. Their arguments, however, did not remain unchallenged, and two supporters of the miasmatic-localistic theory also appeared before the court. As witnesses confirmed that water was taken from the river, the question was whether this actually caused the epidemic. The Pettenkofer disciples argued against Koch that the typhoid fever agent could not be identified in the water, and that epidemiological evidence spoke against a water-borne epidemic, as the epidemic did not appear in all the areas connected to the central water supply. The obvious reason, in their opinion, was because local ground conditions suggested a miasmatic origin of this specific epidemic, just as had been the case with other epidemics. In order to prove this point, one, Emmerich, offered himself as a bio-indicator, and drank water from the severely polluted river. The judges, originally in favour of the generally predominant bacteriological theory, increasingly changed their point of view. In November 1904, after various interruptions to the trial, the verdict was announced. The court ruled that the claim that the waterworks' directors were responsible for the epidemic was dropped, and the sentence for food adulteration alone was reduced to a fine. No causal connection could therefore be found between water supplied from the river and the outbreak of the epidemic. It remained unclear, so the judge announced, whether water-borne epidemics even exist at all (Emmerich and Wolter, 1906, pp. 5–14). However, this was the first time in Germany that water was considered in court as a means of nutrition (Weyer, 1989, p. 61). Moreover, despite their success, the days of the original

---

13 The correlation of daily water consumption per capita and the death rate from typhoid fever in the largest German towns gives the following results:
    1888: r = 0.7233, sig. (two-tailed) = 0.028;
    1912: r = –0.2772, sig. (two-tailed) = 0.470.
    Sources: *Statistisches Jahrbuch Deutscher Städte*, **1** (1890) onwards; *Veröffentlichungen des Kaiserlichen Gesundheitsamtes (Beilagen)* (1889 and 1913).

14 For further details see Grahn (1904b).

15 For further information see Weyer (1989). For a short summary of the events see Howard-Jones (1973).

miasmatic theories were numbered, as scientific evidence against them increased. Supporters of experimental hygiene subsequently developed their theory further, increasingly incorporating aspects of exposure to disease (including social factors). It is clear from this case, however, that outbreaks of epidemics and the causes of disease were no longer taken as a matter of fate, but were now to be explained and analysed by scientific means. By stressing the role of environmental factors, experimental hygiene enabled the towns to protect the health of their inhabitants by providing an adequate sanitary infrastructure.

Appropriate sanitary reform did not only contribute to the reduction of typhoid fever mortality, but also had a positive effect on the death rates from other diseases of the digestive system and therefore on infant mortality. After the installation of the filter plant in Hamburg, the death rate from digestive diseases fell and infant mortality improved, declining to a level never reached before (Fig. 39; Vögele, forthcoming b). On the whole, however, mortality rates from diseases of the digestive system show much wider variation between towns, with a narrowing of the range only after the turn of the century, when mortality from diseases of the digestive system declined in all towns with a population exceeding 15,000 (Fig. 21). In contrast to the trends in typhoid fever mortality, the death rates of the ten largest towns remained both above and below the average for all towns over 15,000 inhabitants. Breslau, Leipzig, Munich and Nuremberg were above the average, and Dresden and Frankfurt am Main below. Health conditions in Düsseldorf and Cologne worsened at the beginning of the 1880s, while in Berlin and Hamburg (as already mentioned, after the installation of the filter plant) the death rate improved and fell below the average for all towns.

The supply of clean water was especially important in areas where breast-feeding was not commonly practised. Artificial food was to a large extent prepared with water and animal milk was often diluted. Furthermore, it was not customary to keep animal milk in a cool place; on the contrary, it was common practice to keep the milk warm over-night. For this purpose it was put in the warmest place in the house or special night-lamps or warming-pans were used (Soxhlet, 1886, p. 255). It is not surprising, therefore, that before appropriate standards in the manufacture and preparation of artificial food were reached, the highest infant mortality rates could be found in non-breast-feeding areas which did not enjoy appropriate sanitary conditions.

Having assessed the impact of central water supply and sewerage systems, the question of whether German sanitary reforms combated disease more effectively than English can finally be evaluated. As health considerations were only one motive (and often only in the background) amongst others for the implementation of sanitary reforms, they certainly cannot be ascribed to a deliberately planned procedure. By contrast, sanitary reforms sometimes fell short of what was required where health aspects were concerned and could have been more effective. However, municipal governments in Germany found easier preconditions for the implementation of sanitary facilities. The well-developed organization of local government, strong police rights and, at least to a certain degree, the possibilities of applying English knowledge and techniques have been mentioned in the previous section. This was equally the case from an epidemiological point of view. Bearing in mind the predominance of the digestive disease complex in Germany, with death rates almost twice as high as in England, the same or a similar strategy to reduce the number of deaths by sanitary reform was likely to have a greater impact on urban health conditions. In other words, the German disease panorama provided a greater potential field for sanitary reforms than was the case in the larger English cities. In this sense, sanitary reform in Germany was likely to have had a more substantial impact than in England. This, however, does not mean that the Germans actively fought disease more effectively. If the test is applied to trends in typhoid fever mortality alone, the pattern is quite similar in both countries (Vögele, 1992). The death rate from typhoid fever declined in urban England from 41 (1871–1880) to 9 (1901–1910) per 100,000 inhabitants, and in urban Germany from 34 (1877–1880) to 4 in the first decade of the twentieth century (1901–1910).[16] This corresponds with a reduction of 78 per cent in English and 88 per cent in German towns. Typhoid fever had become a relatively subordinate cause of death in the contemporary disease panorama. If it is borne in mind that sanitary reforms were initiated some time before the 1870s in England, differences in the course of typhoid fever mortality in both countries were minor and do not confirm a substantially more successful reaction towards disease in the German towns. Similarly, the remaining differences at the beginning of the twentieth century seem to be too small for any far-reaching conclusions to be drawn. National aggregate figures reveal a situation that looks even more advantageous for England. As the complete installation of central water supply and sanitation in Germany remained restricted to the largest towns, with only limited sanitary facilities in small towns and even less in rural areas, the national crude death rates and mortality from typhoid fever and from digestive diseases were consequently higher in Germany than in England, and remained so even at the end of the period under investigation. In this sense, the fight against disease in this area was by no means more effectively prosecuted in Germany than in England.

MUNICIPAL MILK SUPPLY

Sanitary reform or the term '*Städteassanierung*' (urban health reform) used by contemporaries also selectively included disinfection, control of food and especially the introduction of a municipal milk supply for infants and young children. For Britain it has been argued that the substantial fall in infant mortality after the turn of the century could be widely attributed to the improved provision of pasteurized milk, the introduction and popularization of dried milk as an infant food, as well as the widespread use of condensed or evaporated milk (Beaver, 1973). Recent studies, however, are more sceptical concerning the impact of municipal milk supply on the decline of infant mortality. As breast-feeding remained widespread in England, the health of infants was more dependent on relative poverty, the mother's education and

---

16 Sources: *Decennial Supplements to the Annual Reports of the Registrar-General of Births, Deaths, and Marriages in England and Wales* (1871–1880 and 1901–1910); *Veröffentlichungen des Kaiserlichen Gesundheitsamtes (Beilagen)* (1878–1914).

her participation in the labour force, on overcrowded housing, environmental conditions and a general decline in fertility (Woods et al., 1989, pp. 116–120). Others suggest that consumption of poor quality milk contributed to ill health (Atkins, 1992, p. 227), particularly because of its impact on infant deaths from tuberculosis and digestive diseases. In order to clarify these contradictory hypotheses, the quantity and quality of municipal milk supply in England and Germany will be assessed in this section. A further evaluation of this theme can be obtained by epidemiological analysis, namely by following the course of tuberculosis and digestive disease mortality amongst infants and young children, as well as overall infant mortality.

As has been demonstrated, the towns invested very substantial sums of money in the provision of central water supply and sewerage systems, strengthened by official arguments in the battle to combat diseases, such as cholera and typhoid. By contrast, the supply and distribution of municipal milk began with some delay and hesitation. As contemporary doctors complained, high infant mortality rates were regarded as somewhat inevitable (Pfaffenholz, 1902a, pp. 402–03), even though some of the major reasons for these high rates were already known. Contemporaries indicated that differences in infant mortality between urban and rural areas could be mainly attributed to the higher mortality in towns during the hot summer months (Schlossmann, 1897, p. 137). This was substantially supported by the prevalence of digestive diseases in the cause of death panorama. Indeed, the hot period of the year claimed numerous victims amongst infants. In Berlin in 1885, for example, more than 45 per cent of all infant deaths occurred in June, July and August (Würzburg, 1887/88, p. 74). Increasingly fewer experts attributed this to urban housing conditions (see Chapter 10). Instead, the case for adequate infant nutrition increasingly became the focus of their attention. The term children's milk (*Kindermilch*) was coined (Pfaffenholz, 1902b, p. 183), and the supply of adequate animal milk was considered to be a municipal task of the highest priority. These ideas were increasingly taken up by politicians and municipal authorities. In view of the declining birth rate, high infant mortality rates were now seen in a different light. Especially in Germany, where infant mortality rates were extremely high when compared with other Western European countries, the fear of a population decline emerged, and questions were raised as to whether in the future there would be enough workers for the factories, and, above all, whether there would be enough soldiers especially with regard to conflicts with 'the old enemy', France.

As an early form of milk conservation in England and France, soda, natron salycil and boric acid were added to the milk (Wilbert, 1891, p. 30), although the last did more harm than good. In Germany the sale of pasteurized or sterilized milk commenced in the late 1880s with the invention of the so-called Soxhlet apparatus (1886), by which milk was heated within the bottle. As it was not patented, it soon became widespread (Wilbert, 1891, p. 30). Complete sterilization, however, was expensive, and therefore rarely applied in practice. Heating the milk to or beyond its boiling point, of course, caused the loss of a considerable amount of vitamins. Partial sterilization or 'pasteurization' of milk, developed in the 1860s by Louis Pasteur (Dubos, 1988), remained controversial, since it was taken as the cause of various infant diseases, such as infant scurvy (*Säuglingsskorbut*). It was therefore suggested that pasteurized milk should only be used in the hot summer months, with a special treatment of milk regarded as superfluous in the cooler periods of the year (Spiegel, 1908, p. 231). Milk was not amongst the subjects dealt with in the nutrition laws (*Nahrungsmittelgesetz*), and in 1900 only three towns (Berlin, Dresden and Munich) had special regulations concerning children's milk. In general, the quality of milk remained dubious (Flügge, 1894, p. 321). Partly sterilized milk was sold in green or brown bottles in order to make visual quality control impossible for the consumer (Flügge, 1894, p. 321). Condensed milk especially was regarded as a most unsatisfactory product, because it was seldom sterile (Health Department, 1901, p. 142).

Municipal milk was increasingly based on an imported supply as cattle-keeping in the towns declined rapidly. Whereas this was generally seen as a major improvement in the hygiene of towns, long transport distances often led to a deterioration in the quality of milk: '...the railway companies have no financial or other interest in the delivery of clean milk, and therefore very seldom provide proper vans for its conveyance. Fish, paint, petroleum, or any other unsuitable goods are packed along with the milk. The churns from the farms are allowed to stand for hours on platforms of rural stations to be dealt with as ordinary goods, or to await the slow milk train' (Dodd, 1905, p. 11). In the early years, the supply and preparation of milk were completely in the hands of private enterprises and independent tradesmen. By the late nineteenth century, however, many municipalities had established their own management system dealing with milk supply and distribution (Spiegel, 1908, p. 232). Following French models, St Helens was the first English town to put the milk trade into municipal hands by establishing a municipal milk depot in 1899 (Pfaffenholz, 1902a, p. 411; Hawes, 1991, p. 176). Other towns followed: Liverpool, Ashton-under-Lyne and Dukinfield in 1901, Battersea in 1902, Leith and Bradford in 1903, and Burnley, Glasgow and Dundee in 1904 (McCleary, 1904, p. 71; Dwork, 1987, pp. 103–09). Liverpool was again ambitious and acted as a role-model for other towns. In 1910, 11,900 infants were supplied with 'humanized' sterilized milk from milk depots, and 6,431 from dairies (Health Department, 1911, p. 159). Sealed bottles were issued and mothers were instructed as to how to use appropriate feeding practices (Lambertsen, 1989, pp. 70–74).

At the beginning of the twentieth century, however, only a handful of towns in both countries had established municipal milk depots. In Germany the main period of expansion was between 1904 and 1907. By 1907 the number of milk depots had increased to 64, most of them owned or supported by the municipality (Trumpp, 1908, pp. 119–21). Yet many other towns also recognized the importance of regulating milk supply and insisted on certain standards. In England the Manchester Corporation Act 1899 was the first to deal with this issue and functioned as a model for other municipalities. The Milk Clauses increased powers of inspection over all localities purveying milk to the city; they allowed the prohibition of the sale of tuberculous milk within the city, and the isolation of cattle suffering from tuberculosis (Dwork, 1987, p. 73). The number of controlled samples of milk increased steadily, in Liverpool, for example, from 119 in 1896 to 612 in 1910 (Table 40). As

Table 40: Tuberculosis in Liverpool's milk (milk examined bacteriologically for tubercle bacilli), 1896–1910

Year	Number of samples taken	TB milk percentage
1896	119	7.6
1897	150	6.0
1898	112	10.7
1899	352	4.6
1900	560	1.6
1901	566	3.9
1902	595	5.6
1903	582	3.6
1904	571	7.2
1905	560	2.7
1906	530	4.7
1907	451	4.0
1908	528	2.8
1909	600	2.3
1910	612	3.1

Source: Health Department (1911), p. 178.

a consequence, milk quality improved. In Liverpool the percentage of tuberculous milk declined from 7.6 per cent to 3.1 per cent in the same period (Table 40). In Germany, developments were similar. In Düsseldorf, for example, 60 out of 265 official milk examinations were unsatisfactory in 1895; in 1906 only 125 out of 3,743 failed to pass the test (Schrakamp, 1908, p. 110). Police ordinances (*Polizeiverordnungen*) by 1901 included regulations about the quality and the importation of milk from outside the town. Merchants who wanted to sell milk had to register at the police station. Each consignment of milk had to be sealed before being imported, and its origin clearly identified—with name and address on the container—so that, in the case of irregularities, the responsible merchants could be easily found (Schrakamp, 1908, pp. 110–13). Bacteriological examination, however, remained difficult, and hardly feasible in practice, given the expense involved (Pfaffenholz, 1902a, pp. 400). It was for this reason that the amount of specially treated and controlled milk for children available in the towns remained limited, perhaps only 500 litres in a town of 100,000 inhabitants (Pfaffenholz, 1902a, p. 404; Spiegel, 1908, p. 229). Sold at a price of 50–60 *Pfennige* per litre this type of milk was only an option for financially secure sections of the population. In addition, elements of the food industry were, at least at times, not in favour of municipal milk supply and promoted their own artificial products (Wilbert, 1891, p. 24). There were reports from Bonn in 1902 that families, immediately after a child's birth, received a brochure, signed by a paediatrician, promoting the use of powdered infant food, the so-called children's flour (*Kindermehl*) (Cramer, 1902, p. 419).

Despite all these factors, contemporaries were convinced of the success of municipal milk supply in terms of improving the state of health of infants and young children. The Health Department of Liverpool published the following results of its investigations. Out of 11,900 infants coming to the Liverpool milk depots in 1910 whose health conditions were below the average, mortality was 93 per 1,000, as against 147 for the whole city. Infant mortality rates for the years 1906 to 1910 stood at 83 to 102 for the best districts and 225 to 250 for the worst (Health Department, 1911, p. 160). Other milk depots, however, were increasingly reduced in size or completely closed. Whereas in St Helens by the end of the initial year of operation, 120 children received milk and during 1900 over 300 children had been registered with the depot, by 1913 the number had declined rapidly to only 9 (Hawes, 1991, pp. 176, 185). In general, municipal milk was too expensive for those who most needed it, and it was too inconvenient for many mothers to go daily to return the previous day's bottles (Dwork, 1987, p. 124). Developments in Germany were similar. Mothers generally could not be attracted to the centres for the same reasons as in England. They had to clean and return the bottles daily. Broken bottles had to be paid for. Although milk was cheaper than on the free market, this was counterbalanced by the fact that in the big cities such daily visits often required people to travel long distances using expensive public transport. Doctors' expectations that mothers would dutifully set aside three to four hours a day for that purpose (Tugendreich, 1908, p. 72) reflects their unrealistic conception of a working-class mother's life, ignoring the various strains and burdens created by poor working and living conditions, and by large family size. A Berlin mother explained why she no longer attended the milk depot by stating that she had spent 60 *Pfennige* a week on public transport, and that she had increasing difficulties in walking, because a child every year had left her weak. She concluded that her husband suggested that if she spent the same amount of money to feed the child, the baby would be well nourished (Tugendreich, 1908, 72). The final verdict on the milk depots in both countries can therefore only be that they were unsuccessful, because they ignored basic elements of working-class lifestyle and living conditions.

On a larger scale, demographic data confirm the generally poor state of municipal milk provision. An adequate and widespread milk supply should have contributed to a decline in mortality from tuberculosis and digestive diseases amongst infants, as well as weakening the climatic dependency of infant mortality, by reducing the extent of seasonal fluctuation. There is no doubt that especially in cases where breast-feeding was not commonly practised, the quality of milk was of supreme importance in combating tuberculosis and especially the highly feared summer diarrhoea. In view of the declining tendency to breast-feed infants in the large urban areas of Germany (see Chapter 6), the state of municipal milk supply is of special importance and its impact should be most evident in the development of infant mortality in our German sample.

In the German towns, the death rate from tuberculosis amongst infants actually increased from 40.26 per 10,000 in 1877 to 43.17 in 1907, although it decreased in the age-groups from five years onwards (Tables 12 and 18). On the other hand, death rates from digestive diseases both in the average for all towns with a population exceeding

15,000 inhabitants (Fig. 21) and in the ten largest towns (Table 18) registered a strong decline by the beginning of the twentieth century. However, climatic dependency remained. The cold summer of 1902 was accompanied by low infant mortality (Fig. 13; Spiegel, 1908, p. 225; Kruse, 1912, p. 179), but the hot summer of 1911 registered high infant mortality rates (Kruse, 1912; Seidlmayer, 1937, p. 20),[17] not only in Germany, but also in England (*Forty-Second Annual Report*, 1913, pp. 40–41).[18] Seasonal fluctuations persisted, with a pronounced summer peak—much stronger in Germany when compared with England (Figs 43 and 44)[19]—and affected artificially-fed infants (Imhof, 1981b, p. 352). Excellent long-term sources in Hamburg show that summer infant mortality was even higher in the twentieth century, when compared with the preceding hundred years (Fig. 45). In Berlin, the summer peak reached its highest point in 1885, yet in 1900 it was still much higher than in the period 1850–1874, and did not disappear completely until 1926–1928 (Imhof, 1981b, p. 352). A similar development can be observed in Munich, where the summer peak did not vanish until the second decade of the twentieth century (Hecker, 1923, p. 287), in part as a result of increased breast-feeding (Seidlmayer, 1937, pp. 22, 31). Whereas urban infant death rates were already below the corresponding rural figures after 1900, higher urban infant mortality in the hot summer months remained a common feature (Fig. 46). A correlation between air temperature in the ten largest German towns in August 1910–1912 and the corresponding infant mortality rates leaves us with a coefficient of 0.7970 (p=.000; n=30),[20] pinpointing the still strong climatic influence on infant mortality. On the whole, demographic evidence confirms the view that a qualitatively satisfactory milk supply reaching a substantial number of the population, and especially the poor, had still not been developed by the first decade of the twentieth century. Contemporary attempts to provide adequate infant food, however, demonstrate increasing concern over high infant mortality rates. Declining birth rates raised fears about the nation's future in economic and military respects, and led to a concentration of forces in the fight against high infant mortality.

17 A more elaborate statistical test, however, is difficult to achive due to inadequate source material. Some information about climatic conditions in the towns of the sample is only available for a selection of these towns for a small number of years from the *Statistisches Jahrbuch Deutscher Städte*, **1** (1890) onwards. Correlating average annual air temperature with annual overall mortality, infant mortality and death rates from various diseases in the years 1888–1896 leaves us with a rather weak association. Relatively speaking, the strongest, and surprisingly negative correlation is achieved with mortality from digestive diseases (r = –0.5200, sig. = 0.001, n = 67), followed by infant mortality (r = –0.4375, sig.= 0.001, n = 67). A correlation using temperature maxima leaves an even weaker relation. For the period 1907–1911, correlations are weaker. Here the strongest interrelationship is between annual average temperature and deaths from tuberculosis of the lungs (r = –0.5212, sig.= 0.001, n = 49).

18 In 1894 Creighton pointed out for England and Wales that the enormous fluctuations in mortality from diarrhoea and dysentery were to a large extent dependent on the kind of summer they had. In the hot summer of 1893, mortality from infantile diarrhoea almost doubled when compared with the preceding year. See Creighton (1965), p. 760.

19 For climatic influences in English towns see Williams and Mooney (1994), pp. 206–07.

20 Morgenroth (1913), pp. 316–18.

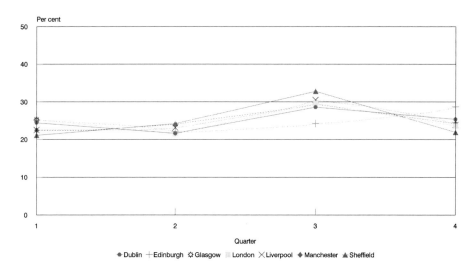

Figure 43: Infant mortality in British towns, 1889–1893—seasonal distribution (per cent)
Source: Silbergleit (1896), especially p. 454.

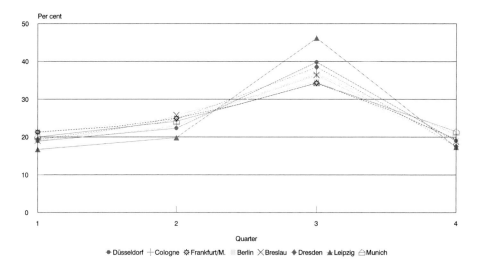

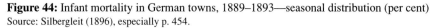

Figure 44: Infant mortality in German towns, 1889–1893—seasonal distribution (per cent)
Source: Silbergleit (1896), especially p. 454.

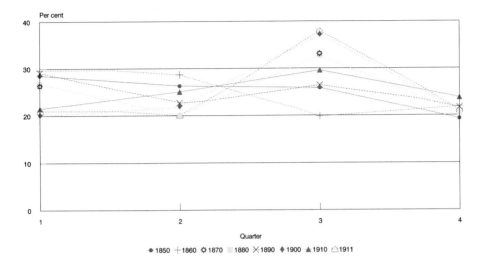

Figure 45: Seasonal distribution of infant mortality rates in Hamburg, 1850–1911 (per cent)
Source: *Statistisches Handbuch für der Hamburgischen Staat* (1921), pp. 48, 70; *Die Gesundheitsuer-haltnisse Hamburgs* (1901), pp. 108, 114

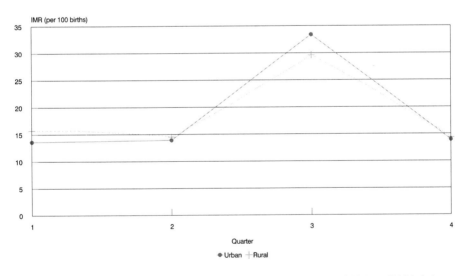

Figure 46: Seasonal distribution of infant mortality rates in Prussia, 1911 (per 100 births)
Source: Kruse (1912), especially p. 178.

CONCLUSION

This chapter has been primarily concerned with the impact of sanitary reform on the urban mortality decline. Central water supply and sewerage systems as well as municipal milk supply were identified as major components of sanitary reform in both countries. In the first part, central water supply and sewerage systems formed the centre of the analysis. As an essential prerequisite, techniques as well as the timing and spatial distribution were discussed, including some comments on the motives behind the specific developments. As a result, a positive effect can be attributed to appropriate central water supply and sewerage systems in two respects:

(a) They provided a guarantee against the further appearance of water- and foodborne epidemics, and therefore helped to make the city a safer place.

(b) They reduced mortality from typhoid fever, as well as to a lesser extent from other diseases of the digestive system, and contributed to a decline in infant mortality.

It has to be borne in mind that there was a wide regional variation in the level of mortality from gastro-intestinal infectious diseases, so that the effects of the 'sanitary revolution' would have been very different depending on the original mortality level. An inadequate sanitary infrastructure, however, increased the risk of disease. Epidemics could be even more easily spread by a central water supply within a specific town, and inadequate sewerage treatment increased health risks for the town and even for neighbouring towns lying downstream.

It is within the framework of demographic evidence that the effectiveness of these health-related infrastructural measures in both countries can be found. Germany followed England after a delay of some twenty years in the implementation of sanitary reform and did not need to pioneer engineering techniques from the very beginning, yet sanitary technology at the end of the nineteenth century was far from being fully developed, as the various types of contemporary sanitary systems show. The liberal bourgeoisie which ruled the German towns, may have realized the commercial benefits of sanitation more clearly and, without a national legislature, sanitary reforms could be more easily carried out in self-governing German towns. Municipalities were in a better position than their English counterparts as they were able to use already established constitutional, legislative and police powers. Sanitary techniques spread quickly, specifically because German towns employed numerous English engineers so that sanitation standards theoretically ought to have been quite similar in the larger towns of both countries. The German urban system, however, did not consciously respond to the need for sanitary reform any more effectively than that in England, and health considerations were seldom the primary motive. Otherwise, given the continuing role of miasmatic theories that stressed the need for the control of groundwater levels, sewerage treatment would have been established at a comparatively early date and not hesitantly after a delay of some decades. An effective response would also have implied that adequate central water supply and sewerage systems would not have been almost exclusively restricted to the largest towns. It seems very likely that Germany imported the sanitary movement from England without the need to combat disease being the primary impetus. But Germany did import the sanitary movement just at the right time, when environmental problems created by industrialization and urbanization required a response in the field of infrastructural measures. Yet these strategies proved to be much more effective in German towns in view of the different disease panorama, with a high prevalence of digestive diseases in Germany. Similar strategies to fight disease by means of sanitary reform, therefore, had different effects in England and Germany because of significant variations in the predominant disease panorama and the relative importance of water-borne diseases.

In addition to the substantial scale of infrastructural measures such as central water supply and sewerage, sanitary reforms also included disinfection, control of food and, especially important in view of the prevalence of digestive diseases amongst infants, municipal milk supply. Many of these enterprises, however, still operated on a small scale; scientific knowledge was still rudimentary, and specific techniques remained controversial and, most of all, expensive. In particular, municipal milk supply for infants rarely reached those sections of the urban population which needed it most. Despite major efforts by individual towns in relation to the organization of milk distribution, the role of municipal milk supply remained marginal. And so did its epidemiological impact where the two major diseases associated with inadequate milk supply, namely tuberculosis and gastro-intestinal disorders, were concerned. The death rates from tuberculosis amongst infants even increased in the German towns. Mortality from digestive diseases declined after the turn of the century, but the persistence of climatic dependency and the seasonal pattern of infant mortality pinpoint the negligible role of these measures with respect to urban mortality change. Yet, seen in a longer-term perspective, public discussions of these issues may have raised awareness of the need to incorporate hygiene measures into everyday life. Such measures, therefore, may have provided a basis for the successful implementation of public health campaigns aimed specifically at improving personal hygiene.

Chapter 12

MEDICINE AND THE CITY

MEDICAL PROVISION AND HEALTH

The historical mortality decline was traditionally attributed to the progress of medical skills and techniques. When McKeown challenged this hypothesis and ascribed a merely subordinate impact to curative medicine, he referred to a large extent to the impact of smallpox vaccination introduced on a larger scale at the beginning of the nineteenth century. The controversial debate arising from this issue may have led to an unjustified neglect of the role of medicine in the second half of the nineteenth and early twentieth century. In an analysis of twentieth-century mortality change in 165 population groups, representing 43 nations, Preston argued that the role of rising living standards has been overestimated and suggested that the medical contribution was stronger in the past than assumed by McKeown (Preston, 1976, pp. 3–83). Yet in the nineteenth century, the situation was completely different as medical knowledge, skills and techniques were less advanced so that a back-projection of twentieth-century conditions might be misleading. Specifically in relation to the German case in the nineteenth century, W. R. Lee and Reinhard Spree at least pinpointed the additional supporting role of medicine in this context (Lee, 1980; Spree, 1981a). All in all, the case remains unclear. The role of medicine, however, becomes especially important when urban health conditions and urban mortality are the focus of attention, for medical provision was far more evident in towns and cities than in rural areas. Medical provision was an urban feature. In Germany in 1898, for example, there were:

- 10.8 doctors per 10,000 inhabitants in towns with a population exceeding 100,000;
- 9.2 in towns with 40,000–100,000 inhabitants;
- 7.6 in towns with 20,000–40,000;
- 6.0 in towns with 5,000–20,000; and only
- 2.4 doctors in towns with less than 5,000 inhabitants (Prinzing, 1906, p. 543).

When the two countries are compared, substantial differences can be elaborated. In terms of quantitative medical provision, England was better served than Germany in relation to the number of doctors and hospitals. In Germany in 1876 there were 3.2 doctors per 10,000 inhabitants; in 1909, 4.8 (Esche, 1954a, p. 374; Statistisches Bundesamt, 1972, p. 124). In German general hospitals the number of beds per 10,000 inhabitants increased from 16.5 in 1877 to 41.5 by 1911, and the number of days spent in hospital increased from 31 to 97 whereas the average length of treatment decreased from 33.3 to 28.0 days during the same period (Esche, 1954b, pp. 387–92). The regional distribution revealed a considerable east–west differential, with poor medical facilities in the less industrialized eastern provinces (*Statistisches Jahrbuch für das Deutsche Reich*, 1881, p. 148; Prinzing, 1906, p. 540). In England and Wales there were 6.5 doctors (physicians, surgeons and registered practitioners) per 10,000 inhabitants in 1871, whereas by 1911 the number was 7.1 (*Published Volumes of the Census of England and Wales*, 1871 and 1911). The level of medical provision in towns was significantly higher than in the country as a whole: in 1901, for example, there were 1,338 persons per physician in urban areas compared with 1,537 in rural areas (*Published Volumes of the Census of England and Wales*, 1901). Yet there were major differences between the towns and registration districts. In 1911 the population per physician, surgeon or registered practitioner ranged from 976 in London to 3,126 in Aston (Table 41), and in general there was a strong south–north gradient, with the northern areas being less well provided (Kearns et al., 1989, p. 18). And it has to be kept in mind that there were immense differences between city-districts (Woodward, 1984, p. 70). In 1901 the inmate population of workhouses was 64 per 10,000 population, and hospitals had 13 in-patients per 10,000 population (*Published Volumes of the Census of England and Wales*, 1901).

Despite this expansion of medical provision in both Germany and England and Wales, its impact on the urban mortality decline remains dubious in view of the problematic relationship between actual medical provision and crude death rates in German and English towns (Tables 41 and 42), which confirm results already gained on a higher aggregate level (Lee, 1980; Spree, 1981a). As the regional distribution pattern reveals, the medical market was clearly structured by more than medical need. The unhealthiest areas, the east of Prussia and northern England, had the poorest medical provision. In the ten largest towns of both countries, this regional distribution of medical facilities is not fully reflected, but the correlation between the doctor:population ratio and the crude death rate remained low even around the turn of the century.[1] This may have been the result of the fact that one major risk group, namely infants, were rarely taken to the doctor. Medical personnel kept complaining that, in the case of an infant's sickness, parents usually asked the midwife and they only consulted the doctor, if at all, when it was too late to apply any successful treatment (Stumpf, 1886). This, however, is hardly surprising as consultation charges were expensive and, above all, in many cases of no avail or even harmful to the health of the infant. In order to treat the widespread diarrhoea or other gastro-intestinal disorders amongst infants, doctors often applied not only useless but also dangerous 'remedies'. A Berlin doctor recommended in 1875, as the common

---

1 The correlation of medical provision (England: population per physician, surgeon, registered practitioner, 1911; Germany: practitioner per 1,000 inhabitants, 1898) and mortality (CDR) gives the following results:
  For the English towns: $r = -0.1007$, sig. (two-tailed) = 0.732;
  For the German towns: $r = -0.0266$, sig. (two-tailed) = 0.935.
  Sources: See Tables 41 and 42.

contemporary treatment of the disease, opium, cold black coffee, wine, ice-cold milk and various kinds of enemas (Baginsky, 1875, p. 329). His complaints about the widespread use of purgatives and patent medicines complete this terrifying picture.

Table 41: Medical provision in large English towns, 1851–1911, crude death rate (per 1,000 inhabitants) and selected causes of death (per 100,000 inhabitants), 1901–1910

City/town	Population per physician, surgeon, registered practitioner				CDR	TB*	Typhoid	Diphtheria
	1851	1871	1891	1911				
London	597	947	970	976	15.8	147.7	6.5	16.6
Bristol	789	1,148	941	1,411	14.9	117.8	6.6	26.6
Birmingham	1,265	1,953	1,875	1,940	22.2	182.9	14.9	30.4
Aston	–	–	2,542	3,126	14.8	115.9	8.4	14.4
Birkenhead	–	–	–	1,677	15.2	113.7	12.9	16.9
Liverpool	1,197	1,707	1,523	1,585	20.0	164.6	12.7	20.7
Bolton	2,549	2,589	2,054	2,010	16.1	110.8	20.4	18.4
Manchester	1,449†	2,066†	2,063	1,709	18.8	176.9	11.7	18.2
Salford	–	–	2,154	2,183	19.6	173.0	23.8	48.5
Bradford	4,417	2,604	1,932	1,885	16.1	135.5	12.4	24.2
Leeds	988	2,041	1,934	1,638	17.9	150.7	14.9	22.3
Sheffield	1,630	2,201	2,014	2,526	17.1	113.5	10.8	17.9
Gateshead	1,162	2,316	2,955	2,657	16.9	126.4	7.5	17.8
Newcastle	905	1,352	1,444	1,367	18.4	162.3	2.6	10.5
England/Wales	1,176	1,547	1,523	1,437	15.4	116.1	9.0	17.8

1851, 1871 physician, surgeon.
1901, 1910 physician, surgeon, registered practitioner.
1851, 1871 principal towns = cities and boroughs having defined municipal limits, except for Manchester (city) and Salford (borough) 1851, 1871 = parliamentary limits; London = registration division.
1891 urban sanitary districts, London = registration division.
1911 principal towns: Bristol, Liverpool, Manchester, Newcastle, Birmingham, Bradford, Leeds, Sheffield = county boroughs (city); Birkenhead, Bolton, Salford, Gateshead = county borough; Aston Manor = municipal borough; London = administrative county.
Mortality rates for London; Bristol; Birmingham; Aston; Birkenhead; Liverpool = Liverpool, Toxteth Park and West Derby; Bolton; Manchester = Manchester, Prestwich and Chorlton; Salford; Bradford; Leeds; Sheffield = Sheffield and Ecclesall Bierlow; Gateshead; Newcastle.
*TB=Pulmonary tuberculosis and phthisis.
† Manchester and Salford.
Sources: *Published Volumes of the Census of England and Wales* (1851, 1871, 1891, 1911); *Decennial Supplement to the Annual Reports of the Registrar-General of Births, Deaths, and Marriages in England and Wales* (1901–1910).

The growing level of medical provision, however, might be taken as an indicator of a rising demand. Yet this only serves as a sign of successful medical treatment if people are assumed to have acted rationally. Looking at the qualitative development of medicine, it has to be stressed that only a limited number of medical inventions and partly improved diagnoses occurred alongside the rise of bacteriology in the 1880s. It

Table 42: Medical and hospital provision in large German towns (per 100,000 population), crude mortality rate (per 1,000 inhabitants) and selected causes of death (per 100,000 inhabitants), 1907

City/ town	Civil practitioners 1898	No. of hospitals	No. of beds	Days of provision	CDR	Mortality TB	Typhoid	Diptheria
	per 100,000		per 100,000		per 1,000		per 100,000	
Berlin	117	84	481	138,848	15.4	220.1	3.6	22.4
Breslau	96	38	754	207,147	22.4	347.2	3.9	21.6
Cologne	81	16	807	238,493	17.9	151.9	3.3	22.0
Dresden	87	31	561	135,621	14.9	208.7	1.9	31.7
Dortmund	57	4	748	202,421	18.6	149.9	3.8	32.4
Düsseldorf	72	10	717	159,480	15.0	172.0	2.3	17.2
Essen	55	5	422	130,097	14.6	156.8	9.1	20.6
Frankfurt	117	24	710	160,040	14.4	199.8	2.0	11.2
Hamburg	72	28	588	171,053	14.8	188.1	2.9	14.8
Leipzig	70	21	448	107,329	15.3	216.7	3.7	20.2
Munich	114	28	636	167,689	18.1	286.2	2.7	7.1
Germany	48*	4,644	602	157,333	18.7†	183.9†	6.0†	27.8†

* 1899.
† 1901–1910.
Sources: *Medizinalstatistische Mitteilungen aus dem Kaiserlichen Gesundheitsamte*, **6** (1901), p. 92; Statistisches Bundesamt (1972), pp. 102, 121, 124–25; *Statistisches Jahrbuch Deutscher Städte*, **17** (1910), pp. 270–77; *Veröffentlichungen des Kaiserlichen Gesundheitsamtes (Beilagen)* (1908); Dornedden (1939), pp. 217, 219, 228.

has to be kept in mind that it took quite some time before such medical improvements found their way into general practice (Spree, 1981a, pp. 110–12). Up to now, our understanding of the average doctor's daily work in the past is minimal. Furthermore, there was no effective therapy for the major killers, namely respiratory and digestive diseases, and all major diseases were already in decline from the beginning of the period under investigation. Tuberculosis, for instance, registered a decline long before the identification of the tubercle bacillus by Robert Koch in 1882 and the start of effective treatment by streptomycin in the 1940s. Still, medicine may have contributed to this decline or even accelerated it. Once developed, medical methods and treatments spread quickly within individual countries and across national borders, so that the pace of change was to some extend independent of the standard of living. Here again a comparative analysis might provide a more detailed understanding of this process. Two examples of medical intervention—the first of a preventive, the second of a curative nature—which are believed to have been successful, shall be discussed briefly: (a) the systematic campaign against typhoid fever in Germany initiated by the bacteriologists around Robert Koch at the beginning of the twentieth century, and (b) the serum-therapy against diphtheria, a childhood disease highly feared because of the danger of complications (Gottstein, 1912, pp. 211–12).

Robert Koch's Campaign against Typhoid Fever

With the rise of bacteriology, attention in the fight against typhoid fever was soon diverted from environmental intervention in the large towns (central water supply and sewerage systems) towards more traditional strategies, focusing on the registration and isolation of the infected person.[2] The official view was that typhoid fever could now be controlled in urban areas—which in view of the (re)occurrence of various epidemics in towns was simply not true—and that attention should now be concentrated on rural areas. This was probably reinforced by the fact that it was still quite difficult to discover and to prove the existence of the typhoid fever agent in water. In any case, the new strategy became increasingly important in Germany and reached its climax with Robert Koch's systematic campaign against typhoid fever in the south-west of Germany after the turn of the century. Koch stressed the importance of monitoring and controlling the infected yet still healthy person, the 'carrier' of typhoid bacilli, and so opened up a new field of preventive medicine, the significance of which had not been realized before to its full extent. He suggested that numerous bacteriological stations should be established in various districts, which would allow close observation of the population at risk. As this procedure corresponded with the classical interventionist approach, Koch sought support not so much from the liberal towns and cities of Germany but from central government. From experiences in the Franco-German war of 1870 the young German Reich was fully aware of the importance of epidemics during military campaigns. At the same time, Koch's approach offered a relatively cheap way to fight the disease in economically less important rural areas—when compared with the enormous sums the municipalities had been forced to spend on environmental improvements. As a consequence, central government agreed to Koch's plans. With substantial financial support from the Reich and the participating states, the campaign was carried out in those south-western parts of Germany where German troops were concentrated against the 'arch-enemy' France (Richter, 1974, p. 54).[3] It was definitely not by chance that Robert Koch delivered his important paper, stressing the need for such a campaign, in front of an audience consisting almost exclusively of military officers, although the military connection was not explicitly referred to. In terms of the success of this campaign, it must be said that mortality from typhoid fever was already at such a low level, that, from an epidemiological point of view, typhoid fever was no longer of major importance. Furthermore, the death rate continued to decline in areas where the campaign was not undertaken systematically. Typhoid fever morbidity declined in Lower Alsace from 8.4 in 1904 to 3.6 in 1909 (per 10,000 inhabitants), but in Upper Alsace, which was not covered by the campaign, it also fell from 8.0 to 4.2 (Kühnemann, 1911, p. 89). By the end of the nineteenth century, typhoid fever had become one of the classic diseases where the sick were isolated in hospital, but this again does not appear to have had a noticeable effect on the mortality trend. No interdependence can be found between hospital provision and typhoid fever mortality in

2 For the following see also Labisch (1992), pp. 139–41 and 265–66; Weindling (1989), pp. 158–68.
3 For contemporary reports see: *Denkschrift* (1912); Fischer (1913); Frosch (1907).

the large German towns (Table 42).[4] The long-term potential effects of Koch's efforts on German troops in times of war remains a different story.

Serum-therapy

Soon after the discovery of the diphtheria agent by Friedrich Löffler in 1885, a blood serum was developed by Emile Roux in Paris and Emil von Behring in Berlin which from 1895 onwards was introduced on a larger scale in both countries under consideration (Grotjahn, 1923, p. 242; Smith, 1979, p. 151). From the mid-1890s onwards, mortality from diphtheria declined drastically in Germany (Fig. 47).[5] This has been taken as an obvious indicator of the quality of the antitoxin and the success of the serum-therapy in general. It has been argued that this was indeed the only successful contribution of the bacteriologists and curative medicine in the late nineteenth century to the secular mortality decline (McKeown, 1976, p. 98; Spree, 1981a, p. 109). In England and Wales, however, where mortality from diphtheria did not play such an important role in the disease panorama—in 1871–1880 only 1.2 deaths per 10,000 inhabitants occurred as a result of diphtheria—the death rate hardly declined at all during the second half of the 1890s (Fig. 48). This might be attributed either to the fact that blood serum-therapy was only rarely administered, because antitoxins were only effective in the first days of the attack, when the symptoms were least clear, or because serum-therapy was very expensive (Smith, 1979, p. 151). The first point, however, cannot explain the differences in the course of diphtheria mortality between England and Germany, as the diagnosis of diphtheria was equally difficult for doctors in both countries. Some evidence against the latter is provided by developments in Birmingham. There were no major changes in diphtheria mortality amongst the inhabitants of the town after the turn of the century, although antitoxin was provided free of charge in the city from 1902 onwards: mortality even increased slightly from 1.7 per 10,000 inhabitants in 1901, to 2.5 in 1902 (in the registration districts of Birmingham and Aston), and remained above two until 1909.[5]

The different development of diphtheria mortality in both countries then leads to the question as to whether serum-therapy was applied more strictly or effectively in Germany. There is indeed some evidence to support this hypothesis. Whereas popular enthusiasm for serum-therapy was overwhelming on the continent, with newspapers organizing public subscriptions to make the antitoxin available to the poor, in England public reaction remained rather limited and the medical profession was

---

4 The correlation coefficients between various indicators of medical provision and mortality from typhoid fever in the largest German towns, 1907, are:
Practitioners/population: 1898: $r = -0.4904$, sig. (two-tailed) = 0.126;
No. of hospitals: $r = -0.2334$, sig. (two-tailed) = 0.490;
No. of beds: $r = -0.4755$, sig. (two-tailed) = 0.139;
Days of provision: $r = -0.1862$, sig. (two-tailed) = 0.584.
Sources: See Table 42.

5 The different scales employed in Figures 47 and 48 demonstrate the extent to which diptheria mortality levels differed in the German and English samples.

6 Sources: *Annual Reports of the Registrar-General of Births, Deaths, and Marriages in England and Wales* (1856–1910).

resistant to the new scientific treatment (Weindling, 1992a, pp. 138–40). In Germany, the discovery and development of the serum created an element of academic and commercial rivalry. Researchers cooperated with various pharmaceutical companies with regard to the commercial exploitation of the serum. In this situation the authorities intervened by establishing a state-sponsored research institute as a supervisory body to maintain serum standards (Weindling, 1992b, pp. 79–82). In July 1896 the Lancet Commission actually complained that German serum was found to be of a much higher strength than the cheaper British product of Burroughs, Wellcome, and Co. ('Report of The Lancet', 1896). This could therefore explain why there is indeed no connection—expressed as a correlation coefficient—between actual medical provision as measured by doctor:population ratio and mortality rates from diphtheria in the selected towns of England and Wales (Tables 41 and 42) around the turn of the century, whereas there is a negative relationship in the German urban sample.[7] That is, the better the doctor: population ratio in German towns, the lower were the mortality rates from diphtheria.

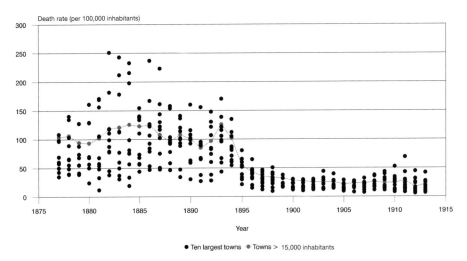

Figure 47: Mortality from diphtheria/croup in German towns, 1877–1913 (per 100,000 inhabitants)

Source: *Veröffentlichungen des kaiserlichen Gesundheitsamtes (Beilagen) 1878–1914.*

---

7 The correlation of medical provision (England: population per physician, surgeon, registered practitioner, 1911; Germany: practitioner per 1,000 inhabitants, 1898) and mortality from diphtheria gives the following results:
For the English towns: r =   0.0505, sig. (two-tailed) = 0.864;
For the German towns: r = –0.5257, sig. (two-tailed) = 0.079.
Sources: See Tables 41 and 42.

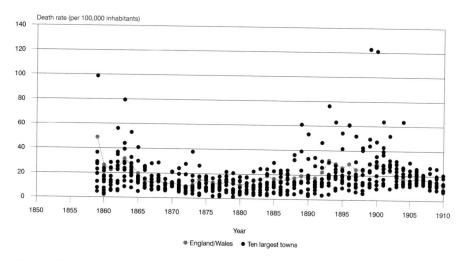

Figure 48: Mortality from diphtheria in English towns, 1859–1910 (per 100,000 inhabitants)
Source: *Annual Reports of the Registrar-General of Births, Deaths, and Marriages in England and Wales* (1856–1910).

There are, however, serious indications that the decline in diphtheria mortality in Germany cannot be attributed mainly to medical invention, but rather to a natural decline in the occurrence and incidence of the disease itself. Mortality from diphtheria tended to increase and fade in intervals throughout the nineteenth century. Like many other endemic childhood infectious diseases (measles, scarlet fever, smallpox) its occurrence followed a cyclical periodicity (Gottstein, 1903; Newsholme 1935, pp. 187–99), with very low death rates in mid-nineteenth-century Europe. In Sir John Simon's Second Report to the Privy Council for the year 1859, he stated that the disease was almost unknown to British doctors until 1855 (Gale, 1959, p. 93). The same is true for Germany. By 1860, Berlin doctors and physicians were reported to know about the disease only from medical literature rather than from direct experience (Gottstein, 1901, p. 607). From the 1860s until the 1890s, however, the death rates increased all over the world (Hirsch, 1886, vol. III, pp. 57–67; Creighton, 1965, vol. 2, pp. 736–46), and diphtheria increasingly constituted a significant element in the overall disease panorama in Germany. In the first half of the 1890s this trend reached a turning point, and a perceptible decline started. This reversal in trend, however, was not a result of the introduction of the antitoxin in 1895, because, as was pointed out by A. Gottstein on the basis of available data, it had already been evident in the previous year. This, however, cannot be taken as too serious an objection to the original hypothesis, as the average mortality rate for all towns with a population exceeding 15,000 in 1894 was indeed lower than in 1893, but still higher than in 1892. Indeed, substantially lower rates occurred only from 1895 onwards. What is more important evidence in this context is that the decline in the death rate from diphtheria was accompanied by a similar fall in morbidity rates (Gottstein, 1901b, p. 611; 1912, p. 214). As preventive treatment was sparse, and

restricted to a few large towns (Prinzing, 1903, p. 451), this clearly indicates a retrogression of the whole disease complex, occurring simultaneously with the introduction of the antitoxin. In Hamburg, for example, diphtheria morbidity declined
from 4.8 per 1,000 inhabitants in 1872–1896 to 2.0 in 1897, 1.7 in 1898 and 1899,
and 1.6 in 1900 (*Die Gesundheits verhältnisse Hamburgs*, 1901, p. 195), despite the
fact that active vaccination was very rarely administered (ibid., p. 197). The proportion of sick people admitted to hospitals declined rapidly in Germany from around
50 per 100,000 inhabitants in 1893 and 1894 to around 40 in the following two years,
and to around 30 thereafter (Loeffler, 1908, p. 128). Based on these figures the morbidity rate in Germany declined from 9.5 (in 1892), 13.5 (1893) and 12.5 (1894) to
5.9 (1895), 4.6 (1896) and 3.8 (1897) (Loeffler, 1908, p. 124). At the same time, the
case fatality rate experienced a decrease of about 50 per cent. If the decline in diphtheria death rates had been exclusively the result of successful curative medical intervention, the morbidity rates would have remained near the previous level until
preventive means were applied on a large scale.

Further evidence can be obtained by leaving the Hamburg example to one side and
returning to the ten largest German towns. The following points need to be stressed
in particular. First of all, mortality declined simultaneously in all towns in the German sample. If this was the result of the introduction of serum-therapy, then it must
have been applied with the same effectiveness in different cities and states of Germany, from Prussia to Bavaria. This seems very doubtful in view of the federal structure of Germany and the major role of local communities with regard to health
policy, which resulted in a variety of public health strategies. As there is no evidence
as to what extent serum-therapy was made available in the individual cities in the
sample, differences in the number of practitioners might serve as a rough indicator
for this specific medical provision. In this respect, there were wide differences within
the sample of towns. In 1898, the number of practitioners per 100,000 inhabitants in
the ten largest towns varied from 70 in Leipzig to 117 in Berlin and Frankfurt am
Main (Table 42). The ratio was even lower in other large towns such as Essen and
Dortmund, with 55 and 57 practitioners per 100,000 inhabitants respectively,
although the decline in diphtheria was similar. Diphtheria mortality rates also
decreased in rural areas, which had significantly lower levels of medical provision
than urban districts. In Prussia, mortality rates decreased in all towns from 3.58
deaths per 100 births in 1892–1894 to 1.51 in 1895–1897, and in all rural communities from 4.55 to 2.42 in the same period (Weissenfeld, 1900, p. 324).[8] Viewed in a
broader perspective, diphtheria mortality also declined in other European countries
with a much poorer doctor:population ratio, e.g. in Galicia, or in other countries
where serum-therapy was rarely administered (Prinzing, 1903, p. 451; Newsholme,
1898, pp. 14–17). Moreover, the decline in German towns affected all age-groups
(Tables 12–19), particularly children aged between 1 and 15 years, but also the very
young and the very old. These were groups which probably benefited less from the

---

8 As population-at-risk figures were not available for the selected years, Weissenfeld used the number of
   births.

new serum-therapy, as they still received minimal medical treatment during sickness. And after all, despite serum-therapy, mortality increased again in Wurtemberg
in 1898–1899, in England at the turn of the century, and in Hamburg at the end of the
first decade of the twentieth century (Prinzing, 1903, p. 451; Gottstein, 1929, p. 71).

Summing up, the available evidence indicates that the introduction of serum-
therapy essentially accompanied a downward move in the cyclical trend of diphtheria mortality and morbidity and that the whole disease complex was in retrogression.
In addition, declining case fatality rates, registered in both countries (Loeffler, 1908,
p. 124; Hardy, 1993, pp. 104–09), indicate that weaker strains of diphtheria types may
have been emerging during that period. Unfortunately, such data are not available for
the individual towns of the German sample. However, the example of Hamburg,
where mortality from diphtheria can be calculated from 1838 onwards, supports this
view from another angle. In Hamburg there were higher death rates in the low-level
mortality period of the 1840s and 1850s than in the period from the late 1890s
onwards—interrupted by a sudden increase in the early 1860s and high mortality in
between these two periods (*Die Gesundheits verhaltnisse Hamburgs*, 1901, p. 194).
The downward cycle at the end of the nineteenth century therefore was accompanied
by lower rates than during the previous cycle in the 1840s and 1850s. Yet medical
intervention may still have reinforced this decline and helped to stabilize mortality at
a low level by curing at least a certain proportion of the sick, and by preventing doctors from applying dangerous traditional methods of scraping off diphtherical furs and
the subsequent cauterization.

HEALTH EDUCATION AND SOCIAL SECURITY

The impact of medical technology, direct preventive intervention (such as vaccination) and curative therapy on the urban mortality decline, therefore, seems to have
been rather limited in the period under consideration. However, the overall contribution may have been greater when medical practice is viewed in a broader perspective.
Measures to control disease and to protect individuals from sickness and its consequences were increasingly incorporated into a legislative framework in both England
and Germany (Labisch and Tennstedt, 1985; Woodward, 1984). Furthermore, traditional forms of poor relief were increasingly replaced by a more comprehensive social
insurance, covering accident, sickness, old age and disability insurance. This was of
particular importance as adverse family circumstances were a major cause of working-class indigence. Rowntree, for example, attributed over twenty per cent of the
cases of primary poverty in York in 1899 to the death, sickness or old age of the head
of the household. Both countries, however, took quite different paths towards the
development of social welfare provision. Whereas England had been more advanced
in relation to sanitary reform, Germany took the lead in creating a modern bureaucratic welfare system. Following the country's tradition of state intervention, a
mandatory sickness insurance system (*gesetzliche Krankenversicherung*), inaugu-
rated in 1883 (*Krankenversicherungsgesetz*, 15 June 1883), was implemented on an
ever-widening scale during the last third of the nineteenth century. Although the initial aim of the scheme was not to guarantee medical treatment in case of sickness but

to provide financial support during any absence from work in order to secure a minimum living standard, this may actually have had a broader effect on general health considering the continuing lack of curative treatments. Although the actual level of support available through the 1883 legislation was rather small, it could nevertheless have prevented the whole family from falling immediately into poverty, and thereby contributed indirectly to the health of other members of the family, who were not covered by the insurance scheme. Given that married women (and younger age-groups) were excluded from the scheme, the inference that there were net family benefits would depend, to some degree, on their distribution within the individual family. Although there is no direct evidence to suggest that non-insured family members benefited to any degree, the fact that improvements in mortality started among the younger age-groups and affected women more strongly than men does, at least, not necessarily contradict the potential impact of the sickness insurance scheme on health conditions. However, the number of people insured was still not large enough to influence the initial urban mortality decline substantially. Their number, however, was constantly increasing. Whereas in Germany 4.29 million people, 10 per cent of the whole population, were members of the statutory sickness insurance scheme in 1884, by 1913 the number had increased to 13.9 million or 25 per cent. If it is estimated that there were on average two or three family members attached to each insured person, financial pressure in case of sickness was arguably ameliorated for 62 per cent of the whole population (Tennstedt, 1981, pp. 169–70). As the scheme was primarily designed out of fear of social upheavel from a socialist workers' movement and in order to counterbalance the increasing influence of the Social Democrats, urban industrial workers were the first target group for social insurance legislation; agricultural labourers, domestic servants and cottage industry workers were only included at a later date. Indeed, agricultural workers were only fully included in the sickness insurance scheme in 1914. Given that three-fifths of the German population lived in communities of 2,000 or more by 1910, the insurance scheme covered a larger proportion of the urban population than average figures for the whole country suggest. Yet, the collective benefits from sickness insurance remained limited as women and children remained disadvantaged in the urban environment. A survey in the Cologne district in 1904 revealed that only 11 per cent of the sickness funds granted family insurance (Tennstedt, 1976, p. 388). Predominant female occupations, such as domestic work, remained largely unregulated.

In England, despite its greater per capita income, a strong tradition of self-help and the dominance of private enterprise led to an expansion of available insurance systems for the working class, particularly in the form of the Friendly Societies and the Trade Union Benefit Funds.[9] Despite Britain's leading role in industrialization, a state welfare system was introduced at a relatively late stage with the National Insur-

---

9 For the Friendly Societies see Riley (1989).

ance Act of 1911.[10] The delayed introduction of a national health insurance system in Britain has been accounted for by basic differences in political motives and existing institutional services (Ritter, 1986, p. 179). After the turn of the century, laissez-faire beliefs were increasingly replaced by the view that the state was the responsible agent for social welfare. The use of social insurance in order to achieve greater productivity from the workers for the benefit of the national economy was an idea which had to be learnt from experience, and so could only guide reform efforts in countries that underwent industrialization at a later date. The main impetus behind Britain's social reforms was less concerned with political and social control, but resulted from the need to solve the problem of mass poverty. This again might be a major reason why Britain's system surpassed the German one in many respects. Whereas in Germany the level of services was largely based on actual contributions paid by the individual into the system, in Britain social security payments were largely calculated on the basis of actual needs. The British system, however, provided access to a general practitioner for all insured workers, male and female, but not for their dependants, that is, mainly women and children (Lewis, 1984, p. 24).

The direct and indirect effects of social insurance on health are difficult to assess. Due to its early introduction, the impact of the German system is of special importance for the period considered in this analysis. The state insurance schemes definitely had a profound impact on the changing role of the medical profession, with the insurance system now being interposed between doctor and patient. It has been argued that the initial neglect of doctors' interest by the social insurance scheme in Germany accelerated the organization of the medical profession (Huerkamp, 1980; Labisch, 1992; Ritter, 1986, p. 112). It has also been argued that the creation of the social insurance scheme with its positive effects on the financing of hospital treatment via an increased number of patients accelerated the evolution of the modern hospital. However, it has to be borne in mind that similar developments also occurred in England, despite the fact that the equivalent scheme was implemented several decades later than in Germany, so that these effects may have been overestimated to a certain degree in the German case. The more direct effects on the health of the population, however, have not yet been analysed in sufficient depth, although the records of the sickness insurance offices (*Krankenkassen*) could be used to extend our knowledge about health conditions in the past because they include not only mortality but also morbidity rates and provide additional information on the theme. The results so far are still largely speculative. For example, the increase in the average number of working days lost per capita from 5.5 in 1888 to 8.7 in 1913 has been taken as an indicator of a deterioration in health (Kuczynski, 1967, p. 407). By contrast, it has been argued that this was not only the result of improved legislation extending the maximum term of benefit payments but also reflected the fact that workers increasingly learnt to make better use of available benefit funds and paid

---

10 Literature on the history of the 'welfare state' is considerable. For a comparative approach to the developments in Britain and Germany and for further literature see Ritter (1983; 1989); Mommsen (1981); Hennock (1987).

more attention to their health (Ritter, 1986, pp. 110–11). This learning process was partly driven forward by direct and indirect educational means, as well as by social control enforced by the state, affecting industrial working conditions and reflecting broader economic needs (Tennstedt, 1983; Labisch, 1992, pp. 180–87). Labisch gives an illustrative example of the extent of official intervention into the private sphere in the case of an urban working-class mother reported to be ill from tuberculosis. Social insurance, if the family was covered, or municipal poor relief, financed her isolation in hospital and later her long-term treatment in a sanatorium. Her husband, children and other people with whom she potentially had contact were also subject to medical control. The family's dwelling was inspected and disinfected. As the father was working, the children had to be taken to a children's home. In this way, the family was systematically monitored and subjected to various social provision schemes, whereas the case might have remained unnoticed in agricultural labourer families in the eastern provinces (Labisch, 1992, pp. 186–87). This direct intervention was certainly one method by which the perception of health and disease was increased. This, in turn, influenced actual health conditions.

A further potential impact on urban health came from another area. Health-promotion measures, created in the period under investigation, formed the essential base for a health-preserving way of life. The role of the recipients of health care, however, was of equal importance. Many contemporary reports pinpointed the fact that the state of personal hygiene was extremely poor. The bath after birth was often the first and the last (Maier, 1871, p. 193). Ignorance about the feeding and care of infants was almost universal. The provision of satisfactory hygienic milk, for instance, was of little value, if the purchaser did not keep it cool, and instead stored it in the warmest place in the house (Soxhlet, 1886, p. 255), failed to wash his or her hands before preparing the milk, and didn't clean the bottles after use. In other words, the potential benefits of an improved health-related infrastructure remained to a large extent under-utilized in the absence of a corresponding improvement in personal hygiene. The evolution of a collectively rooted personal hygiene regime was therefore a prerequisite for enjoying to the full the health benefits made possible by sanitary reform. This in turn was the result of an increasingly rational approach to life, based on the assumption that one could mould one's own destiny. Essential in this context was the attempt to adopt a health-preserving way of life. Corresponding mentalities and norms of behaviour pervaded society from top to bottom. Within this process, medicine increasingly took over the educating and controlling tasks (Labisch, 1992; Spree, 1980). As already mentioned, nineteenth-century doctors, for the most part, remained excluded from access to the sick infant. Medical guides and handbooks on infant care required a certain level of education and therefore did not receive a wide circulation and distribution before literacy was common amongst the working class. Also, specific hygiene education found its way to the general population via school attendance. In England, elementary education became compulsory for all children between the ages of five and fourteen in 1870. For the next generations this meant an increased ability to read, some basic acquisition of personal hygiene through specific education in activities and behaviour, and first hand experience of school hygiene, reinforced through social pressure on families to present their children to a certain decent standard. Moreover, the girls who were in school in the 1870s and 1880s became the mothers of infants in the first decade of the twentieth century, when infant mortality declined drastically. In most of the German states, elementary school education was already compulsory in the seventeenth and eighteenth centuries. Although it was a long process until this was actually realized, Germany had a higher level of literacy than England in the mid-nineteenth century, female literacy rates improved significantly over time, and towards the end of the nineteenth century illiteracy was almost eradicated—except for some eastern provinces of Prussia (Flora, 1973; 1975). However, standards were often low, especially in rural areas, where the one-class schools dominated. In urban areas, elementary school education lasted several years, although hygiene matters were not a part of the official curriculum. Even in the training of elementary school teachers, health and hygiene played only a marginal part (Krei, 1995). There are some qualitative contemporary judgements that aspects of infant feeding and infant care were taught in the last classes of urban girls' schools within the framework of housekeeping lessons (Dietrich, 1908, p. 47). There is, however, no information available as to whether or to what degree children accepted this. Overall, the component of hygiene education via school-teaching seems to have been rather limited.

This educational momentum was reinforced and expanded by an increasing number of health visits, and by 'advancing infant care' (called in Germany *zugehende Säuglingsfürsorge*), that was developed systematically in both countries in the early twentieth century.[11] This enabled doctors or medical personnel to be in direct contact with mothers and children through house-visits. And, as a consequence, this enabled doctors to transmit these new values, which spread amongst working-class people and affected contemporary views on hygiene and health. In the towns of the English sample, the percentage of infants born who were visited once by a health visitor or woman sanitary inspector varied from 25 per cent in Manchester to 91 per cent in Newcastle (*Forty-Second Annual Report*, 1913, pp. 106–11). In most of the towns, municipal child welfare work was supported by voluntary societies, like, for instance, the Infant's Health Society, and Women's Settlement in Birmingham (*Forty-Second Annual Report*, pp. 384–86). The following quotation will give an impression of the existing child welfare work in the city of Liverpool:[12]

> Both municipal and voluntary agencies are at work in Liverpool. Broadly speaking, the visiting of infants is carried out by the municipality, and the infant consultation work, which is not extensive, by voluntary societies. Municipal Work. —Notification of Birth Act adopted in 1908. About 87 per cent. of all births are notified. There are 25 health visitors, who are termed lady inspectors. The city is

11 For an overview of the developments in England see Dwork (1987). For Germany, unfortunately, there is no comprehensive study available at present. For some regional evidence see Stöckel (1986).
12 A systematic overview of the voluntary services' work in the 242 urban areas of England and Wales can be obtained from the *Forty-Second Annual Report of the Local Government Board, 1912–13* (1913), pp. 106–391; this paragraph appears on pp. 263–64.

divided into 21 districts with a lady inspector to each. The babies are visited after the midwife or doctor has ceased attending, about 70 per cent. of all infants being thus visited. About 13 per cent. of all cases are re-visited, the total number of re-visits in 1911 amounting to 1,673. Some of the health visitors work also under the school medical inspectors, but many of them give their whole time to the baby work. After 12 month the babies' names are no longer kept on the books. One day in the week is devoted by the health visitors to house-to-house visitation, when advice is given to mothers and any insanitary conditions noted. Leaflets on the care of infants and allied subjects are distributed. In summer special measures are taken as to the babies suffering from diarrhoea. Some doctors notify cases of diar-rhoea, and the visitors also go to the dispensaries and collect the addresses of the diarrhoeal patients who are attending. All the cases are visited ... Voluntary Work.—There are several agencies at work in this direction. The dispensary for women and children holds an infant consultation for the babies connected with the dispensary patients. The attendance varies from 20 to 30. The consultation is held weekly. Suitable garments for infants are shown.

However, the immediate direct impact of the health visiting movement on infant mortality seems to have been rather small. J. Lewis provided evidence from qualita-tive sources that the health visitors were not very popular amongst working-class mothers. The visits were perceived as offensive, and a sharp communication divide could not be crossed. Moreover, even if middle-class values of bringing up children were accepted, this often asked the impossible in terms of both material provision and infant care schedules (Lewis, 1986, pp. 111–12). Quantitative material supports this pessimistic view. Specific data are available for the 72 largest towns of England and Wales which offered this service. The coefficient of correlation between the per-centage of children visited and the infant mortality rate in 1907 in these towns is as low as −.0132 (p=.912), and with infant deaths from diarrhoea −.1006 (p=.401).[13]

The situation in Germany was almost certainly similar. Health visiting was initi-ated with great enthusiasm. Infant welfare centres were created by the municipali-ties, often connected to the local milk depots, or by private associations (*Vereine*), supported by municipal authorities. By 1907 there were 101 infant welfare centres, 17 of which included health visiting (Trumpp, 1908, pp. 119–20). Figure 49 shows the German cities and towns with such a centre in the same year. From the sample, all towns except Nuremberg had such an institution. Regulations were usually strict: mothers had to agree to be visited (*Hauskontrolle*), they had to present themselves at the centre once a week or once a fortnight. Their eligibility to receive financial sup-port for breast-feeding (*Stillprämien*) had to be proved by a demonstration of the breast-feeding procedure in front of the doctor. As with the milk depots, the success of these facilities was rather limited. Local practitioners were often in opposition to the centres, as they feared that the free advice on offer would reduce their income (Dietrich, 1908, p. 51; Trumpp, 1908, p. 129). Even in 1927 there were complaints

---

13 Source: *Forty-Second Annual Report of the Local Government Board, 1912–13* (1913), pp. 106–11, 329–95.

that despite house visits and financial support for breast-feeding, many mothers could not be dealt with by the local advisory centres. The proud claims that 60 to 80 per cent of all the mothers in a town had been officially contacted must be treated with scepticism and great caution.[14] Medical experts involved in health visiting conceded that even in the industrial town of Dortmund, the rate did not surpass 60 to 70 per cent despite very substantial efforts (Engel and Behrendt, 1927, p. 97). And this refers to single visits, and provides no indication concerning the intensity or frequency of contacts.

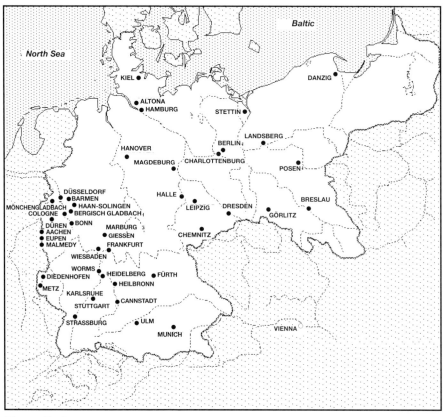

Figure 49: German towns with infant welfare centres, 1907
Source: Trumpp (1908), p. 120

14 For a more optimistic view see Frevert (1984).

Table 43: *Personal hygiene: British soap consumption per inhabitant (lb)*

1791	3.1		
1801	3.6		
1811	4.2		
1821	4.6		
1831	4.5		
1841	6.4		
1851	7.0	duty removed in 1853	
1861	8.0		
1871	9.0		
1881	10.0/14.0	-	France 6

Source: Mulhall (1886), p. 419; (1903), p. 542.

Yet, there are numerous indications that these various efforts to explain and promote health care as well as personal and public hygiene may have made people more susceptible and receptive to health issues. For example, whereas breast-feeding campaigns in the nineteenth century obviously remained without any substantial impact in Germany, as declining breast-feeding rates in the towns demonstrate, similar campaigns in the early twentieth century had greater success. Breast-feeding rates rose generally in German towns during the war years. In Munich, for instance, an investigation of the *Bezirksverband* (local committee) for infants reveals that 70 per cent of the 30,000 infants surveyed were breast-fed between 1916 and 1919. The average duration was between 18 and—for illegitimate infants—10 weeks (Hecker, 1923, p. 292). Yet, even after the war, breast-feeding remained at a relatively high level. Personal hygiene and health became an increasingly important aspect of everyday life. For example, British soap consumption per inhabitant rose enormously during the nineteenth century (Table 43); in Germany, private expenditure on health and hygiene took off after the turn of the twentieth century (Fig. 50). An analysis of the housekeeping books of blue- and white-collar workers and civil servants indicates, however, that there remained substantial differences in expenditures on health and personal care between the classes (*2. Sonderheft zum Reichsarbeits-blatte*, 1909, pp. 56–57). This implies that these indicators may simply be a proxy for higher income or improved living standards rather than reflecting an increased hygiene consciousness.

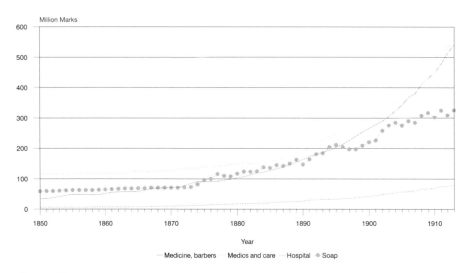

Figure 50: Private expenditures for health and hygiene in Germany at 1913 prices (million Marks), 1850–1913

Source: Hoffmann (1965), pp. 676–77.

CONCLUSION

All in all, the direct impact of medicine on the urban mortality decline of the late nineteenth and early twentieth centuries seems to have been rather limited. Potentially successful medical intervention often concentrated on diseases of minor importance in the disease panorama, yet there was no cure for the main killers. Even medical campaigns and methods traditionally perceived as being effective, such as the systematic control of typhoid fever and the introduction of serum-therapy, left no clear epidemiological evidence. Infants, as an age-group at particular risk, especially in the urban environment, received the least medical attention or treatment. With respect to preventive health care, medicine and medical personnel often played a subordinate role. The driving forces behind the major environmental reforms of the nineteenth century were engineers, bureaucrats or government officials, rather than medical practitioners. It was during this period, however, that medicine improved its prestige with both state officials and the public as a result of major improvements in diagnosis, surgery and medical theory. This, in turn, provided the basis for its important role during the course of the twentieth century. And it was precisely as a result of these changes that medicine may have made a more indirect contribution towards health improvements which cannot be analysed on the basis of mortality statistics. The ability of the urban working class to participate in the labour market may have been sustained or rebuilt through hospital treatment. In the end, they may have died from diseases completely unrelated to those for which they received hospital treatment, after having survived an additional number of productive years.

A broader impact on the registered mortality decline might also be attributed to medicine in relation to health education, for instance in the case of the health visiting movement, developed in both England and Germany in the first decade of the twentieth century. Yet this was only one element within a broader concept of training the urban population to adopt a self-preserving and more rational lifestyle, including aspects of health. A more successful transmission and implementation of these new values may have been facilitated by school attendance, which reached a broader audience for a longer period of time. This resulted in increased literacy, some basic acquisition of personal hygiene through specific education, as well as an active experience of school hygiene through teachers and fellow pupils, reinforced through social pressure on families to present their children to a certain decent standard.

A final comment on the present-day situation might be of use and will conclude this section. Although modern medicine is based on a much more elaborate scientific framework, similarities to the late nineteenth and early twentieth centuries are still quite striking. Today, there is no guaranteed curative therapy for many of the most feared contemporary killers, for instance, cancer and AIDS. In this respect, as in past decades, preventive medicine is likely to be the most successful approach embedded in a broad range of socio-economic efforts to preserve life.

IV CONCLUSION

Chapter 13

SUMMARY AND CONCLUDING REMARKS

Life expectancy has increased substantially during the last 200 years. It has risen from
between 20 and 40 years to 70 or 80 years and even higher. The main causes of death
have shifted from acute and chronic infectious diseases to degenerative illnesses. This
dramatic mortality change has affected all areas of human life, and influenced economic and social development towards a modern industrialized society. With the relative certainty of living through such an extended timespan, values and behaviour
have changed, including views on religion. However, our understanding of the mechanisms behind this development still remains far from complete. Historians of medicine have often tried, in a self-congratulatory manner, to ascribe these achievements
to the medical profession. But despite this, social and economic historians as well as
historical demographers have been more sceptical concerning the role medicine
played within this process. Their criticisms, however, were widely disregarded, as
their competence in the medical field was rigorously denied. In the 1950s and 1960s
Thomas McKeown, himself a trained medical practitioner, was more successful in
challenging the traditional view. He hypothesized that curative medical treatment
contributed only marginally towards the historical decline in mortality, and identified
instead rising living standards in the course of industrialization as the true driving
force behind declining death rates. His arguments were not new; neither was his
methodology very elaborate. Yet, set against the background of the post-1945 economic boom with its widespread belief in the deftness of the market's invisible hand,
his ideas fell on fruitful ground. Although McKeown's arguments still influence present-day health campaigns, criticism has mounted over recent years. One major
objection concerns his use of aggregated data at the national level, which thereby
obscure the immense difference between urban and rural mortality to the disadvantage of towns and cities. Towards the end of the nineteenth century this gap began to
close, as urban mortality rates declined faster than those of rural areas or the national
aggregate. As the decrease coincided with a period of major sanitary reform in many
Western European countries, it has been argued that the impact of environmental
intervention on the historical decline in mortality has been underestimated.

The present study has attempted to expand this perspective with a view to
analysing the role of towns and cities as social agents. It has aimed to reassess the
historical mortality decline by analysing the ten largest English and German towns.
First of all, urban mortality change was differentiated according to age-, sex- and
cause-specific trends, taking into consideration the temporal, spatial and social distribution of the major diseases. Thereafter, the determinants of urban mortality
change were examined within the framework of economic development, housing
conditions, sanitary reform, as well as medical and social provision. The compara-

tive approach adopted in the study sought to delineate more general processes as well as discerning the truly distinctive features of each country within the context of the European mortality decline.

In terms of mortality, the general health conditions in Germany at the beginning of the period under consideration were much worse than in England, with German death rates well above the English figures. The conditions in urban areas were particularly adverse. All the ten largest towns in England also registered substantially higher mortality rates than the average for the country as a whole. By contrast, the 'urban penalty' in Germany was not as unequivocal as in England, became attenuated earlier, and disappeared after the turn of the century. Indeed, the 'urban penalty' in Germany corresponded chronologically with the early stages of large-scale urbanization, so that the highest death rates were registered in the 1860s and 1870s. Thereafter, a steady decline set in. In England, improvements in urban health conditions started earlier in the century, but progressed more slowly, and by the end of the period under investigation towns still showed higher death rates than rural areas or the national aggregate. After the turn of the century urban health conditions in both countries were on a similar level, whereas the aggregate national death rates were lower in England and Wales. These improvements in the death rates were not equally distributed among the population. Infants and men in the higher age-groups constituted the high-risk sector. The younger age-groups in particular benefited from the urban mortality decline, whereas in relative terms the situation for the latter group even deteriorated. Infant mortality, however, was on the decline in large towns, whereas the national rates did not improve substantially before the beginning of the twentieth century. Correspondingly, the main causes of death were still diseases of the respiratory and digestive systems, with similar rates in England and Germany for the former, and much higher death rates from digestive diseases in Germany. The 'urban penalty' was especially marked in relation to these diseases, although almost all important diseases registered higher rates in an urban context.

The chronology of events suggests that a rise in the standard of living had a strong impact on the mortality decline, with towns in particular profiting from accelerated industrialization in Germany. Yet, in view of the changing disease panorama, an improvement in living standards does not explain the mortality decline completely. The medical contribution seems to have been rather small in the sense that curative medical treatment was rare and not available for the major killers. Traditional methods like isolation of the sick concentrated on diseases of minor importance from an epidemiological point of view. Serum-therapy against diphtheria, commonly believed to be one of the rare successful medical interventions during this period, seems to have reinforced a natural fall in diphtheria mortality in Germany, whereas there were no changes in English diphtheria mortality rates despite the simultaneous introduction of the antitoxin. Rather than providing actual therapies, the medical impact on mortality change tended to be in the promotion of individual and public hygiene measures. An essential prerequisite for this phenomenon, however, was the provision of adequate central water supply and sewerage systems. Adequate sanitary measures definitely contributed to an improvement in urban health conditions, especially with respect to the decline of the gastro-intestinal disease complex. However, they served primarily as a form of prevention against the reoccurrence of epidemics and supported the actual secular decline in mortality, rather than directly causing the decrease. It remains unclear, however, whether, or indeed to what extent, sanitary reform may have had an impact on diseases unrelated to the digestive system. On the one hand, certain diseases of the lungs are transmitted via water. Legionnaires' disease, described for the first time in 1977, is most likely to prefer an aerosol form of transmission. On the other hand, a reduction in morbidity from digestive diseases may have increased resistance to other diseases completely unrelated to water. In this sense it might be worth questioning whether the Anglo-Saxon distinction between water- and air-borne diseases is not misleading. In any case, however, sanitary reform during urbanization clearly indicates that a sensible intervention in environmental conditions offered the opportunity of positively influencing health conditions. Finally, housing conditions and overcrowding in particular may have been responsible to a certain degree for the rise of the 'urban penalty'. A high population density was ideal for the transmission of the prevalent infectious diseases. As no substantial improvements in housing conditions were discovered during the period under examination, either in quantitative or qualitative terms, any improvement in urban health conditions, particularly in relation to the decline in infant mortality and tuberculosis deaths, cannot be attributed to this factor.

Evaluating the impact of the various determinants of urban mortality change in both countries remains a difficult task for various reasons. First of all, England as a frontrunner of the industrial revolution was the first country to be confronted with the new threats to health created by industrialization and large-scale urbanization. The development and implementation of strategies to combat disease required capital, knowledge, bureaucratic infrastructure and time. Consequently, England was affected most severely by high urban death rates. The industrial revolution in Germany followed with a perceptible time-lag. Although England led the world in initiating public health legislation, the actual systematic implementation of different public health strategies suggests a high degree of simultaneity in both countries. Medical inventions and therapies spread quickly over national borders. Similarly, knowledge and techniques for the expansion of water supply and sewerage systems were rapidly exchanged. In this instance Germany assimilated English knowledge and engineering techniques, despite the lack of a legislative framework and in the absence of state interference. The self-governing German municipalities had strong financial powers, a corps of trained bureaucrats, and far-reaching police rights that enabled them to intervene in private property rights and to regulate municipal building policies. Owing to the three-class electoral system, municipal political power in Germany remained in the hands of a minority of residents, who very probably gained the most substantial net economic benefits from sanitary reform. By contrast, in England middle-class rate-payers often became alarmed at plans for prospective local sanitary investments and were often successful in blocking reform. From a historical point of view, the expansion of central water supply and sanitation was by no means a straightforward and steady progression. The adoption of water-closets can only be termed a step towards improved hygiene, once there was actually enough water available. On the other hand, in the experimental phase of early sanitation, systems were being tested but not applied on a large scale, which from a retrospective point of view had obvious advantages. For example, the use of two different water systems, one for consumption and personal hygiene, and the other for sanitary facilities (*Brauchwasser*) could be a prospective model for economizing with one of today's most precious natural resources—clean water. However, as the preservation of health was not the primary motive for sanitary reform, these facilities often remained inappropriate with respect to their impact on health. Whereas in England sewerage systems were often implemented before the instigation of a central water supply, the German municipal authorities had learned from the English example that only the latter lived up to the expectations of profit-making. Contrary to dominant medical theories, sewerage systems were therefore generally delayed for some decades. Without a completely integrated system, sanitary provision remained unsatisfactory, and in some cases was even counterproductive, so that various typhoid fever epidemics still occurred as a consequence around the turn of the century. All in all, Germany may have been more efficient in establishing central water supplies, but was certainly not in implementing appropriate sanitary reforms, aimed at preserving and ameliorating the health of the population. This view is amply supported by the fact that in Germany these facilities remained restricted to the large cities, while smaller towns and rural areas remained without them for several decades. Consequently, when comparing the national death rates, Germany still registered worse health conditions than England and Wales, especially where diseases of the digestive system were concerned.

Secondly, similar strategies to fight disease in both countries confronted different disease panoramas. Furthermore, the strategies developed and applied during this period were more appropriate for improving urban health conditions in Germany. Diphtheria, for example, did not play an important role in the English disease panorama, whereas in Germany it was one of the major killers in the infectious disease group, affecting mainly children. More to the point, sanitary reforms had a much greater impact on German urban mortality, characterized to a much higher degree than England by deaths from digestive diseases.

Thirdly, since various determinants of urban mortality change were interactive and operated in combination, an evaluation in the sense of McKeown's precise percentage figures regarding the contribution of each factor appears rather speculative. The analysis indicates that in the long run, the urban-industrial world has had a positive impact on health conditions. The required basis for improved health seems to have been the attainment of a certain standard of living, whereby the pace of the mortality decline was perceptibly accelerated if the rise in living standards occurred as a quantum leap rather than as a gentle incremental progression. This in turn allows for the implementation of an appropriate health-related infrastructure, particularly in the late nineteenth century in terms of the costly expansion of central water supply and sewerage systems. Consequently, the 'new industrial towns' played a leading role in the implementation of these facilities. In England, these towns also registered very high death rates at the start of the period under examination. In Germany, the more industrialized towns in the western parts of the country, for example Düsseldorf, were also frontrunners in the development of sanitary reform—despite their low mortality rates. As a result of the creation of health-preserving environmental conditions and rising living standards, urban populations lost their disadvantage in terms of survival chances when compared with rural areas. This reached the point whereby even traditional risk factors were largely eliminated. Despite a decrease in breast-feeding in towns, infant mortality rates started to decline earlier and more rapidly in urban areas in comparison with the national average. When adequate drinking-water was available, differences in the survival chances between breast-fed and artificially nourished infants vanished. For infants in families at the lower end of the income scale, their survival chances were further enhanced by additional income provided by the participation of the mother in the labour market, although this was associated with non-breast-feeding. By implementing an increasing number of ancillary measures in the following decades, these highly organized industrial societies created a health-preserving system which counterbalanced traditional urban health risks and improved those created by industrialization. These measures included, for example, the expansion of the health sector in general, municipal housing, statutory sickness insurance as well as an 'advancing infant care' system. At the same time, many of these components included an important element of health education and social control. The working class was partly forced to adopt a new rationalistic value system incorporating a more health-conscious behaviour pattern, although in part it deliberately adopted middle-class lifestyles.

In conclusion, it is clear that a variety of often interdependent factors determined the level and trend of mortality in English and German towns in the period under consideration. Some of them have been investigated thoroughly, while others are more difficult to assess, partly due to the available source material, and partly because of the complexity of the subject. As a result, it is clear that studies restricting themselves to the use of single hard indicators or variables tend to provide rather limited results. On the other hand, from a broader perspective, it seems clear that both England and Germany, as well as several other Western European countries, showed very similar characteristics despite having followed individual paths towards attaining the status of modern industrial societies. This point is reinforced, for example, by the fact that the secular mortality decline started among the younger age-groups in both countries, and that infant mortality rates fell simultaneously in England and Germany at the beginning of the twentieth century. These phenomena highlight the need for further comparative multi-national studies. One of the ways of gaining a further insight into the mechanisms of the secular mortality decline in future research would be to combine the advantages of micro-level studies and cross-national comparative analysis by selecting an English and a German town as case studies, further extending the analysis down to a micro-level on the basis of city-districts or even streets, and then drawing comparisons.

APPENDICES

CLASSIFICATION OF DISEASES IN GERMANY

CAUSES OF DEATH IN THE ANNUAL SERIES

Deaths from the following causes have been selected, grouped and computerized on an annual basis. The sources of this annual series are the *Veröffentlichungen des Kaiserlichen Gesundheitsamtes* (*Publications of the Imperial Health Office*) for the period 1877 to the First World War, where deaths from a selection of diseases in towns with more than 15,000 inhabitants are registered.

Measles and Rubella:
    1877–1913

Scarlet fever:
    1877–1913

Diphtheria and croup:
    1877–1913

Childbirth:
    1877–1913

Pulmonary tuberculosis:
    1877–1913 except
    1905 and 1907–1913: tuberculosis

Diseases of the respiratory system:

1877	other acute diseases of the respiratory system, whooping cough
1878–1884	other acute diseases of the respiratory system, pneumonia and bronchitis, whooping cough
1885–1904	acute diseases of the respiratory system
1905	diseases of the respiratory system, whooping cough
1906	acute diseases of the respiratory system, whooping cough
1907–1913	diseases of the respiratory system, whooping cough

Typhoid:

1877–1904	typhoid, gastric fever, nervous fever
1905	'Typhus' (which in Germany became equivalent to typhoid fever)
1906	typhoid, gastric fever, nervous fever
1907–1913	'Typhus' (which in Germany became equivalent to typhoid fever)

Diseases of the digestive system:

1877–1884	catarrh of the intestines and enteritis, diarrhoea
1885	catarrh of the intestines and diarrhoea
1886–1904	acute diseases of the digestive system including diarrhoea
1905	catarrh of stomach and intestines and diarrhoea
1906	acute diseases of the digestive system including diarrhoea
1907–1913	catarrh of stomach and intestines and diarrhoea

AGE- AND SEX-SPECIFIC DISEASE PANORAMA

For the sake of comparison over time and between the towns, the following diseases had to be grouped together for the age- and sex-specific disease panorama. Rarely occurring diseases (below one per cent), which could not be subsumed into the main categories, have been grouped under the 'other diseases' category (the letters refer to the categories in the tables).

1877

Berlin, Breslau, Cologne, Düsseldorf, Frankfurt, Prussia, 1877:

L=cholera nostras, diarrhoea, convulsions;

Q=diseases of the heart, dropsy;

R=diseases of the brain, apoplexy, stroke;

S=bronchitis, catarrh of the lungs, pneumonia, pleurisy, other diseases of the lungs.

Dresden, 1876:

N/O=pulmonary tuberculosis.

Hamburg, 1875:

B=childbirth and puerperal fever;

L=diseases of the stomach and the intestines, diarrhoea and dysentery, convulsions of children, diseases of the digestive system;

Q=diseases of the heart and vascular system, dropsy;

R=cerebral apoplexy, acute and chronic inflammation of the central nervous system;

S=inflammation of the respiratory system, acute and chronic inflammation of the respiratory system, pneumonia, pleurisy, other diseases of the respiratory system;

T=diseases of the urinary system, venereal diseases.

Leipzig, 1875:

B=childbirth and puerperal fever;

L=diseases of the stomach and the intestines, catarrh of stomach and intestines, diarrhoea and dysentery, convulsions, atrophy (children);

Q=diseases of the heart and circulatory system, inflammation of the heart, organic disease of the heart, dropsy, vascular disease;

R=brain and nerves, stroke, other diseases of the nervous system;

S=diseases of the respiratory system, bronchitis, catarrh of the lungs, diseases of the respiratory organs;

T=diseases of the kidneys and urinary system.

1885

Berlin, Breslau, Cologne, Frankfurt, Prussia, 1885:
> L=cholera nostras, diarrhoea (children), convulsions;
> Q=diseases of the heart, dropsy;
> R=diseases of the brain, apoplexy, stroke;
> S=bronchitis, catarrh of the lungs, pneumonia, pleurisy, other diseases of the lungs.

Hamburg, 1885:
> F=measles;
> L=convulsions (children), diarrhoea and dysentery, diseases of the digestive system;
> Q=diseases of the heart and vascular system, dropsy;
> R=brain and nerves, cerebral apoplexy, acute and chronic inflammation of the central nervous system;
> S=acute and chronic inflammation of the respiratory organs, pneumonia, pleurisy, other diseases of the respiratory system;
> U=catarrh and influenza.

Leipzig, 1885:
> B=childbirth and puerperal fever;
> L=catarrh of stomach and intestines, diarrhoea and dysentery, atrophy (children), convulsions, peritonitis, other diseases of the digestive organs;
> Q=diseases of the heart and circulatory system, other diseases of the heart and vascular system;
> R=brain and nerves, apoplexy, stroke, diseases of the brain and nervous system;
> S=bronchitis, inflammation of the trachea, catarrh of the lungs, diseases of the respiratory organs, other diseases of the respiratory organs, pneumonia, pleurisy.

Munich, 1885:
> L=diarrhoea and dysentery, catarrh of intestines;
> S=bronchitis, catarrh of the lungs, pneumonia.

1900

Berlin, Breslau, Cologne, Düsseldorf, Frankfurt, Prussia, 1900:
> L=cholera nostras, diarrhoea (children), convulsions;
> Q=diseases of the heart, dropsy;
> R=diseases of the brain, apoplexy, stroke;
> S=bronchitis, catarrh of the lungs, pneumonia, pleurisy, other diseases of the lungs.

Dresden, 1900:
> F=measles only;
> L=catarrh of stomach and intestines, diarrhoea and dysentery;
> S=bronchitis, pneumonia;
> T=venereal and urinary diseases.

Hamburg, 1900:
> L=diseases of the digestive organs, diarrhoea and dysentery, convulsions of children, peritonitis;
> N=pulmonary tuberculosis;

O=other tuberculosis;

Q=diseases of the heart and vascular system;

R=diseases of the brain, stroke, other diseases of the nervous system and brain;

S=inflammation of the respiratory system, other inflammations of the respiratory system, pneumonia, catarrh, influenza, other diseases of the respiratory organs;

T=diseases of the urinary system, venereal diseases.

Munich, 1900:

F=measles only;

L=acute catarrh of stomach and intestines, diarrhoea, peritonitis;

N=pulmonary tuberculosis;

O=other tuberculosis;

Q=diseases of the heart, dropsy, heart failure;

R=diseases of the brain, stroke, other diseases of the nervous system;

S=inflammation of the respiratory organs, pneumonia.

1907

Berlin, Breslau, Cologne, Düsseldorf, Frankfurt, Prussia, 1907:

L=diseases of the digestive organs, diarrhoea, diarrhoea (children), convulsions, appendicitis;

Q=diseases of the heart and circulatory system, heart, dropsy, diseases of the circulatory system;

R=diseases of the brain, stroke, apoplexy, cerebral apoplexy, other diseases of the nervous system;

S=bronchitis, catarrh of the lungs, pneumonia, pleurisy, other diseases of the lungs;

T=diseases of the kidneys, diseases of the urinary system, venereal diseases.

Dresden, 1910:

L=catarrh of stomach and intestines, other diseases of the digestive organs, atrophy (children), appendicitis;

Q=diseases of circulatory system, diseases of the heart;

R=diseases of the brain and nerves, cerebral apoplexy, other diseases of the nervous system;

S=diseases of the respiratory organs, pneumonia;

T=nephritis, other diseases of the urinary system, venereal diseases.

Hamburg, 1910:

L=diseases of the digestive organs, catarrh of stomach and intestines, diarrhoea, diarrhoea (children), convulsions, appendicitis;

Q=diseases of the heart, dropsy, diseases of the circulatory system;

R=diseases of the brain, stroke, apoplexy, cerebral apoplexy, other diseases of the nervous system;

S=bronchitis, catarrh of the lungs, pneumonia, pleurisy, other diseases of the lungs.

Leipzig, 1912:

L=diseases of the digestive organs, catarrh of stomach and intestines, diarrhoea, diarrhoea (children), convulsions, appendicitis, atrophy (children);

Q=diseases of the heart, dropsy, arteriosclerosis;

R=diseases of the brain, stroke, apoplexy, cerebral apoplexy, other diseases of the nervous system;

S=bronchitis, catarrh of the lungs, pneumonia, pleurisy, other diseases of the lungs.

Munich, 1910:

B=puerperal fever, childbirth;

L=other diseases of the digestive organs, catarrh of stomach and intestines, peritonitis;

Q=diseases of the heart and circulatory system, dropsy;

R=brain and nerves, diseases of the brain, stroke, apoplexy, cerebral apoplexy, other diseases of the nervous system;

S=pneumonia, pleurisy, bronchitis, catarrh of the lungs, other diseases of the respiratory organs;

T=kidneys, urinary, liver.

APPENDIX 2

SOURCES OF DATA ON AGE- AND SEX-SPECIFIC MORTALITY IN GERMANY

Town	Sources
Berlin:	*Preußische Statistik*. Vol. **50**, 184cont *Preußische Statistik*, Vol. **91**, 44cont. *Preußische Statistik*, Vol. **171**, 44. *Preußische Statistik*, Vol. **214**, 46cont.
Breslau:	*Preußische Statistik*, Vol. **50**, 198cont. *Preußische Statistik*, Vol. **91**, 44cont. *Preußische Statistik*, Vol. **171**, 44cont. *Preußische Statistik*, Vol. **214**, 46cont.
Cologne:	*Preußische Statistik*, Vol. **50**, 228cont. *Preußische Statistik*, Vol. **91**, 46cont. *Preußische Statistik*, Vol. **171**, 46cont. *Preußische Statistik*, Vol. **214**, 48cont.
Dresden:	*Mittheilungen des Statistischen Bureaus der Stadt Dresden*, Heft V., Dresden, 1877, 21. *Mittheilungen des Statistischen Bureaus der Stadt Dresden*, Heft 4a, Dresden, 1877, 48cont. *Statistisches Jahrbuch für die Stadt Dresden, 1900*, Dresden, 1901, 22. *Statistisches Jahrbuch für die Stadt Dresden, 1901*, Dresden, 1902, 10cont. *Statistisches Jahrbuch der Stadt Dresden*, **12** (1910), Dresden, 1912, 23. *Statistisches Jahrbuch der Stadt Dresden*, **14** (1912). *Verwaltungsstatistischer Anhang*, Dresden, 1913, 8.
Düsseldorf:	*Preußische Statistik*, Vol. **50**, 184cont. *Preußische Statistik*, Vol. **171**, 50cont. *Preußische Statistik*, Vol. **214**, 50cont.
Frankfurt:	*Preußische Statistik*, Vol. **50**, 224cont. *Preußische Statistik*, Vol. **91**, 48cont. *Preußische Statistik*, Vol. **171**, 46cont. *Preußische Statistik*, Vol. **214**, 48cont.
Hamburg:	*Statistik des Hamburgischen Staates*, **8** (1876), 94cont. and 112cont. *Statistik des Hamburgischen Staates*, **14**, 2. Abteilung (1887), 122cont. *Statistik des Hamburgischen Staates*, **22** (1904), 50cont.

Statistik des Hamburgischen Staates, **27** (1918), 100cont.

Statistisches Handbuch für den Hamburgischen Staat, ed. Statistisches Bureau der Steuer-Deputation, 4. Ausgabe, Hamburg, 1891, 26.

Statistisches Handbuch für den Hamburgischen Staat, ed. Statistisches Landesamt, 5. Ausgabe 1920, Hamburg, 1921, 18.

Leipzig: *Mittheilungen des statistischen Bureaus der Stadt Leipzig*, 10. Heft, Leipzig 1876, 6cont.

Mittheilungen des statistischen Bureaus der Stadt Leipzig, 11. Heft, Leipzig 1877, 18cont. and 45.

Mittheilungen des statistischen Amtes der Stadt Leipzig, 18. Heft, Leipzig 1887, 6cont.

Verwaltungsbericht des Rathes der Stadt Leipzig für das Jahr 1886, Leipzig 1888, 48cont. and 92cont.

Statistisches Jahrbuch der Stadt Leipzig, **2** (1912), Leipzig, 1914, 18cont. and 52cont.

Munich: *Mittheilungen des Statistischen Bureaus der Stadt München*, Band II, Munich, 1880, 25cont. and 13.

Mittheilungen des Statistischen Bureaus der Stadt München, Band VIII, Munich, 1887.

Mittheilungen des Statistischen Bureaus der Stadt München, Band IX, Munich, 1886–1888, 33.

Mittheilungen des Statistischen Amtes der Stadt München, Band XVII, Munich, 1900–1902, Heft 1, 138cont. and Heft 3, 44cont.

Mitteilungen des Statistischen Amtes der Stadt München, Band XXII, Munich, 1910–1913, Heft 1, 22cont.

Mitteilungen des Statistischen Amtes der Stadt München, Band XXIII, Munich, 1910–1911, Heft 2, 18.

Prussia: *Preußische Statistik*, Vol. **50**, 140cont.

Preußische Statistik, Vol. **91**, 2cont.

Preußische Statistik, Vol. **171**. 2cont.

Preußische Statistik, Vol. **214**, 2cont.

APPENDIX 3

ANNUAL CAUSES OF DEATH IN ENGLAND AND WALES, 1856–1910

In the annual series of the Registrar-General, deaths from the following causes have been registered, grouped and computerized.

No.	Disease	Period	Grouped with no.
1	Smallpox	1856–1910	
2	Measles	1856–1910	
3	Scarlet fever	1856–1910	
4	Whooping cough	1856–1910	12,14,30,31
5	Typhus	1856–1910	17,18
6	Childbirth	1856–1910	10
7	Phthisis	1856–1910	32
8	Diarrhoea	1856–1910	15,24
9	Violence	1856–1910	
10	Metria/puerperal fever	1856–1900	6
11	Cholera	1856–1900	
12	Dis. respiratory system	1856–1900	4,14,30,31
13	Erysipelas	1856–1880	
14	Influenza	1856–1880	4,12,30,31
15	Dysentery	1856–1880	8,24
16	Diphtheria	1859–1910	
17	Enteric fever	1869–1910	5,18
18	Simple continued fever	1869–1900	5,17
19	Cancer	1881–1910	
20	Tabes mesenterica	1881–1910	21,33,34
21	Other tuberculosis	1881–1910	20,33,34
22	Dis. nervous system	1881–1910	
23	Dis. circulatory system	1881–1910	
24	Dis. digestive system	1881–1900	8,15
25	Dis. urinary system	1881–1900	
26	Dis. generative system	1881–1900	
27	Other causes	1881–1900	
28	Septic disease	1901–1910	
29	Rheumatic fever	1901–1910	
30	Pneumonia	1901–1910	4,12,14,31
31	Bronchitis	1901–1910	4,12,14,30
32	Pulmonary tuberculosis	1901–1910	7
33	TB meningitis	1901–1910	20,21,34
34	TB peritonitis	1901–1910	20,21,33
35	Pyrexia	1901–1910	

The causes of death classification system changed twice (1881, 1900) in the annual series.

REGISTRATION DISTRICT NUMBER AND BOUNDARY CHANGES IN THE ENGLISH SAMPLE OF TOWNS

The numbers of the Registration Districts change slightly over time. Some of the Registration Districts covered in the analysis were created in the course of the period under research.

City/town and RDs	Registration District no. in the year/period				Comments on boundary changes
	1870	1871–1880	1881–1908	1909–1910	
Bristol:					
Bristol	329	320	320	319	
Clifton	330	321	321	–	Since 1878 called Barton Regis. Boundary changes Bristol/Barton on 1.1.1902 and 1.7.1903. Dissolved on 1.1.1905.
Birmingham:					
Birmingham	394	387	386	384	
Aston	395	388	387	385	
Liverpool:					
Birkenhead	460b	454	452	452	
Liverpool	461	455	453	453	
Toxteth Park	–	–	454	454	Created on 1.1.1881 from W. Derby.
West Derby	462	456	455	455	
Bolton:					
Bolton	468	462	461	461	
Manchester:					
Chorlton	471	465	464	464	
Salford	472	466	465	465	Boundary changes on 1.7.1890.
Manchester	473	467	466	466	
Prestwich	–	467a (1874)	467	467	Detached from Manchester on 1.10.1874.

Bradford:					
Bradford	499	496	497	498	Boundary changes in 1883, 1892, 1894. Without North Bierley.
Leeds:					
Leeds	501	500	501	500	
Sheffield:					
Ecclesall Bierlow	507	507	508	509	
Sheffield	508	508	509	510	Boundary Changes 1.10.1902.
Newcastle:					
Gateshead	551	552	555	557	Boundary Changes 1.10.1902.
Newcastle	552	553	556	558	Boundary Changes 1.1.1905.

London:
Registration Division

POPULATION IN THE SELECTED REGISTRATION DISTRICTS OF ENGLAND AND WALES, 1871–1880 AND 1901–1910

Selected towns	Registration District	Population 1871	Mean population 1871–1880	Mean population 1901–1911
London	London*	3,254,260	3,535,372	4,529,630
Bristol	Bristol	62,662	60,070	347,439
	Clifton	128,984	147,110	–
Birmingham	Birmingham	231,015	238,684	235,995
	Aston	146,818	178,352	329,539
Liverpool	Birkenhead	79,463	91,445	186,299
	Liverpool	238,411	224,288	138,668
	Toxteth Park	–	–	136,188
	West Derby	342,925	409,613	568,665
Bolton	Bolton	158,408	175,406	266,142
Manchester	Chorlton	211,384	234,805	365,778
	Salford	128,890	155,208	234,988
	Manchester	251,956	254,576†	123,663
			157,619‡	
Bradford	Bradford	257,713	284,647	231,801
Leeds	Leeds	162,421	176,634	258,802
Sheffield	Ecc. Bierlow	87,432	100,925	191,776
	Sheffield	162,271	172,703	252,907
Newcastle	Gateshead	80,271	92,841	187,849
	Newcastle	131,198	140,725	241,664

* Registration Division.
† 1871–30.9.1874.
‡ 1.10.1874–1880 (see Appendix 4).

Sources: *Decennial Supplement to the Annual Reports of the Registrar-General of Births, Deaths, and Marriages in England and Wales* (1871–1880 and 1901–1910).

APPENDIX 6

AGE- AND SEX-SPECIFIC DISEASE PANORAMA IN GERMAN TOWNS, IN PRUSSIA, IN ENGLISH TOWNS AND IN ENGLAND AND WALES

Age-, sex- and cause-specific mortality (per 10,000 inhabitants)
LARGEST GERMAN TOWNS 1877

Male

	Causes of death	All	0–1	1–5	5–15	15–30	30–40	40–60	> 60
A	Weakness of life	31.82	910.04	27.65	1.13	0.00	0.00	0.00	0.00
B	Childbirth	0.00	0.00	0.00	0.00	0.00	0.00	0.00	0.00
C	Infirmity	7.61	0.33	0.38	0.60	0.31	1.0	1.24	170.47
D	Smallpox	0.15	1.30	0.38	0.07	0.03	0.06	0.20	0.26
E	Scarlet fever	5.98	9.76	42.54	13.29	0.34	0.06	0.13	0.00
F	Measles and rubella	2.37	26.35	17.42	0.39	0.01	0.00	0.07	0.00
G	Diphtheria and croup	9.81	29.28	75.37	15.89	0.40	0.13	0.20	0.77
H	Whooping cough	2.41	47.18	10.48	0.14	0.00	0.00	0.00	0.00
I	Typhoid fever	4.73	3.90	8.08	3.74	4.71	4.77	3.91	6.39
J	Typhus	0.02	0.00	0.00	0.00	0.00	0.06	0.07	0.00
K	Dysentery	1.44	19.52	5.05	1.06	0.09	0.13	0.59	2.04
L	Digestive system	77.63	2,094.03	107.18	2.82	0.68	1.38	1.56	2.81
M	Scrofula	1.25	14.64	8.58	0.42	0.00	6.27	0.00	0.00
N+O	Tuberculosis	46.00	56.29	26.51	6.45	36.25	63.41	81.78	79.48
P	Cancer	4.41	0.00	0.25	0.14	0.24	2.26	12.64	46.00
Q	Heart	9.58	21.80	5.18	4.58	2.18	5.90	20.79	66.70
R	Brain and nerves	27.45	182.85	70.70	7.75	3.35	11.85	35.51	133.41
S	Lungs	28.95	326.66	71.58	3.49	4.10	10.10	28.09	104.53
T	Urinary system	9.09	26.68	11.36	2.15	3.13	8.03	17.72	38.85
U	Influenza	0.64	0.33	0.63	0.21	0.09	0.31	2.15	2.81
V	Other communicable diseases	0.12	0.65	0.00	0.00	0.00	0.06	0.26	1.02
W	Violence	10.12	7.16	6.19	3.45	8.56	12.23	17.79	15.59
X	Other causes	31.97	264.19	26.13	7.65	7.34	18.50	50.04	152.07
	All causes	313.54	4,042.95	521.64	75.41	71.78	146.5	274.73	823.2

Sources: See Appendix 2.

For the classification and grouping of the diseases, see Appendix 1.

Age-, sex- and cause-specific mortality (per 10,000 inhabitants)
LARGEST GERMAN TOWNS 1877
Female

	Causes of death	All	0–1	1–5	5–15	15–30	30–40	40–60	> 60
A	Weakness of life	24.70	729.54	19.59	1.38	0.00	0.00	0.00	0.00
B	Childbirth	3.39	0.00	0.00	0.07	5.82	7.46	1.30	0.00
C	Infirmity	12.12	0.34	0.29	0.52	0.37	0.57	0.77	186.55
D	Smallpox	0.09	0.67	0.19	0.00	0.06	0.00	0.00	0.50
E	Scarlet fever	5.61	6.71	27.91	13.65	0.47	0.63	0.00	0.00
F	Measles and rubella	2.20	22.83	12.52	0.59	0.03	0.06	0.00	0.17
G	Diphtheria and croup	8.96	27.19	51.03	15.25	0.45	0.19	0.12	0.50
H	Whooping cough	3.07	50.69	13.67	0.26	0.00	0.00	0.00	0.00
I	Typhoid fever	4.95	3.02	6.69	4.33	5.61	3.92	3.14	6.12
J	Typhus	0.00	0.00	0.00	0.00	0.00	0.00	0.00	0.00
K	Dysentery	1.53	23.17	3.15	0.59	0.19	0.32	0.83	2.15
L	Digestive system	66.07	1,834.75	72.44	1.97	1.81	2.15	2.19	5.62
M	Scrofula	1.09	12.09	6.12	0.39	0.00	0.00	0.00	0.17
N+O	Tuberculosis	32.25	39.95	21.98	9.28	30.41	47.49	40.76	36.88
P	Cancer	8.66	0.34	0.19	0.26	0.47	5.44	25.26	50.44
Q	Heart	10.99	14.44	4.01	3.61	2.30	5.44	19.29	72.93
R	Brain and nerves	21.55	143.69	50.56	6.40	2.76	5.31	19.58	87.82
S	Lungs	28.78	286.04	73.68	3.31	4.13	9.17	18.16	88.48
T	Urinary system	2.67	6.71	2.20	1.84	1.15	2.28	4.14	7.44
U	Influenza	0.00	0.00	0.00	0.00	0.00	0.00	0.00	0.00
V	Other communicable diseases	0.10	0.00	0.00	0.00	0.06	0.00	0.00	0.00
W	Violence	2.65	1.01	0.10	0.72	2.40	2.28	0.06	0.50
X	Other causes	27.80	211.84	19.40	5.67	7.49	18.34	35.79	105.35
	All causes	269.22	3,422.08	388.68	70.10	65.98	111.04	174.4	656.08

Sources: See Appendix 2.

For the classification and grouping of the diseases, see Appendix 1.

Age-, sex- and cause-specific mortality (per 10,000 inhabitants)
LARGEST GERMAN TOWNS 1885

Male

	Causes of death	All	0–1	1–5	5–15	15–30	30–40	40–60	> 60
A	Weakness of life	29.06	969.52	20.57	0.12	0.00	0.00	0.00	0.00
B	Childbirth	0.00	0.00	0.00	0.00	0.00	0.00	0.00	0.00
C	Infirmity	6.81	0.26	0.24	0.39	0.21	0.51	0.95	136.74
D	Smallpox	0.10	1.28	0.08	0.00	0.02	0.09	0.12	0.31
E	Scarlet fever	3.13	6.16	19.02	6.11	0.37	0.13	0.04	0.00
F	Measles and rubella	3.28	40.79	21.96	0.89	0.00	0.09	0.12	0.00
G	Diphtheria and croup	12.28	40.28	85.38	18.55	0.40	0.17	0.16	0.00
H	Whooping cough	2.30	39.25	13.14	0.19	0.00	0.00	0.00	0.00
I	Typhoid fever	2.59	0.77	1.39	1.75	3.49	3.40	1.86	3.24
J	Typhus	0.00	0.00	0.00	0.00	0.00	0.00	0.00	0.00
K	Dysentery	0.35	3.34	1.31	0.31	0.09	0.00	0.21	0.46
L	Digestive system	54.52	1,672.48	62.28	1.56	0.77	1.91	4.12	10.64
M	Scrofula	1.33	14.62	9.71	0.31	0.00	0.00	0.00	0.00
N+O	Tuberculosis	44.43	39.77	23.43	6.53	36.01	72.89	76.38	70.30
P	Cancer	6.12	0.26	0.24	0.08	0.33	2.51	15.67	60.12
Q	Heart	9.21	12.31	1.88	2.41	2.36	6.94	18.89	65.06
R	Brain and nerves	23.11	109.04	41.38	6.61	3.58	11.7	31.80	139.67
S	Lungs	32.32	319.92	80.81	3.15	4.85	14.42	32.29	129.49
T	Urinary system	4.88	4.62	4.98	2.18	1.40	3.32	8.50	30.52
U	Influenza	2.39	56.96	8.90	0.00	0.00	0.00	0.00	0.15
V	Other communicable diseases	0.20	3.34	0.16	0.00	0.05	0.04	0.16	0.92
W	Violence	9.88	3.85	5.06	2.68	9.06	12.98	16.58	19.89
X	Other causes	27.64	226.28	32.32	6.49	6.39	18.64	41.70	103.44
	All causes	275.92	3,565.09	434.25	60.32	69.39	149.73	249.56	770.95

Sources: See Appendix 2.

For the classification and grouping of the diseases, see Appendix 1.

Age-, sex- and cause-specific mortality (per 10,000 inhabitants)
LARGEST GERMAN TOWNS 1885
Female

	Causes of death	All	0–1	1–5	5–15	15–30	30–40	40–60	>60
A	Weakness of life	21.46	772.56	18.34	0.34	0.00	0.00	0.00	0.00
B	Childbirth	2.78	0.00	0.00	0.00	4.12	7.37	1.59	0.00
C	Infirmity	11.07	0.00	0.16	0.31	0.26	0.20	0.55	154.93
D	Smallpox	0.05	0.52	0.08	0.04	0.00	0.04	0.00	0.29
E	Scarlet fever	2.81	5.21	18.90	5.62	0.31	0.16	0.00	0.00
F	Measles and rubella	2.95	36.50	22.14	0.69	0.09	0.00	0.04	0.29
G	Diphtheria and croup	11.24	27.64	81.11	20.39	0.44	0.16	0.22	0.29
H	Whooping cough	2.56	48.76	15.51	0.08	0.00	0.00	0.00	0.00
I	Typhoid fever	1.91	1.56	2.59	1.64	2.32	1.73	1.22	2.12
J	Typhus	0.00	0.00	0.00	0.00	0.00	0.00	0.00	0.00
K	Dysentery	0.29	3.39	0.81	0.15	0.00	0.08	0.18	0.87
L	Digestive system	43.00	1,410.06	55.74	1.64	1.49	1.81	2.62	8.09
M	Scrofula	1.05	10.43	8.73	0.31	0.00	0.00	0.04	0.00
N+O	Tuberculosis	30.09	35.46	23.19	10.71	28.41	45.69	37.61	32.18
P	Cancer	8.96	0.26	0.24	0.08	0.48	5.03	23.35	53.09
Q	Heart	9.43	8.87	2.18	2.79	2.30	5.27	14.52	61.95
R	Brain and nerves	17.57	82.65	37.32	6.43	2.19	4.83	16.96	95.58
S	Lungs	26.00	276.64	86.44	3.21	3.22	5.96	15.59	90.85
T	Urinary system	3.46	4.17	4.60	1.38	1.34	3.10	5.17	12.43
U	Influenza	2.29	56.84	9.78	0.00	0.00	0.00	0.00	0.29
V	Other communicable diseases	0.14	2.61	0.16	0.00	0.04	0.04	0.04	0.48
W	Violence	2.83	6.52	3.55	0.77	2.45	2.86	3.18	5.97
X	Other causes	22.12	190.34	27.95	4.97	6.09	14.25	25.31	74.86
	All causes	224.08	2,980.99	419.53	61.55	55.56	98.59	148.21	594.55

Sources: See Appendix 2.

For the classification and grouping of the diseases, see Appendix 1.

Age-, sex- and cause-specific mortality (per 10,000 inhabitants)
LARGEST GERMAN TOWNS 1900
Male

	Causes of death	all	0–1	1–5	5–15	15–30	30–40	40–60	> 60
A	Weakness of life	22.42	840.26	5.83	0.11	0.00	0.00	0.00	0.00
B	Childbirth	0.00	0.00	0.00	0.00	0.00	0.00	0.00	0.00
C	Infirmity	5.89	0.00	0.11	0.48	0.18	0.42	0.54	116.74
D	Smallpox	0.01	0.00	0.00	0.00	0.00	0.00	0.03	0.20
E	Scarlet fever	1.90	1.98	13.20	3.50	0.19	0.14	0.00	0.00
F	Measles and rubella	3.00	40.30	20.31	0.81	0.06	0.03	0.05	0.00
G	Diphtheria and croup	2.37	11.87	16.49	3.25	0.07	0.11	0.10	0.00
H	Whooping cough	1.83	36.34	9.55	0.25	0.00	0.00	0.00	0.00
I	Typhoid fever	0.68	0.00	0.64	0.36	1.00	0.61	0.72	0.20
J	Typhus	0.00	0.00	0.00	0.00	0.00	0.00	0.00	0.00
K	Dysentery	0.04	0.36	0.11	0.00	0.00	0.06	0.03	0.10
L	Digestive system	44.19	1,503.33	37.12	1.48	0.75	1.33	3.37	8.14
M	Scrofula	1.78	29.32	11.30	0.11	0.00	0.00	0.00	0.00
N+O	Tuberculosis	34.47	62.24	30.70	7.92	26.39	43.14	59.28	48.13
P	Cancer	9.53	0.36	0.85	0.25	0.82	3.50	23.61	89.0
Q	Heart	12.06	11.15	1.38	2.55	2.17	5.88	25.30	102.04
R	Brain and nerves	15.42	69.26	20.89	3.75	2.11	5.72	24.48	105.66
S	Lungs	32.24	372.19	65.97	2.46	3.34	10.07	32.28	159.97
T	Urinary system	6.28	5.04	2.23	1.15	1.55	2.94	14.05	46.07
U	Influenza	0.35	0.72	0.11	0.00	0.06	0.03	0.57	4.12
V	Other communicable diseases	0.28	9.89	0.05	0.00	0.03	0.00	0.03	0.00
W	Violence	9.84	6.84	6.15	3.22	8.27	10.79	16.96	20.78
X	Other causes	17.11	139.23	7.48	3.44	4.43	9.52	29.78	80.18
	All causes	221.69	3,140.67	250.45	35.11	51.43	94.27	231.19	781.30

Sources: See Appendix 2.

For the classification and grouping of the diseases, see Appendix 1.

Age-, sex- and cause-specific mortality (per 10,000 inhabitants)
LARGEST GERMAN TOWNS 1900

Female

	Causes of death	All	0–1	1–5	5–15	15–30	30–40	40–60	> 60
A	Weakness of life	16.53	684.06	4.65	0.13	0.00	0.00	0.00	0.00
B	Childbirth	1.79	0.00	0.00	0.00	2.89	4.75	0.74	0.00
C	Infirmity	10.63	0.37	0.16	0.61	0.20	0.22	0.51	146.84
D	Smallpox	0.01	0.00	0.00	0.00	0.00	0.00	0.00	0.06
E	Scarlet fever	1.70	2.02	11.18	3.90	0.22	0.05	0.00	0.00
F	Measles and rubella	2.74	40.58	20.48	0.50	0.01	0.00	0.00	0.00
G	Diphtheria and croup	2.04	8.26	14.68	3.40	0.17	0.11	0.00	0.06
H	Whooping cough	2.03	42.05	12.23	0.21	0.00	0.00	0.04	0.00
I	Typhoid fever	0.55	0.37	0.42	0.40	0.73	0.62	0.42	0.31
J	Typhus	0.00	0.00	0.00	0.00	0.00	0.00	0.00	0.00
K	Dysentery	0.04	0.00	0.10	0.00	0.01	0.05	0.07	0.12
L	Digestive system	34.05	1,261.06	33.75	1.29	1.13	1.11	2.17	5.42
M	Scrofula	1.39	25.16	9.56	0.05	0.00	0.00	0.00	0.00
N+O	Tuberculosis	22.71	49.95	28.68	9.99	21.99	27.48	22.78	27.30
P	Cancer	11.62	0.73	0.52	0.18	1.01	6.46	26.69	71.48
Q	Heart	12.31	8.63	2.30	2.53	2.99	6.33	17.80	87.19
R	Brain and nerves	11.85	48.85	19.02	3.77	1.33	3.64	12.22	73.33
S	Lungs	27.52	305.21	65.88	2.50	3.34	5.97	16.44	132.36
T	Urinary system	4.01	5.69	1.78	1.00	1.34	2.20	6.97	20.64
U	Influenza	0.31	0.00	0.10	0.03	0.03	0.11	0.27	3.14
V	Other communicable diseases	0.20	7.35	0.10	0.03	0.03	0.00	0.04	0.00
W	Violence	2.74	8.26	3.60	1.26	2.21	2.01	2.35	8.32
X	Other causes	14.73	126.16	8.57	2.32	5.66	10.05	16.30	58.91
	All causes	181.50	2,624.78	237.76	34.10	45.30	71.16	125.81	635.49

Sources: See Appendix 2.

For the classification and grouping of the diseases, see Appendix 1.

Age-, sex- and cause-specific mortality (per 10,000 inhabitants)
LARGEST GERMAN TOWNS 1907
Male

	Causes of death	All	0–1	1–5	5–15	15–30	30–40	40–60	> 60
A	Weakness of life	11.04	485.65	0.00	0.00	0.00	0.00	0.00	0.00
B	Childbirth	0.00	0.00	0.00	0.00	0.00	0.00	0.00	0.00
C	Infirmity	3.31	0.00	0.00	0.04	0.00	0.02	0.02	65.72
D	Smallpox	0.00	0.00	0.00	0.00	0.00	0.00	0.00	0.00
E	Scarlet fever	0.83	1.75	5.73	1.73	0.10	0.02	0.00	0.00
F	Measles and rubella	1.99	32.10	15.06	0.43	0.01	0.00	0.00	0.00
G	Diphtheria and croup	2.76	11.58	19.32	4.82	0.23	0.12	0.11	0.08
H	Whooping cough	1.61	39.64	8.82	0.04	0.00	0.00	0.00	0.08
I	Typhoid fever	0.46	0.00	0.05	0.16	0.85	0.52	0.32	0.32
J	Typhus	0.00	0.00	0.00	0.00	0.00	0.00	0.00	0.00
K	Dysentery	0.00	0.00	0.00	0.00	0.00	0.00	0.00	0.00
L	Digestive system	26.46	830.82	17.14	2.22	2.78	4.77	14.21	30.03
M	Scrofula	0.00	0.00	0.00	0.00	0.00	0.00	0.00	0.00
N+O	Tuberculosis	24.62	43.15	24.19	5.00	20.15	29.11	40.93	38.64
P	Cancer	10.70	1.58	0.71	0.67	1.01	3.61	24.41	99.98
Q	Heart	18.80	45.08	4.16	2.18	2.97	7.00	32.28	178.29
R	Brain and nerves	13.35	96.11	14.25	2.06	1.91	4.86	20.62	88.03
S	Lungs	24.00	300.62	46.35	1.75	2.97	6.95	24.15	131.85
T	Urinary system	5.12	8.07	1.17	0.85	1.20	2.84	10.48	37.52
U	Influenza	1.18	4.03	0.61	0.25	0.22	0.26	1.65	11.55
V	Other communicable diseases	1.59	40.34	1.42	0.70	0.48	0.49	0.94	0.48
W	Violence	10.54	8.94	7.35	3.39	8.56	10.82	17.91	25.57
X	Other causes	13.03	245.19	13.94	1.70	2.42	5.45	14.91	31.71
	All causes	171.38	2,194.65	180.27	27.98	45.86	76.83	202.95	739.85

Sources: See Appendix 2.

For the classification and grouping of the diseases, see Appendix 1.

Age-, sex- and cause-specific mortality (per 10,000 inhabitants)
LARGEST GERMAN TOWNS 1907
Female

	Causes of death	All	0–1	1–5	5–15	15–30	30–40	40–60	> 60
A	Weakness of life	8.19	382.83	0.00	0.00	0.00	0.00	0.00	0.00
B	Childbirth	2.38	0.00	0.00	0.00	3.86	6.33	0.90	0.00
C	Infirmity	6.93	0.00	0.00	0.02	0.00	0.02	0.00	99.16
D	Smallpox	0.00	0.00	0.00	0.00	0.00	0.00	0.00	0.00
E	Scarlet fever	0.77	1.25	5.83	1.58	0.08	0.05	0.02	0.00
F	Measles and rubella	1.69	24.65	14.32	0.91	0.03	0.00	0.00	0.00
G	Diphtheria and croup	2.45	8.93	16.00	4.82	0.29	0.24	0.08	0.22
H	Whooping cough	1.79	42.52	11.45	0.13	0.00	0.00	0.00	0.00
I	Typhoid fever	0.30	0.18	0.20	0.22	0.39	0.43	0.22	0.16
J	Typhus	0.00	0.00	0.00	0.00	0.00	0.00	0.00	0.00
K	Dysentery	0.00	0.00	0.00	0.00	0.00	0.00	0.00	0.00
L	Digestive system	21.87	695.45	17.59	2.78	2.83	4.39	8.84	27.47
M	Scrofula	0.00	0.00	0.00	0.00	0.00	0.00	0.00	0.00
N+O	Tuberculosis	19.35	35.91	25.00	6.48	20.32	23.63	19.71	23.53
P	Cancer	13.43	1.61	0.77	0.27	1.29	6.52	31.06	83.51
Q	Heart	18.19	40.02	3.07	2.11	3.36	6.59	23.99	142.17
R	Brain and nerves	11.64	68.96	12.94	1.49	1.50	3.35	13.35	76.45
S	Lungs	20.88	261	46.17	2.11	2.24	4.68	13.04	107.64
T	Urinary system	3.89	8.04	1.53	0.69	1.55	2.65	6.70	18.06
U	Influenza	1.22	2.32	0.41	0.04	0.11	0.33	0.88	12.53
V	Other communicable diseases	1.07	30.01	0.66	0.38	0.21	0.52	0.61	0.66
W	Violence	4.14	7.15	3.58	1.40	3.32	3.69	4.91	13.02
X	Other causes	9.78	201.33	12.53	2.04	1.69	3.57	7.76	24.02
	All causes	149.96	1,812.14	172.05	27.46	43.06	66.98	132.06	628.62

Sources: See Appendix 2.

For the classification and grouping of the diseases, see Appendix 1.

Age-, sex- and cause-specific mortality (per 10,000 inhabitants)
PRUSSIA 1877
Male

	Causes of death	All	0–1	1–5	5–15	15–30	30–40	40–60	> 60
A	Weakness of life	22.17	507.18	31.92	3.54	0.00	0.00	0.00	0.00
B	Childbirth	0.00	0.00	0.00	0.00	0.00	0.00	0.00	0.00
C	Infirmity	22.99	0.11	0.11	0.27	0.38	0.54	0.94	335.84
D	Smallpox	0.00	0.00	0.00	0.00	0.00	0.00	0.00	0.00
E	Scarlet fever	8.23	31.68	43.32	10.33	0.65	0.09	0.03	0.06
F	Measles and rubella	4.75	39.58	24.97	2.69	0.11	0.02	0.02	0.01
G	Diphtheria and croup	17.42	103.79	94.01	14.91	0.44	0.18	0.20	0.32
H	Whooping cough	6.19	106.87	20.26	0.78	0.02	0.00	0.05	0.25
I	Typhoid fever	6.14	4.85	6.13	4.37	5.82	5.78	8.31	8.69
J	Typhus	0.11	0.04	0.01	0.01	0.11	0.16	0.24	0.19
K	Dysentery	1.15	12.10	3.71	0.64	0.15	0.18	0.34	0.81
L	Digestive system	54.91	1,249.39	79.30	3.48	1.22	1.67	2.70	5.18
M	Scrofula	0.98	8.13	4.82	0.76	0.00	0.00	0.00	0.00
N+O	Tuberculosis	35.68	22.85	11.23	4.18	30.72	44.55	68.62	99.40
P	Cancer	2.25	0.13	0.12	0.07	0.16	0.79	5.95	14.96
Q	Heart	8.29	6.33	5.69	2.76	0.15	4.57	14.48	45.98
R	Brain and nerves	18.10	99.16	22.33	5.41	3.70	9.08	22.25	71.15
S	Lungs	18.66	81.28	22.69	3.01	5.44	12.07	29.95	63.90
T	Urinary system	1.59	1.34	1.46	0.60	0.58	1.18	2.16	8.39
U	Influenza	–	–	–	–	–	–	–	–
V	Other communicable diseases	–	–	–	–	–	–	–	–
W	Violence	10.21	4.00	7.14	3.33	9.22	12.22	16.59	18.99
X	Other causes	33.97	261.14	43.33	8.39	8.60	15.13	41.56	93.29
	All causes	273.79	2,539.94	422.55	69.53	69.46	108.21	214.39	767.4

Sources: See Appendix 2.

For the classification and grouping of the diseases, see Appendix 1.

Age-, sex- and cause-specific mortality (per 10,000 inhabitants)
PRUSSIA 1877
Female

	Causes of death	All	0–1	1–5	5–15	15–30	30–40	40–60	> 60
A	Weakness of life	18.67	420.32	33.42	4.91	0.00	0.00	0.00	0.00
B	Childbirth	4.74	0.00	0.00	0.00	7.34	15.96	4.03	0.00
C	Infirmity	27.70	0.11	0.11	0.37	0.32	0.37	0.79	368.74
D	Smallpox	0.00	0.00	0.00	0.00	0.00	0.00	0.00	0.00
E	Scarlet fever	7.31	25.68	39.28	10.06	0.54	0.16	0.05	0.02
F	Measles and rubella	4.43	36.54	24.63	2.68	0.12	0.04	0.01	0.00
G	Diphtheria and croup	15.48	84.35	87.88	15.05	0.44	0.21	0.18	0.13
H	Whooping cough	6.69	109.23	26.06	1.10	0.03	0.02	0.08	0.19
I	Typhoid fever	5.63	3.89	6.09	4.94	5.46	5.39	6.29	7.05
J	Typhus	0.07	0.00	0.04	0.02	0.05	0.12	0.15	0.14
K	Dysentery	1.02	11.30	3.11	0.59	0.15	0.14	0.37	0.89
L	Digestive system	44.15	1,011.19	76.59	3.38	1.39	1.86	2.39	5.27
M	Scrofula	0.91	6.13	4.87	0.89	0.00	0.00	0.00	0.00
N+O	Tuberculosis	28.44	20.54	12.39	6.50	25.89	37.96	46.51	64.95
P	Cancer	3.07	0.18	0.13	0.09	0.22	1.90	8.51	15.55
Q	Heart	10.94	4.90	4.65	2.46	2.75	6.03	19.50	63.03
R	Brain and nerves	13.15	78.22	20.20	4.73	2.71	4.93	12.98	49.28
S	Lungs	13.96	67.34	23.81	2.78	3.36	7.19	17.13	49.00
T	Urinary system	0.80	1.37	0.82	0.43	0.46	0.79	1.09	2.06
U	Influenza	–	–	–	–	–	–	–	–
V	Other communicable diseases	–	–	–	–	–	–	–	–
W	Violence	2.41	3.03	4.89	1.24	1.77	1.79	2.68	4.18
X	Other causes	30.71	226.29	43.06	8.64	8.55	15.92	35.65	78.02
	All causes	240.29	2,110.61	412.02	70.85	61.57	100.78	158.37	708.5

Sources: See Appendix 2.

For the classification and grouping of the diseases, see Appendix 1.

Age-, sex- and cause-specific mortality (per 10,000 inhabitants)
PRUSSIA 1885
Male

	Causes of death	All	0–1	1–5	5–15	15–30	30–40	40–60	>60
A	Weakness of life	21.57	571.89	25.12	2.57	0.00	0.00	0.00	0.00
B	Childbirth	0.00	0.00	0.00	0.00	0.00	0.00	0.00	0.00
C	Infirmity	22.34	0.13	0.11	0.39	0.33	0.41	1.09	303.69
D	Smallpox	0.00	1.00	0.00	0.00	0.00	0.00	0.00	0.00
E	Scarlet fever	6.53	24.31	33.52	9.34	0.32	0.07	0.04	0.04
F	Measles and rubella	5.82	49.26	33.47	3.14	0.07	0.02	0.02	0.01
G	Diphtheria and croup	19.63	101.62	109.39	20.24	0.82	0.27	0.25	0.25
H	Whooping cough	4.59	88.31	15.12	0.61	0.01	0.01	0.07	0.25
I	Typhoid fever	3.46	2.65	2.86	2.60	3.62	3.36	4.09	5.45
J	Typhus	0.03	0.07	0.03	0.01	0.03	0.02	0.05	0.01
K	Dysentery	0.67	7.59	2.00	0.39	0.09	0.12	0.28	0.59
L	Digestive system	51.36	1,308.2	72.56	3.31	0.99	1.39	2.05	3.30
M	Scrofula	1.06	10.86	5.30	0.68	0.00	0.00	0.00	0.00
N+O	Tuberculosis	33.66	25.00	11.66	4.62	28.49	45.19	65.19	84.91
P	Cancer	3.09	0.18	0.16	0.07	0.19	1.09	7.96	20.69
Q	Heart	7.40	4.96	3.44	2.37	2.06	4.09	12.79	42.66
R	Brain and nerves	18.39	86.85	21.96	6.39	3.94	9.53	23.55	76.79
S	Lungs	24.67	124.01	35.95	3.86	6.56	14.42	36.38	86.50
T	Urinary system	2.38	2.12	2.15	1.08	0.69	1.76	3.58	11.32
U	Influenza	–	–	–	–	–	–	–	–
V	Other communicable diseases	–	–	–	–	–	–	–	–
W	Violence	10.17	4.42	6.70	3.31	9.64	12.51	17.23	19.41
X	Other causes	29.30	232.84	33.21	7.38	7.09	15.13	38.05	86.85
	All causes	266.24	2,646.59	415.01	72.45	65.00	109.44	212.75	742.77

Sources: See Appendix 2.

For the classification and grouping of the diseases, See Appendix 1.

Age-, sex- and cause-specific mortality (per 10,000 inhabitants)
PRUSSIA 1885
Female

	Causes of death	All	0–1	1–5	5–15	15–30	30–40	40–60	> 60
A	Weakness of life	17.90	480.54	25.32	3.73	0.00	0.00	0.00	0.00
B	Childbirth	4.45	0.00	0.00	0.00	6.60	16.00	3.70	0.00
C	Infirmity	27.57	0.05	0.08	0.28	0.26	0.29	0.89	337.25
D	Smallpox	0.14	1.45	0.29	0.09	0.06	0.06	0.11	0.05
E	Scarlet fever	5.89	20.42	31.07	9.15	0.46	0.14	0.03	0.04
F	Measles and rubella	5.39	42.83	32.70	3.58	0.10	0.06	0.02	0.01
G	Diphtheria and croup	18.01	87.70	103.81	21.24	0.83	0.28	0.17	0.18
H	Whooping cough	4.92	91.97	19.16	0.79	0.03	0.02	0.08	0.31
I	Typhoid fever	3.33	2.18	3.00	2.92	3.68	3.42	3.35	4.03
J	Typhus	0.02	0.02	0.01	0.01	0.02	0.01	0.03	0.00
K	Dysentery	0.55	6.00	1.66	0.37	0.10	0.09	0.20	0.58
L	Digestive system	41.23	1,074.70	68.88	3.27	1.09	1.46	1.73	3.84
M	Scrofula	0.96	8.68	5.25	0.79	0.00	0.00	0.00	0.00
N+O	Tuberculosis	27.95	22.24	12.65	7.52	26.39	38.67	43.08	58.62
P	Cancer	3.96	0.11	0.14	0.08	0.27	2.32	10.43	20.74
Q	Heart	10.04	4.07	3.08	2.39	2.51	4.85	17.22	58.14
R	Brain and nerves	14.03	70.14	20.36	6.10	3.14	4.99	13.98	56.27
S	Lungs	19.25	105.53	37.03	4.30	4.49	8.57	21.10	65.96
T	Urinary system	1.40	1.61	1.64	0.82	0.62	1.37	1.91	4.02
U	Influenza	–	–	–	–	–	–	–	–
V	Other communicable diseases	–	–	–	–	–	–	–	–
W	Violence	2.36	2.98	4.36	1.17	1.74	1.96	2.69	4.72
X	Other causes	25.74	192.32	31.72	7.08	7.65	14.27	31.27	70.61
	All causes	235.10	2,215.54	402.21	75.70	60.03	98.86	151.99	685.37

Sources: See Appendix 2.

For the classification and grouping of the diseases, see Appendix 1.

Age-, sex- and cause-specific mortality (per 10,000 inhabitants)
PRUSSIA 1900
Male

	Causes of death	All	0–1	1–5	5–15	15–30	30–40	40–60	> 60
A	Weakness of life	20.78	617.32	12.44	0.87	0.00	0.00	0.00	0.00
B	Childbirth	0.00	0.00	0.00	0.00	0.00	0.00	0.00	0.00
C	Infirmity	21.60	0.08	0.12	0.34	0.27	0.31	0.84	306.73
D	Smallpox	0.02	0.21	0.01	0.00	0.01	0.00	0.03	0.03
E	Scarlet fever	3.76	13.03	19.72	5.37	0.25	0.07	0.02	0.01
F	Measles and rubella	2.13	24.07	11.66	0.61	0.02	0.01	0.01	0.02
G	Diphtheria and croup	5.16	37.71	27.34	4.57	0.23	0.08	0.03	0.11
H	Whooping cough	3.90	86.58	10.67	0.28	0.01	0.02	0.02	0.07
I	Typhoid fever	1.46	0.76	0.83	0.96	2.26	1.57	1.38	1.18
J	Typhus	0.00	0.02	0.00	0.00	0.01	0.00	0.00	0.00
K	Dysentery	0.21	2.52	0.51	0.11	0.05	0.04	0.09	0.30
L	Digestive system	54.56	1,504.84	59.51	2.80	0.66	0.86	1.40	2.36
M	Scrofula	1.39	17.58	6.76	0.58	0.00	0.00	0.00	0.00
N+O	Tuberculosis	23.14	25.69	9.29	4.29	21.93	28.90	42.91	47.89
P	Cancer	5.74	0.37	0.23	0.10	0.38	1.91	14.21	41.49
Q	Heart	7.63	8.04	1.83	1.70	2.06	3.79	14.34	47.47
R	Brain and nerves	16.71	77.37	16.78	5.05	3.13	6.67	22.12	84.66
S	Lungs	33.62	221.70	49.56	4.19	6.56	13.00	40.40	146.00
T	Urinary system	3.42	4.51	2.63	1.16	0.99	1.95	5.78	17.64
U	Influenza	–	–	–	–	–	–	–	–
V	Other communicable diseases	–	–	–	–	–	–	–	–
W	Violence	10.28	4.21	6.44	3.37	9.43	11.87	17.67	21.14
X	Other causes	22.10	186.92	14.89	3.55	5.46	10.20	31.02	82.18
	All causes	237.59	2,833.54	251.22	39.91	53.70	81.24	192.28	799.28

Sources: See Appendix 2.

For the classification and grouping of the diseases see, Appendix 1.

Age-, sex- and cause-specific mortality (per 10,000 inhabitants)
PRUSSIA 1900
Female

	Causes of death	All	0–1	1–5	5–15	15–30	30–40	40–60	> 60
A	Weakness of life	16.37	501.16	12.37	1.16	0.00	0.00	0.00	0.00
B	Childbirth	2.40	0.00	0.00	0.00	3.64	8.42	1.81	0.00
C	Infirmity	27.96	0.14	0.12	0.33	0.22	0.28	0.73	340.91
D	Smallpox	0.01	0.08	0.01	0.00	0.01	0.00	0.02	0.01
E	Scarlet fever	3.45	11.19	17.95	5.66	0.32	0.10	0.02	0.02
F	Measles and rubella	1.95	21.78	11.33	0.71	0.02	0.01	0.00	0.00
G	Diphtheria and croup	4.51	29.63	24.30	5.10	0.24	0.10	0.07	0.06
H	Whooping cough	4.07	86.31	13.97	0.36	0.00	0.01	0.03	0.07
I	Typhoid fever	1.31	0.97	0.87	1.16	1.78	1.55	1.09	0.94
J	Typhus	0.00	0.00	0.01	0.00	0.00	0.00	0.01	0.00
K	Dysentery	0.22	2.70	0.58	0.09	0.03	0.07	0.11	0.30
L	Digestive system	43.56	1,230.99	57.35	2.65	0.84	0.88	1.03	1.77
M	Scrofula	1.19	14.83	6.14	0.62	0.00	0.00	0.00	0.00
N+O	Tuberculosis	19.19	20.33	9.80	6.71	20.98	25.96	25.95	31.28
P	Cancer	6.48	0.26	0.22	0.12	0.56	3.23	15.73	37.02
Q	Heart	9.72	7.48	1.90	1.98	2.57	5.06	15.28	58.86
R	Brain and nerves	13.35	61.34	14.99	4.87	2.69	4.33	13.76	64.23
S	Lungs	28.48	174.99	48.32	5.16	5.52	9.74	25.62	122.49
T	Urinary system	2.20	3.09	1.98	0.94	0.91	1.72	3.44	7.58
U	Influenza	–	–	–	–	–	–	–	–
V	Other communicable diseases	–	–	–	–	–	–	–	–
W	Violence	2.50	4.24	4.09	1.32	1.78	1.75	2.90	5.44
X	Other causes	20.17	155.09	14.85	3.55	6.18	11.61	24.75	69.72
	All causes	209.11	2,326.59	241.11	42.50	48.30	74.84	132.36	740.71

Sources: See Appendix 2.

For the classification and grouping of the diseases, see Appendix 1.

Age-, sex- and cause-specific mortality (per 10,000 inhabitants)
PRUSSIA 1907

Male

	Causes of death	All	0–1	1–5	5–15	15–30	30–40	40–60	> 60
A	Weakness of life	13.34	466.84	0.00	0.00	0.00	0.00	0.00	0.00
B	Childbirth	0.00	0.00	0.00	0.00	0.00	0.00	0.00	0.00
C	Infirmity	16.83	0.00	0.00	0.00	0.00	0.00	0.00	246.43
D	Smallpox	–	–	–	–	–	–	–	–
E	Scarlet fever	2.28	8.12	11.35	3.57	0.19	0.06	0.02	0.01
F	Measles and rubella	1.90	23.90	10.41	0.59	0.02	0.01	0.00	0.01
G	Diphtheria and croup	2.56	13.63	14.13	2.84	0.17	0.08	0.03	0.03
H	Whooping cough	2.24	53.17	6.49	0.15	0.00	0.00	0.01	0.11
I	Typhoid fever	0.59	0.21	0.23	0.35	0.86	0.79	0.69	0.39
J	Typhus	–	–	–	–	–	–	–	–
K	Dysentery	–	–	–	–	–	–	–	–
L	Digestive system	22.77	527.88	20.65	2.27	2.23	3.53	11.63	28.71
M	Scrofula	–	–	–	–	–	–	–	–
N+O	Tuberculosis	18.13	29.96	10.29	4.09	18.02	21.98	31.42	31.02
P	Cancer	6.80	1.07	0.42	0.20	0.55	1.99	15.62	52.42
Q	Heart	14.16	36.00	3.52	1.83	2.99	6.26	23.96	96.98
R	Brain and nerves	12.31	56.25	11.35	3.50	2.56	5.39	17.24	63.85
S	Lungs	28.24	246.96	43.07	3.45	5.06	10.62	59.51	113.16
T	Urinary system	3.35	5.50	1.98	0.96	0.98	2.04	5.57	18.77
U	Influenza	1.36	3.89	0.55	0.16	0.22	0.40	1.58	11.20
V	Other communicable diseases	0.77	9.13	1.72	0.60	0.44	0.24	0.22	0.16
W	Violence	9.96	5.22	6.43	3.00	9.70	11.64	16.80	20.90
X	Other causes	32.39	715.99	35.46	3.59	3.00	5.21	15.33	48.24
	All causes	190.03	2,203.72	178.04	31.17	47.01	70.24	171.71	732.37

Sources: See Appendix 2.

For the classification and grouping of the diseases, see Appendix 1.

Age-, sex- and cause-specific mortality (per 10,000 inhabitants)
PRUSSIA 1907
Female

	Causes of death	All	0–1	1–5	5–15	15–30	30–40	40–60	>60
A	Weakness of life	10.13	373.76	0.00	0.00	0.00	0.00	0.00	0.00
B	Childbirth	1.96	0.00	0.00	0.00	3.11	6.77	1.48	0.00
C	Infirmity	22.26	0.00	0.00	0.00	0.00	0.00	0.00	268.16
D	Smallpox	–	–	–	–	–	–	–	–
E	Scarlet fever	2.20	6.48	10.72	3.93	0.28	0.10	0.01	0.01
F	Measles and rubella	1.75	20.90	10.27	0.68	0.03	0.02	0.00	0.01
G	Diphtheria and croup	2.35	12.30	12.61	3.16	0.19	0.06	0.04	0.03
H	Whooping cough	2.42	55.37	8.72	0.18	0.00	0.01	0.01	0.04
I	Typhoid fever	0.55	0.35	0.28	0.41	0.76	0.63	0.60	0.45
J	Typhus	–	–	–	–	–	–	–	–
K	Dysentery	–	–	–	–	–	–	–	–
L	Digestive system	19.19	438.98	20.01	2.48	2.53	4.07	8.61	24.29
M	Scrofula	–	–	–	–	–	–	–	–
N+O	Tuberculosis	16.22	24.55	10.10	6.21	19.93	22.06	18.96	20.53
P	Cancer	7.97	1.11	0.35	0.13	0.62	3.60	18.43	47.22
Q	Heart	13.99	30.10	3.12	2.02	3.37	7.11	18.87	86.80
R	Brain and nerves	10.60	44.85	10.34	3.37	2.30	3.73	11.38	53.87
S	Lungs	23.03	204.62	41.14	3.89	4.25	7.50	17.84	87.04
T	Urinary system	2.66	4.42	1.61	0.89	1.21	2.32	4.40	9.27
U	Influenza	1.55	2.81	0.47	0.19	0.19	0.39	1.39	12.44
V	Other communicable diseases	0.58	7.46	1.31	0.55	0.21	0.21	0.18	0.15
W	Violence	2.65	4.31	4.61	1.21	1.88	1.90	2.96	6.49
X	Other causes	27.29	578.40	33.15	3.26	2.72	4.51	12.98	47.66
	All causes	169.34	1,810.76	168.82	32.56	43.59	64.98	118.16	664.47

Sources: See Appendix 2.

For the classification and grouping of the diseases, see Appendix 1.

Age-, sex- and cause-specific mortality (per 10,000 inhabitants)
ENGLAND AND WALES 1901–1910
Male

	Causes of death	All	0–1	1–2	2–5	5–10	10–15	15–20
A	Smallpox	0.16	0.49	0.12	0.14	0.08	0.06	0.07
B	Measles	3.28	32.49	61.12	13.83	1.60	0.10	0.04
C	Scarlet fever	1.11	2.06	5.63	7.28	2.75	0.60	0.34
D	Typhus	0.01	0.00	0.00	0.01	0.00	0.01	0.01
E	Influenza	2.16	5.06	1.83	0.64	0.30	0.23	0.55
F	Whooping cough	2.55	54.26	33.32	6.42	0.56	0.01	0.00
G	Diphtheria	1.78	4.00	10.24	11.38	4.93	0.88	0.20
H	Pyrexia	0.01	0.13	0.06	0.02	0.02	0.01	0.01
I	Enteric fever	1.09	0.11	0.19	0.43	0.52	0.71	1.37
J	Diarrhoea and dysentery	6.26	195.53	38.14	2.44	0.29	0.08	0.07
K	Pulmonary tuberculosis	5.84	3.43	4.01	1.51	0.74	0.77	3.07
L	Phthisis (not otherwise defined)	7.83	1.64	1.71	0.73	0.63	0.94	4.49
M	Tuberculous meningitis	1.89	19.62	16.78	6.64	2.68	1.14	0.64
N	Tuberculous peritonitis	1.08	15.18	8.01	2.14	0.86	0.58	0.46
O	Tabes mesenterica	0.53	14.19	4.58	0.75	0.15	0.08	0.02
P	Other tuberculous diseases	1.85	13.88	8.50	2.57	1.30	1.13	1.29
Q	Cancer	7.73	0.34	0.36	0.36	0.18	0.17	0.31
R	Septic diseases	1.01	6.37	0.77	0.28	0.24	0.29	0.42
S	Rheumatic fever	0.70	0.18	0.08	0.25	0.69	0.92	0.88
T	Pneumonia	14.67	148.30	90.06	17.12	3.16	1.24	2.54
U	Bronchitis	11.76	135.87	37.76	4.79	0.52	0.14	0.18
V	Childbirth and puerperal fever	0.00	0.00	0.00	0.00	0.00	0.00	0.00
W	Violence	8.27	29.01	9.12	7.46	3.29	2.62	4.47
X	Other causes	82.16	988.82	99.92	22.21	9.56	7.83	9.46
	All causes	163.73	1,670.97	432.30	109.40	35.04	20.54	30.89

Male

	Causes of death	20–25	25–35	35–45	45–55	55–65	65–75	>75–
A	Smallpox	0.11	0.16	0.25	0.27	0.18	0.17	0.17
B	Measles	0.02	0.02	0.02	0.01	0.00	0.00	0.01
C	Scarlet fever	0.17	0.10	0.05	0.02	0.01	0.00	0.01
D	Typhus	0.01	0.01	0.03	0.02	0.01	0.00	0.00
E	Influenza	0.67	0.98	1.70	3.07	6.29	12.91	28.02
F	Whooping cough	0.00	0.00	0.00	0.00	0.00	0.01	0.03
G	Diphtheria	0.11	0.07	0.06	0.05	0.05	0.07	0.07
H	Pyrexia	0.01	0.00	0.01	0.01	0.01	0.02	0.02
I	Enteric fever	1.79	1.78	1.42	1.04	0.80	0.40	0.17
J	Diarrhoea and dysentery	0.11	0.20	0.30	0.57	1.44	4.04	12.01
K	Pulmonary tuberculosis	6.19	8.21	10.36	11.50	9.96	6.44	2.42
L	Phthisis (not otherwise defined)	9.01	11.45	14.10	16.03	13.83	8.77	3.25
M	Tuberculous meningitis	0.39	0.27	0.20	0.14	0.08	0.05	0.01
N	Tuberculous peritonitis	0.39	0.32	0.32	0.33	0.37	0.26	0.10
O	Tabes mesenterica	0.02	0.01	0.01	0.01	0.01	0.01	0.00
P	Other tuberculous diseases	1.44	1.33	1.23	1.33	1.48	1.34	0.90
Q	Cancer	0.53	1.09	4.14	15.49	39.04	66.83	78.74
R	Septic diseases	0.50	0.56	0.90	1.45	2.27	3.90	6.86
S	Rheumatic fever	0.57	0.61	0.72	0.78	0.94	1.24	1.16
T	Pneumonia	3.68	5.31	9.60	15.34	24.94	37.61	55.45
U	Bronchitis	0.26	0.57	1.91	7.33	26.63	74.49	185.70
V	Childbirth and puerperal fever	0.00	0.00	0.00	0.00	0.00	0.00	0.00
W	Violence	5.55	6.77	9.14	12.57	16.23	18.18	26.21
X	Other causes	10.27	15.84	35.07	74.80	173.48	411.73	1,123.24
	All causes	41.80	55.65	91.54	162.17	318.06	648.47	1,524.54

Source: Decennial Supplement to the Annual Reports of the Registrar-General of Births, Deaths and Marriages in England and Wales (1901–1910).

Age-, sex- and cause-specific mortality (per 10,000 inhabitants)
ENGLAND AND WALES 1901–1910

Female

	Causes of death	All	0–1	1–2	2–5	5–10	10–15	15–20
A	Smallpox	0.10	0.59	0.18	0.13	0.07	0.06	0.06
B	Measles	2.90	27.67	55.46	14.31	1.88	0.10	0.05
C	Scarlet fever	1.01	1.72	5.28	6.93	2.73	0.69	0.25
D	Typhus	0.01	0.00	0.00	0.00	0.00	0.00	0.01
E	Influenza	2.12	3.66	1.39	0.63	0.32	0.25	0.43
F	Whooping cough	2.97	60.83	43.56	9.60	0.91	0.03	0.01
G	Diphtheria	1.78	3.27	9.89	11.41	6.03	0.95	0.20
H	Pyrexia	0.02	0.11	0.06	0.05	0.02	0.01	0.01
I	Enteric fever	0.74	0.08	0.19	0.42	0.59	0.81	1.00
J	Diarrhoea and dysentery	5.12	164.28	35.63	2.47	0.35	0.09	0.06
K	Pulmonary tuberculosis	3.86	2.85	3.44	1.31	0.98	1.61	3.88
L	Phthisis (not otherwise defined)	5.83	1.39	1.40	0.72	0.95	2.34	6.00
M	Tuberculous meningitis	1.63	15.62	14.70	6.38	2.66	1.25	0.68
N	Tuberculous peritonitis	0.98	11.81	6.69	1.83	0.93	0.68	0.64
O	Tabes mesenterica	0.40	10.80	3.97	0.67	0.16	0.07	0.03
P	Other tuberculous diseases	1.52	11.17	7.43	2.32	1.28	1.14	1.27
Q	Cancer	10.27	0.25	0.28	0.31	0.13	0.15	0.27
R	Septic diseases	0.78	6.23	0.85	0.31	0.20	0.22	0.32
S	Rheumatic fever	0.72	0.14	0.07	0.23	0.78	1.12	0.89
T	Pneumonia	10.56	112.22	80.58	16.38	3.09	1.23	1.61
U	Bronchitis	11.56	106.50	36.81	4.82	0.57	0.16	0.18
V	Childbirth and puerperal fever	2.11	0.00	0.00	0.00	0.00	0.00	0.67
W	Violence	3.33	27.32	7.37	5.82	2.26	0.81	1.03
X	Other causes	73.75	761.48	87.94	20.22	9.21	7.86	9.38
	All causes	144.04	1,329.98	403.17	107.27	36.12	21.66	28.92

Female

	Causes of death	20–25	25–35	35–45	45–55	55–65	65–75	<75–
A	Smallpox	0.07	0.10	0.12	0.08	0.06	0.07	0.04
B	Measles	0.03	0.03	0.03	0.01	0.01	0.01	0.01
C	Scarlet fever	0.18	0.13	0.06	0.02	0.01	0.01	0.0
D	Typhus	0.00	0.01	0.02	0.01	0.01	0.00	0.00
E	Influenza	0.50	0.75	1.25	2.23	5.25	13.52	30.12
F	Whooping cough	0.00	0.00	0.00	0.00	0.01	0.01	0.02
G	Diphtheria	0.10	0.09	0.07	0.06	0.08	0.07	0.04
H	Pyrexia	0.01	0.01	0.01	0.01	0.01	0.02	0.03
I	Enteric fever	0.99	0.97	0.86	0.67	0.50	0.29	0.10
J	Diarrhoea and dysentery	0.09	0.16	0.29	0.49	1.35	3.82	10.89
K	Pulmonary tuberculosis	4.70	5.69	6.02	4.99	4.02	2.85	1.38
L	Phthisis (not otherwise defined)	7.65	9.07	9.49	8.11	6.45	4.70	2.19
M	Tuberculous meningitis	0.38	0.23	0.17	0.11	0.06	0.02	0.02
N	Tuberculous peritonitis	0.49	0.50	0.43	0.36	0.29	0.19	0.12
O	Tabes mesenterica	0.01	0.01	0.01	0.01	0.01	0.01	0.01
P	Other tuberculous diseases	1.03	1.02	0.99	0.91	1.03	1.15	1.23
Q	Cancer	0.39	1.70	8.46	23.21	44.10	66.58	79.01
R	Septic diseases	0.39	0.45	0.62	0.89	1.42	2.45	4.50
S	Rheumatic fever	0.60	0.53	0.62	0.80	0.96	1.22	1.14
T	Pneumonia	1.99	3.02	5.01	7.47	14.40	27.86	46.65
U	Bronchitis	0.22	0.48	1.82	6.22	22.91	70.22	185.77
V	Childbirth and puerperal fever	3.66	6.07	5.19	0.26	0.00	0.00	0.00
W	Violence	1.11	1.35	1.98	3.07	4.23	7.52	22.87
X	Other causes	10.40	15.10	31.77	65.11	141.30	336.66	975.88
	All causes	34.99	47.44	75.29	125.08	248.48	539.28	1,362.04

Source: *Decennial Supplement to the Annual Reports of the Registrar-General of Births, Deaths and Marriages in England and Wales* (1901–1910).

Age-, sex- and cause-specific mortality (per 10,000 inhabitants)
ALL ENGLISH TOWNS 1901-1910
Male

	Causes of death	All	0–1	1–2	2–5	5–10	10–15	15–20
A	Smallpox	0.08	0.31	0.06	0.04	0.03	0.01	0.03
B	Measles	4.80	44.20	91.02	20.59	1.79	0.07	0.02
C	Scarlet fever	1.51	2.89	8.29	10.38	3.54	0.78	0.38
D	Typhus	0.03	0.00	0.00	0.01	0.01	0.02	0.02
E	Influenza	1.73	3.34	1.21	0.45	0.23	0.15	0.43
F	Whooping cough	3.23	59.12	45.12	9.27	0.79	0.01	0.00
G	Diphtheria	1.94	5.99	14.84	12.16	4.70	0.65	0.15
H	Pyrexia	0.01	0.14	0.03	0.02	0.02	0.01	0.00
I	Enteric fever	1.15	0.12	0.17	0.39	0.51	0.76	1.42
J	Diarrhoea and dysentery	8.89	269.54	60.12	3.63	0.35	0.10	0.08
K	Pulmonary tuberculosis	9.81	4.64	6.49	2.41	1.08	0.96	4.13
L	Phthisis (not otherwise defined)	9.11	1.46	1.67	0.82	0.65	0.92	4.38
M	Tuberculous meningitis	2.40	24.31	22.87	9.15	3.23	1.12	0.60
N	Tuberculous peritonitis	1.20	16.67	9.10	2.66	1.02	0.61	0.44
O	Tabes mesenterica	0.58	15.23	4.79	0.87	0.15	0.06	0.02
P	Other tuberculous diseases	2.15	16.56	11.65	3.86	1.76	1.35	1.35
Q	Cancer	8.85	0.50	0.62	0.54	0.30	0.30	0.52
R	Septic diseases	1.35	8.32	1.31	0.44	0.28	0.43	0.60
S	Rheumatic fever	0.70	0.27	0.07	0.26	0.80	1.01	0.80
T	Pneumonia	18.68	175.98	121.58	23.20	4.03	1.54	2.97
U	Bronchitis	14.25	146.78	42.75	5.41	0.61	0.20	0.25
V	Childbirth and puerperal fever	0.00	0.00	0.00	0.00	0.00	0.00	0.00
W	Violence	8.87	51.74	11.21	9.36	3.90	2.66	3.46
X	Other causes	81.81	1,032.97	117.97	25.05	10.65	9.59	11.39
	All causes	183.14	188,1.09	572.95	140.99	40.43	23.32	33.46

Male

	Causes of death	20–25	25–35	35–45	45–55	55–65	65–75	>75–
A	Smallpox	0.06	0.07	0.14	0.15	0.08	0.07	0.06
B	Measles	0.01	0.01	0.01	0.01	0.01	0.00	0.00
C	Scarlet fever	0.16	0.12	0.06	0.02	0.01	0.00	0.03
D	Typhus	0.03	0.04	0.08	0.05	0.02	0.00	0.00
E	Influenza	0.56	0.86	1.56	2.95	5.69	11.69	23.79
F	Whooping cough	0.00	0.00	0.00	0.00	0.00	0.00	0.00
G	Diphtheria	0.08	0.07	0.06	0.04	0.05	0.06	0.06
H	Pyrexia	0.00	0.00	0.00	0.01	0.00	0.02	0.03
I	Enteric fever	1.83	1.92	1.54	1.01	0.80	0.33	0.15
J	Diarrhoea and dysentery	0.11	0.21	0.34	0.60	1.61	4.40	12.50
K	Pulmonary tuberculosis	7.89	11.78	18.36	22.18	19.54	13.48	5.97
L	Phthisis (not otherwise defined)	8.35	11.74	17.35	20.88	18.04	11.15	4.45
M	Tuberculous meningitis	0.37	0.26	0.21	0.13	0.07	0.07	0.00
N	Tuberculous peritonitis	0.31	0.30	0.30	0.33	0.41	0.31	0.12
O	Tabes mesenterica	0.01	0.01	0.01	0.01	0.01	0.00	0.00
P	Other tuberculous diseases	1.27	1.19	1.24	1.45	1.58	1.50	0.97
Q	Cancer	0.71	1.52	5.71	21.78	49.79	77.57	83.91
R	Septic diseases	0.71	0.84	1.24	2.05	3.13	5.11	9.13
S	Rheumatic fever	0.53	0.55	0.77	0.75	0.97	1.12	1.17
T	Pneumonia	4.29	6.72	12.68	20.64	33.23	50.17	82.57
U	Bronchitis	0.42	0.95	3.22	11.83	40.86	111.19	263.44
V	Childbirth and puerperal fever	0.00	0.00	0.00	0.00	0.00	0.00	0.00
W	Violence	4.43	6.05	8.92	13.01	17.44	20.33	36.18
X	Other causes	11.39	17.59	40.17	86.38	192.61	428.82	1,064.54
	All causes	43.54	62.82	113.97	206.27	385.95	737.40	1,589.05

Source: *Decennial Supplement to the Annual Reports of the Registrar-General of Births, Deaths and Marriages in England and Wales* (1901–1910).

Age-, sex- and cause-specific mortality (per 10,000 inhabitants)
ALL ENGLISH TOWNS 1901-1910
Female

	Causes of death	All	0–1	1–2	2–5	5–10	10–15	15–20
A	Smallpox	0.05	0.39	0.13	0.07	0.03	0.03	0.02
B	Measles	4.11	38.63	82.25	20.95	2.17	0.06	0.02
C	Scarlet fever	1.31	2.25	7.52	9.79	3.48	0.84	0.25
D	Typhus	0.02	0.00	0.01	0.01	0.01	0.01	0.02
E	Influenza	1.73	2.37	1.10	0.41	0.28	0.16	0.29
F	Whooping cough	3.73	67.47	59.46	13.65	1.27	0.03	0.00
G	Diphtheria	1.86	4.88	14.58	12.67	5.46	0.72	0.17
H	Pyrexia	0.01	0.08	0.04	0.04	0.02	0.01	0.00
I	Enteric fever	0.73	0.11	0.23	0.38	0.53	0.81	0.89
J	Diarrhoea and dysentery	7.05	227.19	55.35	3.87	0.42	0.10	0.08
K	Pulmonary tuberculosis	5.11	4.08	5.39	2.11	1.32	1.82	4.25
L	Phthisis (not otherwise defined)	5.77	1.07	1.40	0.76	1.03	1.87	4.84
M	Tuberculous meningitis	1.98	20.30	20.49	8.79	3.15	1.13	0.49
N	Tuberculous peritonitis	1.00	12.70	7.52	2.30	1.07	0.64	0.53
O	Tabes mesenterica	0.43	12.00	4.16	0.68	0.20	0.07	0.02
P	Other tuberculous diseases	1.66	13.81	9.99	3.46	1.72	1.34	1.10
Q	Cancer	10.65	0.36	0.39	0.45	0.22	0.22	0.35
R	Septic diseases	1.02	8.25	1.40	0.41	0.29	0.32	0.52
S	Rheumatic fever	0.74	0.14	0.08	0.30	0.91	1.28	0.85
T	Pneumonia	13.26	138.63	110.27	22.34	3.95	1.58	1.76
U	Bronchitis	14.20	118.45	42.22	5.63	0.63	0.19	0.24
V	Childbirth and puerperal fever	1.95	0.00	0.00	0.00	0.00	0.00	0.56
W	Violence	4.44	48.91	9.72	7.80	3.07	0.98	0.99
X	Other causes	71.80	794.26	103.83	22.57	10.38	9.23	10.10
	All causes	154.60	1,516.35	537.52	139.43	41.60	23.44	28.36

Female

	Causes of death	20–25	25–35	35–45	45–55	55–65	65–75	>75–
A	Smallpox	0.03	0.05	0.07	0.03	0.04	0.04	0.03
B	Measles	0.02	0.03	0.03	0.02	0.00	0.01	0.03
C	Scarlet fever	0.19	0.12	0.05	0.01	0.02	0.01	0.02
D	Typhus	0.01	0.03	0.06	0.04	0.04	0.00	0.02
E	Influenza	0.36	0.60	1.12	2.14	4.97	12.54	27.96
F	Whooping cough	0.00	0.00	0.00	0.00	0.00	0.02	0.02
G	Diphtheria	0.07	0.07	0.08	0.04	0.09	0.05	0.03
H	Pyrexia	0.00	0.00	0.01	0.00	0.00	0.01	0.00
I	Enteric fever	0.88	0.99	0.91	0.69	0.44	0.19	0.13
J	Diarrhoea and dysentery	0.08	0.12	0.24	0.45	1.39	4.14	11.93
K	Pulmonary tuberculosis	4.85	6.43	8.72	8.03	6.10	4.40	2.34
L	Phthisis (not otherwise defined)	6.00	7.98	10.50	9.49	7.42	4.91	2.65
M	Tuberculous meningitis	0.27	0.19	0.12	0.11	0.05	0.01	0.00
N	Tuberculous peritonitis	0.37	0.36	0.34	0.34	0.24	0.21	0.08
O	Tabes mesenterica	0.01	0.01	0.01	0.01	0.00	0.01	0.00
P	Other tuberculous diseases	0.82	0.82	0.87	0.77	0.87	1.20	1.71
Q	Cancer	0.51	2.22	10.37	27.02	48.91	69.42	79.43
R	Septic diseases	0.60	0.59	0.81	1.16	1.88	3.24	6.00
S	Rheumatic fever	0.62	0.55	0.63	0.83	0.87	1.33	1.21
T	Pneumonia	2.07	3.45	6.36	10.30	19.55	35.91	61.96
U	Bronchitis	0.22	0.68	3.05	10.67	36.52	100.17	250.26
V	Childbirth and puerperal fever	3.28	5.36	4.44	0.21	0.00	0.00	0.00
W	Violence	1.10	1.54	2.47	4.05	5.81	10.45	30.02
X	Other causes	10.64	16.09	36.72	74.68	151.68	335.90	915.61
	All causes	33.00	48.27	87.97	151.09	286.88	584.20	1,391.43

Source: *Decennial Supplement to the Annual Reports of the Registrar-General of Births, Deaths and Marriages in England and Wales* (1901–1910).

MORTALITY PROFILE AND DISEASE PANORAMA IN THE LARGEST TOWNS IN ENGLAND AND WALES AND IN GERMANY

England and Wales

LONDON

1871–1880: London's health conditions were better than most of the ten English largest towns, with the death rates of almost all diseases being below the average for all towns in the sample. Having the densest net of medical provision, London registered the lowest death rate of 'other causes'.

1901–1910: London had kept its favourable status. Pulmonary tuberculosis and cancer were the only diseases which registered obviously higher death rates than the average of all towns in the English sample. The latter may not have been the result of environmental conditions or of the effects of big city lifestyle, but rather be attributed to the frequency of professional diagnosis resulting from the better doctor: population ratio in comparison with the other towns, which might also have been responsible for the continuing low death rate from 'other causes'.

BRISTOL

1871–1880: South-eastern Bristol was the healthiest town of the English sample, with an especially low death rate in the registration district of Clifton (Bristol RD: 25.5; Clifton RD: 20.0 deaths per 1,000 inhabitants). This status resulted mainly from the low rates in the main killer groups of phthisis, diarrhoea and dysentery, and especially from diseases of the respiratory system. The death rate from scarlet fever was also much lower than in the northern towns of England and was quite similar to the London death rates. Diseases of the nervous and of the circulatory system as well as cancer registered higher rates than the ten-city average. In an inner-city comparison the most striking difference between the registration districts of Bristol and Clifton lay in the death rate from diseases of the respiratory system, with 52.31 deaths per 10,000 inhabitants in the Bristol RD and 36.25 in the Clifton RD, followed by violence, with 15.13 deaths per 10,000 inhabitants in the Bristol RD and only 3.48 in the Clifton RD.

1901–1910: Bristol remained the healthiest city, even becoming the only city in the sample with a death rate lower than for the whole of England and Wales. Only the death rate from diphtheria surpassed the average for the ten cities.

BIRMINGHAM

1871–1880: The city of Birmingham, situated in the Midlands, was the 'average town' of the English sample. The death rate was 23.6 per 1,000 inhabitants, again with poor conditions in the inner-city district in comparison with the surrounding area (25.8 deaths per 1,000 inhabitants in the registration district of Birmingham, 20.7 in the Aston RD). Birmingham RD was unhealthier in any respect, but again the differences were predominantly marked by diseases of the respiratory system, followed by phthisis, violence, 'other causes', diseases of the nervous system and diarrhoea and dysentery.

1901–1910: The 'best governed city in the world' had lost its average position due to the bad health conditions in the Birmingham registration district. In the inner-city, the death rates had not improved as much as in the neighbouring Aston RD. The differences between the two registration districts were in relation to all diseases, but are still predominantly marked by respiratory diseases, violence, cancer and to a lesser degree by diarrhoea and dysentery as well as measles.

LIVERPOOL

1871–1880: The world harbour city of Liverpool was the town with the second highest death rates in the English sample (after Manchester), with especially poor conditions in the registration district of Liverpool (33.6 per 1,000 inhabitants) in contrast to much better rates in the West Derby RD (23.4) and, beyond the Mersey, in the Birkenhead RD (20.4). Almost all diseases were implicated in for these conditions. Especially high death rates occurred from typhus, diarrhoea and dysentery, diseases of the nervous system, phthisis, violence, 'other causes' and a very high rate from diseases of the respiratory system, which was only comparable with the rate in the Manchester RD.

1901–1910: Liverpool had taken over the role of the unhealthiest city in the sample from Manchester, with a still extraordinarily high crude death rate in the Liverpool RD of 30.5 deaths per 1,000 inhabitants. This constituted only a slight improvement in comparison with the period of 1871–1880. Especially predominant causes of death in comparison with the other towns in the English sample were pneumonia, bronchitis, diarrhoea and dysentery, violence and 'other causes'. The death rate from diarrhoea and dysentery was even worse than in the first period selected for the analysis.

BOLTON

1871–1880: Bolton registered the typical disease panorama of the northern English towns, with especially high death rates from lung diseases and gastro-intestinal disorders.

1901–1910: The death rates in Bolton had improved substantially, yet the rates were still above the average of the towns in the English sample. All diseases had contributed to this picture.

MANCHESTER

1871–1880: Manchester, the archetype for the inhumane conditions in the early phase of industrialization, was the unhealthiest town in the English sample during the selected period. In comparison with the other unhealthy place in the north, Liverpool, these high rates resulted mainly from the key killers of the respiratory and digestive group, followed by diseases of the nervous system (diseases of the respiratory system: 57.89 deaths per 10,000 inhabitants; phthisis: 30.10; diarrhoea and dysentery: 18.39; diseases of the nervous system: 33.02). And again the inner-city, the registration district of Manchester, was the place with the worst living conditions.
1901–1910: Manchester, however, was the town which showed the biggest improvements in health conditions, resulting from a vast reduction in mortality from the main killers. The inner-city remained a bad place to live in, and, worthy of note, the number of deaths from violence had even increased. With a death rate of 19.04 per 10,000 inhabitants it constituted one of the most predominant single causes of death in Manchester registration district, only surpassed by the death rate from pneumonia (25.71).

BRADFORD

1871–1880: Bradford registered the typical disease panorama of the northern English towns, with a high prevalence of lung diseases and gastro-intestinal disorders.
1901–1910: Health conditions in Bradford had improved quite substantially, as a consequence of which it had become one of the rare northern towns with a lower mortality rate than the average for all English towns in the sample. This, however, has to be taken with a pinch of salt, as due to major boundary changes in the Bradford registration district the city, together with Leeds, is one of the problem cases in the English sample (see Chapter 3).

LEEDS

1871–1880: Leeds was almost as unhealthy a place as Liverpool and Manchester, even surpassing the two where the crude mortality rates from digestive and nervous diseases were concerned.
1901–1910: Substantial improvements in the death rates had occurred in Leeds, referring to all disease groups, yet, just like in the case of Bradford, this again has to be considered within the context of major boundary changes concerning the registration district.

SHEFFIELD

1871–1880: Sheffield was an unhealthy northern town with a typically high risk of dying from respiratory diseases, showing the average improvement by 1901–1910.

NEWCASTLE

1871–1880: Newcastle was another unhealthy northern town, despite a comparatively lower death rate from diseases of the respiratory system. The town had kept its relative standing in the period 1901–1910.

Germany

BERLIN

1877: The capital Berlin was one of the unhealthiest places in the German sample due in large degree to a high mortality rate from intestinal diseases, whereas the death rates from respiratory disease were almost average when compared with the other towns in the German sample.

1885: By 1885 the situation had improved, and Berlin had become one of the healthier towns in the sample. Despite this, Berlin registered the highest death rate from diphtheria in the sample.

1900: Berlin managed to maintain its good position, although there was a rise in the death rate from various diseases, especially in the death rates from cancer and diseases of the circulatory system. On the other hand, there was a sharp decline in diphtheria mortality, and further slight improvements in the death rates from digestive diseases.

1907: In 1907 this advantage had been completely lost, and Berlin registered quite average rates from all causes of death, even in the death rate from digestive diseases.

BRESLAU

1877: Breslau, situated in the east, was the unhealthiest town of the sample, resulting from very high death rates from intestinal diseases, respiratory diseases—but not tuberculosis with rates below the average—diseases of the brain and nerves as well as from 'weakness of life'.

1885: By 1885 the situation in Breslau had improved only slightly, and the town kept its position as the unhealthiest town of the sample.

1900: Breslau maintained this position until the end of the century. Very high infant mortality rates, resulting from a high mortality from digestive diseases and 'weakness of life', were accompanied by high mortality rates from tuberculosis and from diseases of the respiratory system in all age-groups. In addition there was also a high death rate from the degenerative diseases complex.

1907: Mortality from digestive diseases and 'weakness of life' had been reduced substantially. Breslau remained, however, an unhealthy town. The high death rates from tuberculosis and respiratory diseases were now accompanied by high death rates from diseases of the circulatory system.

COLOGNE

1877: Cologne, an old commercial town, had an average overall death rate. The high death rates from intestinal diseases were counterbalanced by low rates of respiratory diseases and 'weakness of life'.

1885: Improvements in the death rate from numerous diseases were counterbalanced by a deterioration of the death rate from 'weakness of life', so that the overall death rate remained quite stable.

1900: In Cologne CDR improved with a strong decline in the tuberculosis death rate from 42.83 deaths per 10,000 inhabitants in 1885 to 29.04, whereas the death rate from digestive diseases even increased from 50.89 to 64.82 per 10,000 inhabitants.

1907: The most substantial improvement occurred after the turn of the century. This affected all age-groups, but especially infants. Correspondingly there was a strong decline in the death rate from digestive diseases.

DRESDEN

1877: For Dresden in 1877 only eleven causes of death were registered. Of the main killers only tuberculosis can be compared with the other towns of the sample, showing quite average rates.

1900: The average health conditions in Dresden were confirmed by a more complete disease panorama in 1900.

1910: By this time Dresden had become the healthiest town in the sample with relatively low death rates from almost all diseases, but especially the main killers.

DÜSSELDORF

1877: Düsseldorf was the healthiest town in the sample in 1877. A tuberculosis death rate above the average for all towns was counterbalanced by especially low rates of respiratory diseases and 'weakness of life'.

1900: The CDR decreased, a result to a large extent of a sharp decline in tuberculosis mortality from 40.58 to 21.05 per 10,000 inhabitants. The death rate from respiratory diseases increased, however, from 19.80 to 29.69 deaths per 10,000 inhabitants. Very predominant were the diseases of the digestive system, with 50.18 deaths per 10,000 inhabitants.

1907: Düsseldorf registered quite an average CDR, yet the death rates from intestinal diseases were still above the average for the sample.

FRANKFURT

1877: Frankfurt was amongst the healthier towns in the sample, as a result mainly of a low death rate of infants and children from digestive diseases and weakness. Together with Hamburg and Leipzig, it belongs to the group of towns with better death rates than the Prussian average, resulting in this case from low death rates from infirmity and from intestinal diseases.

1885: There was quite a strong improvement in health conditions by 1885, as a result of a reduction in mortality from almost all diseases with special emphasis on 'other causes', digestive, brain and respiratory diseases, whereas tuberculosis, measles and rubella, whooping cough and cancer registered higher rates.

1900: Frankfurt had a relatively low mortality rate as a result of very low rates of digestive diseases, whereas the death rates from tuberculosis and respiratory diseases were quite average. The infant mortality rate was very low in comparison with the other towns of the German sample, but almost all other age-groups registered lower rates as well.

1907: This development continued more slowly, with strongest improvements in infant mortality from digestive diseases and 'weakness of life'.

HAMBURG

1877: The port city registered death rates below the Prussian average, merely a result from the low death rate from infirmity.

1885: The situation in Hamburg remained almost stable. Strong improvements in the death rate from respiratory diseases may have been a consequence of changes in registration as the rate from influenza registered a substantial increase.

1900: By this time, health conditions in Hamburg had improved, diphtheria had been conquered, and the death rates from almost all diseases had reduced (especially the main killers), with the exception of the degenerative diseases (cancer and circulatory system).

1907: Mortality continued to improve due to a reduction in the death rate from almost all diseases, but especially from the main killers, diseases of the digestive and the respiratory system.

LEIPZIG

1877: In Leipzig again the low death rate from infirmity is responsible for the crude death rate being below the average for Prussia. In comparison with the other towns of the sample, almost all the main killers showed better death rates.

1885: Leipzig managed to maintain this good position.

1912: By 1912, it was amongst the healthiest towns of the sample.

MUNICH

1885: Munich was an unhealthy town with high death rates from digestive and respiratory diseases as well as from infirmity. This has to be taken with caution as there was an exceptionally high death rate from 'other causes' (50.17 per 10,000 inhabitants).

1900: As this category decreased substantially, down to 14.70 per 10,000 inhabitants), with hardly any change in the CDR, the disease panorama of Munich reveals a predominance of digestive diseases and deaths from 'weakness of life', which burdened infants especially. The degenerative diseases (cancer, circulatory system) as well as infirmity had strongly increased by 1900.

1907: The major improvement occurred after the turn of the century, with substantially decreased mortality rates from intestinal diseases, reducing infant mortality, whereas the death rate from tuberculosis, diseases of the respiratory system and infirmity even increased. The latter, however, might be attributed at least in some degree to the strong decline in the 'other causes' group, which became especially low in the higher age-groups.

NUREMBERG

1877–1913: Nuremberg's high death rate from digestive disease is comparable with Munich. In addition, however, there were also extraordinarily high death rates from diseases of the respiratory system and from tuberculosis.

APPENDIX 8

ECONOMIC CLASSIFICATION OF THE LARGEST ENGLISH CITIES AND REGISTRATION DISTRICTS ACCORDING TO GREENHOW AND WELTON

	Greenhow, 1858	Welton, 1911
Aston	hardware manufacture	metal working, engineering
Birmingham	hardware manufacture	metal working, engineering
Barton Reg.	–	–
Bolton	–	cotton, engineering
Bradford	–	woollen
Bristol	commerce	commerce, boots, engineering
Chorlton	cotton manufacture	–
Ecclesall Bierlow	cutlery	–
Gateshead	mining, iron, glass manufacture	engineering, colliery
Leeds	woollen manufacture	engineering, commerce, woollen
Liverpool	commerce	commercial
Manchester	cotton manufacture	engineering, commerce, cotton
Newcastle upon Tyne	commerce	engineering, shipbuilding, commerce
Prestwich	–	cotton
Preston	cotton manufacture	–
Salford	cotton manufacture	engineering, cotton, commerce
Sheffield	hardware	tools, steel, metal working
West Derby	commerce	–
Toxteth Park	–	–
London	commerce	–

Sources: Greenhow, 1858; Welton, 1911.

THE EXPANSION OF CENTRALIZED WATER SUPPLY AND SEWERAGE SYSTEMS IN THE TEN LARGEST GERMAN AND ENGLISH TOWNS

Germany

Town	Timing; system
Berlin	Waterworks opened in 1856; intensive expansion phase at the end of 1870s–80s (1876/77/88), r., lake, f.; sewerage scheme commenced in 1852 (gutters), comprehensive sewerage scheme since 1873; centralized canalization; mixed system; purification: irrigation farms.
Breslau	Waterworks opened in 1871, r., f.; commencement of sewerage scheme: 1881; centralized canalization; mixed system; purification: irrigation farms.
Cologne	Waterworks opened in 1871, gr., commencement of sewerage scheme: 1881; centralized canalization; mixed and separate system; purification: filter bed (test).
Dresden	Waterworks opened in 1875, gr., sp.; commencement of sewerage scheme: 1890; centralized canalization; mixed system; purification: rake.
Düsseldorf	Waterworks opened in 1870, gr.; commencement of sewerage scheme: 1884; centralized canalization; mixed and separate system; purification: filter bed.
Frankfurt	Waterworks opened in 1873 (sp.), 1885 (gr.) and 1885 (f.); commencement of sewerage scheme: 1867; centralized canalization; mixed system; purification: rake and filter bed.
Hamburg	Centralized water supply since 1849, filter plant since 1893, r.; commencement of sewerage scheme: 1842; centralized canalization; mixed system; purification: rake, biological '*Füllverfahren*' without septic tank treatment, tests: biological '*Tropfverfahren*' without septic tank treatment.
Leipzig	Waterworks opened in 1866 and 1887, gr.; commencement of sewerage scheme: 1860; centralized canalization; mixed sys-

tem with flush faeces; purification: filter bed and chemical-mechanical purification.

Munich   Waterworks opened in 1883, sp.; sewerage scheme since 1880/81; centralized canalization; mixed system; purification: none.

Nuremberg   Waterworks opened in 1865 and 1885, gr.; commencement of sewerage scheme: 1874; centralized canalization; mixed system without faeces; purification: none.

Sewerage scheme: system and purification 1907. Water supply (1890): sp.=spring water; gr.=ground water; r.=river; f.=artificially filtered.

Sources: *Statistisches Jahrbuch Deutscher Städte*, **1** (1890) onwards; Grahn, 1883; 1898–1902; Brix et al., 1934; Salomon, 1907; 1911.

England and Wales

Town	**Timing; system**
Birmingham	*water supply*: constant supply of 8.5 million gallons daily for 483,923 inhabitants in 15 square miles (1880s); three-quarters from wells described by the Rivers Pollution Commissioners as of a 'uniformly excellent quality'; one-quarter from river water. *sewerage*: start of construction in 1852; sewage untreated in Rivers Tame and Rea; 1859 first sedimentation tank; 59.3 km sewers in use by 1903; precipitation, 18 tanks; borough and 8 other districts: 13 million gallons daily.
Bolton	*water supply*: waterworks corporation established in 1824 two service reservoirs, four storage reservoirs; constant supply of 2,625,000 gallons in the borough (1880s); works carried out under Bolton Improvement Acts, 1854, 1864, and 1865; no filtering beds. *sewerage*: date of the sewage scheme 1872 and 1884/1886; precipitation chiefly by lime; system of sewers is single; no pumping of sewage; volume 3.5 million gallons/24h; 9 tanks; privy and ashpit town, but 1,640 closets; system is considered satisfactory.
Bradford	*water supply*: derived from various gathering-grounds; supply in Bradford is 24 gallons per head for domestic purposes and 20 gallons for trade purposes, or from 8.25 to 8.5 million

gallons per day (1880s); works were carried out under the Bradford Corporation Water Works Act, 1854; Amendment Act, 1855; Acts of 1858, 1862; Waterworks and Improvement Act, 1868, 1873, 1875 and 1878, Waterworks Act, 1869.
sewerage: precipitation by lime since 1885; sewage is pumped; 8.45 million gallons daily; 4,000 water-closets; separate tank system.

Bristol

water supply: works carried out under Bristol Waterworks Act, 1862; Amendment Acts, 1865 and 1872; 1851: 4 million gallons daily; little rain in the winters of 1861–1863, so 1864 only 350,000 gallons per day; additional store reservoirs built.
sewerage: discharged by gravitation; houses generally have water-closets or privies; houses generally drain into the sewers.

Leeds

water supply: from gathering-grounds at Eccup, and from the River Washburn; water is filtered; yield is about 14,000,000 gallons, half the quantity is used; Waterwork Acts 1852, 1862, 1867, 1874, and 1877; the works cost £535,620.
sewerage: lime precipitation, 11 tanks; system of sewers single; 9 million gallons daily; the effluent flows into the river; 10 million gallons daily; population 320,000; 12 tanks; effluent water was to be found fairly clear.

Liverpool

water supply: First Waterworks Act in 1709; 1847 Corporation Waterworks Act; the works cost £256,808; 1879 average supply estimated 672,00 gallons, which is equal to 22.8 gallons per head for all purposes; various gathering-grounds; million gallons daily: 11 (early 1880s: 16); gallons per inhabitant: 20.
sewerage: Sanitary Act, 1846; by 1858 costs £215,231, saving £10,000 per annum; 1876 'victory of the water-closet'.

London

water supply: million gallons daily: 145; gallons per inhabitant: 38; 8 waterworks: East London, New River, Southwark and Vauxhall, Lambeth, West Middlesex, Grand Junction, Kent, Chelsea.
sewerage: 16 km of sewers by 1832; by 1853 construction of sewers completed (64.8 km); severe pollution, since sewers discharged directly into Thames; tons of sewage discharged weekly: 777,000; construction of storage tanks.

Manchester

water supply: 1847 Corporation Waterworks Act; 1851 first supply from Longdendale; 1894 first supply from Thirlmere; 1904 second pipe from Thirlmere; 1915 third pipe from

Thirlmere; million gallons daily: 11 (early 1880s: 19); gallons per inhabitant: 20.

sewerage: population 380,000; principally pail system; single system of sewers;v 9 million gallons daily; precipitation intended; 1851 privy midden, drainage to rivers; 1868 improved middens; 1879 drainage system proposed and abandoned; 1878 precipitation (Salford); 1885 scheme renewed; 1889 scheme sanctioned; 1894 work completed, problems with filters and presses; 1895 faults found in construction; filter experiments; 1896 problems over capacity and construction; 1897 sludge disposal in Irish Sea; 1898 construction of percolating filters (Salford); 1899 experiments: bacteria beds, septic tanks, Roscoe filters; 1902 building of contact beds begins; 1904 septic tanks installed; 1907 secondary contact beds installed; 1911 second drainage scheme sanctioned; 1914 experiments with activated sludge (Salford); Salford 12 tanks similar to those in Leeds; tons of sewage discharged weekly: 777,000.

Newcastle   *water supply*: 1868 5.5 million gallons per day, 27.5 per head; original gravitation work constructed in 1846–48 with 1.5 million gallons per day; additional reservoirs were constructed, but still insufficient supply, so that the River Tyne had to be pumped; 1880s supply 9 million gallons daily for 145,228 inhabitants (Newcastle); 1.8 million gallons for 65,873 inhabitants (Gateshead).

sewerage: drainage very defective (1844); sewage into the sea; irrigation farm (1893).

Sheffield   *water supply*: supply by private company; 4,858,584 gallons delivered daily to 50,000 houses and 700 works; service 12 hours every day (1860s); Sheffield Waterworks Act 1853, 1860, 1864, 1867, 1873.

sewerage: date of sewerage scheme 1883; single system of sewers; no pumping of sewage; 10 million gallons daily, 30 tanks; 75% use privies, 25% water closets; lime precipitation.

Sources: Baldwin-Wiseman, 1909; *First Report*, 1844; *Manchester Corporation, Council Proceedings 1884–85*; Midwinter, 1969; Mulhall, 1886; de Rance, 1882; *Report of the Royal Sanitary Commission*, 1874; Royal Commission on Water Supply, 1869; Silverthorne, 1884; Stanbridge, 1976; Wardle, 1893; Wilson, 1990.

BIBLIOGRAPHY

ABEL, W. (1981), *Stufen der Ernährung. Eine historische Skizze*, Göttingen.

AMBROSIUS, G. (1987), 'Die wirtschaftliche Entwicklung von Gas-, Wasser- und Elektrizitätswerken (ab ca. 1850 bis zur Gegenwart)', in H. Pohl (ed.), *Kommunale Unternehmen. Geschichte und Gegenwart*, Zeitschrift für Unternehmensgeschichte, Beiheft 42, Stuttgart, 125–53.

Annual Reports of the Registrar-General of Births, Deaths, and Marriages in England and Wales (1851–1910).

ASCHROTT, P. F. (1886), 'Die Arbeiterwohnungsfrage in England', *Schriften des Vereins für Socialpolitik*, **30**, Vol. 1, 93–146.

ASHTON, J. (ed.) (1992), *Healthy Cities*, Milton Keynes.

ASHLEY, J. and T. DEVIS (1992), 'Death Certification from the Point of View of the Epidemiologist', *Population Trends*, **67**, 22–28.

ASHLEY, W. J. (1904), *The Progress of the German Working Classes in the Last Quarter of a Century*, London.

ASMUS, G. (ed.) (1982), *Hinterhof, Keller und Mansarde. Einblicke in Berliner Wohnungselend 1901–1920*, Reinbek bei Hamburg.

ATKINS, P. J. (1992), 'White Poison?: The Social Consequences of Milk Consumption in London, 1850–1939', *Social History of Medicine*, **5**, 207–28.

AYERS, P. (1990), 'The Hidden Economy of Dockland Families: Liverpool in the 1930s', in P. Hudson and W.R. Lee (eds.), *Women's Work and the Family Economy in Historical Perspective*, Manchester, 271–90.

AYERS, P. and J. LAMBERTZ (1986), 'Marriage Relations, Money and Domestic Violence in Workingclass Liverpool, 1919–39', in J. Lewis (ed.), *Labour and Love. Women's Experience of Home and Family, 1850–1940*, Oxford, 195–219.

BAGINSKY, A. (1875), 'Ueber den Durchfall und Brechdurchfall der Kinder', *Jahrbuch für Kinderheilkunde und physische Erziehung*, **8**, 310–30.

BALDWIN-WISEMAN, W. R. (1909), 'The Increase in the National Consumption of Water', *Journal of the Royal Statistical Society*, **72**, 248–92.

BALLOD, C. (1899), *Die mittlere Lebensdauer in Stadt und Land*, Leipzig.

BALLOD, C. (1906), 'Die Fortschritte der Sterblichkeitsforschung in Preussen', in A. Manes (ed.), *Berichte, Denkschriften und Verhandlungen des Fünften Internationalen Kongresses für Versicherungs-Wissenschaft zu Berlin vom 10. bis 15. September 1906, Vol. 2: Denkschriften*, Berlin, 7–16.

BALLOD, C. (1913), *Grundriss der Statistik*, Berlin.

BANKS, J. A. (1978), 'The Social Structure of Nineteenth Century England as seen through the Census', in R. Lawton (ed.), *The Census and Social Structure. An Interpretative Guide to Nineteenth Century Censuses for England and Wales*, London, 179–223.

BAUM, M. (1912), 'Lebensbedingungen und Sterblichkeit der Säuglinge im Kreise Grevenbroich', *Zeitschrift für Säuglingsfürsorge*, **6**, 197–208, 309–16.

BEAVER, M. W. (1973), 'Population, Infant Mortality and Milk', *Population Studies*, **27**, 243–54.

BEETZ, F. (1882), *Die Gesundheitsverhältnisse der K.B. Haupt- und Residenzstadt München. Ein hygienischer Führer für Einheimische und Fremde*, Munich.

BEIER, R. (1982), 'Leben in der Mietskaserne. Zum Alltag Berliner Unterschichtsfamilien in den Jahren 1900 bis 1920', in G. Asmus (ed.), *Hinterhof, Keller und Mansarde. Einblicke in Berliner Wohnungselend 1901–1920*, Reinbek bei Hamburg, 244–70.

BLEICHER, H. (1895), *Statistische Beschreibung der Stadt Frankfurt am Main und ihrer Bevölkerung* Beiträge zur Statistik der Stadt Frankfurt am Main, **1**, Part II, Frankfurt am Main.

BLEKER, J. (1983), 'Die Stadt als Krankheitsfaktor. Eine Analyse ärztlicher Auffassungen im 19. Jahrhundert', *Medizinhistorisches Journal*, **18**, 118–36.

BLOTEVOGEL, H. H. (1979), 'Methodische Probleme der Erfassung städtischer Funktionen und funktionaler Städtetypen anhand quantitativer Analysen der Berufsstatistik 1907', in W. Ehbrecht (ed.), *Voraussetzungen und Methoden geschichtlicher Städteforschung*, Vienna.

BÖCKH, R. (1887a), 'Tabellen betreffend den Einfluss der Ernährungsweise auf die Kindersterblichkeit', *Bulletin de l'Institute International de Statistique*, **2**, 14–24.

BÖCKH, R. (1887b), 'Die statistische Messung des Einflusses der Ernährungsweise der kleinen Kinder auf die Sterblichkeit derselben', *VI. Internationaler Congress für Hygiene und Demographie zu Wien 1887, Heft 28: Arbeiten der Demographischen Section*, Vienna, 3–48.

BOOTH, C. (1889 and 1891), *Life and Labour of the People*, 2 vols, London and Edinburgh. Second edition (1892–1897), *Life and Labour of the People in London*, London and New York.

BRAND, J. L. (1965), *Doctors and the State: The British Medical Profession and Government Action in Public Health, 1870–1912*, Baltimore.

BRANDLMEIER, K. P. (1942), *Medizinische Ortsbeschreibung des 19. Jahrhunderts im deutschen Sprachgebiet*, Berlin.

BRÄNDSTRÖM, A. (1993), 'Infant Mortality in Sweden—1750–1950. Past and Present Research into its Decline', in C. A. Corsini and P. P. Viazzo (eds), *The Decline of Infant Mortality in Europe, 1800–1950. Four National Case Studies*, Florence, 19–34.

BRANDT, O. (1902), *Studien zur Wirtschafts- und Verwaltungsgeschichte der Stadt Düsseldorf im 19. Jahrhundert*, Düsseldorf.

BREYER, H. (1980), *Max von Pettenkofer*, Leipzig.

BRIX, J., K. IMHOFF and R. WELDERT (1934), *Die Stadtentwässerung in Deutschland, Vol. 1*, Jena.

BROCKINGTON, C. F. (1965), *Public Health in the Nineteenth Century*, Edinburgh and London.

BROCKINGTON, C. F. (1966), *A Short History of Public Health*, London.

BROWN, J. C. (1987), 'Reforming the Urban Environment: Sanitation, Housing, and Government Intervention in Germany, 1870–1910', unpublished PhD thesis, Ann Arbor.

BROWN, J. C. (1989), 'Public Reform for Private Gain? The Case of Investments in Sanitary Infrastructure: Germany, 1870–1887', *Urban Studies*, **26**, 2–12.

BROWN, J. C. (forthcoming), 'Public Health Reform and the Decline in Urban Mortality. The Case of Germany, 1876–1912', in G. Kearns, W. R. Lee, M. C. Nelson and J. Rogers (eds), *Improving the Public Health: Essays in Medical History*, Liverpool.

BRÜCKNER, N. (1890), 'Die Entwicklung der grossstädtischen Bevölkerung im Gebiete des Deutschen Reiches', *Allgemeines Statistisches Archiv*, **1**, 135–84, 615–72.

BUDD, W. (1873), *Typhoid Fever*, London.

BÜLLER, F. (1887), 'Ursachen und Folgen des Nichtstillens in der Bevölkerung Münchens', *Jahrbuch für Kinderheilkunde*, **16**, 313–40.

BURGDÖRFER, F. (1914), 'Geburtenhäufigkeit und Säuglingssterblichkeit mit besonderer Berücksichtigung der bayerischen Verhältnisse, *Allgemeines Statistisches Archiv*, **7**, 63–154.

BURNETT, J. (1966), *Plenty and Want: A Social History of Diet in England from 1815 to the Present Day*, London.

BURNETT, J. (1978), *A Social History of Housing*, Newton Abbot.

BUSSE, E. (1908), 'Die Gemeindebetriebe Münchens', *Schriften des Vereins für Socialpolitik*, **129**, Part 1, Vol. 2, Leipzig.

CARTER, H. (1983), *An Introduction to Urban Historical Geography*, London.

CHADWICK, E. (1842, repr. 1965), *Report on the Sanitary Condition of the Labouring Population of Great Britain*, edited with an introduction by M. W. Flinn, Edinburgh.

Charles Booth's London. A Portrait of the Poor at the Turn of the Century, Drawn from his 'Life and Labour of the People in London', (1969), selected and edited by A. Fried and R. M. Elman, London.

CONDRAN, G. A. and R. A. CHENEY (1982), 'Mortality Trends in Philadelphia: Age- and Cause-specific Death Rates, 1870–1930', *Demography*, **19**, 97–127.

CONDRAN, G. A. and E. CRIMMINS (1980), 'Mortality Differentials between Rural and Urban Areas of States in the Northeastern United States 1890–1900', *Journal of Historical Geography*, **6**, 179–202.

CONDRAN, G. A. and E. CRIMMINS-GARDNER (1978), 'Public Health Measures and Mortality in US Cities in the Late Nineteenth Century', *Human Ecology*, **6**, 27–54.

'Cost of Living in German Towns. Report of an Enquiry by the Board of Trade into Working Class Rents, Housing and Retail Prices, Together with the Rates of Wages in Certain Occupations in the Principal Industrial Towns of the German Empire' (1908), in British Parliamentary Papers, *Accounts and Papers*, Vol. 108, London.

'Cost of Living of the Working Classes. Report of an Enquiry by the Board of Trade into Working Class Rents, Housing and Retail Prices, Together with the Standard Rates of Wages Prevailing in Certain Occupations in the Principal Industrial Towns of the United Kingdom' (1908), in British Parliamentary Papers, *Accounts and Papers*, Vol. 107, London.

CRAMER (1902), contribution to the discussion of Pfaffenholz, 1902a.

CREIGHTON, C. (1894; 2nd edn 1965), *A History of Epidemics in Britain*, 2 vols, London.

CRONJÉ, G. (1984), 'Tuberculosis and Mortality Decline in England and Wales, 1851–1900', in R. Woods and J. Woodward (eds), *Urban Disease and Mortality in Nineteenth-Century England*, London, 79–101.

CULLEN, M. J. (1974), 'The Making of the Civil Registration Act of 1936', *Journal of Ecclesiastical History*, **25**, 39–59.

CURSCHMANN (1888), 'Statistisches und Klinisches über den Unterleibstyphus in Hamburg', *Deutsche medicinische Wochenschrift*, **16**, 361–62.

DAUNTON, M. J. (1983), *House and Home in the Victorian City: Working-Class Housing, 1850–1914*, London.

DAUNTON, M. J. (1990), 'Introduction', in M. J. Daunton (ed.), *Housing the Workers, 1850–1914. A Comparative Perspective*, London, 1–32.

DAWSON, W. H. (1914), *Municipal Life and Government in Germany*, London.

Decennial Supplements to the Annual Reports of the Registrar-General of Births, Deaths, and Marriages in England and Wales (1851–1860, 1871–1880, 1901–1910).

Denkschrift über die seit dem Jahre 1903 unter Mitwirkung des Reichs erfolgte systematische Typhusbekämpfung im Südwesten Deutschlands (1912). Arbeiten aus dem Kaiserlichen Gesundheitsamte, Bd. 41, Berlin.

Denkschrift zur ersten Wohnung—Enquete der Orts-krankerkassen in Breslau (1906), Breslau.

DENNIS, R. (1984), *English Industrial Cities of the Nineteenth Century: A Social Geography*, Cambridge.

DICKLER, R. A. (1975), 'Labour Market Pressure Aspects of Agricultural Growth in the Eastern Region of Prussia, 1840–1914: A Case Study of Economic-Demographic Interrelations during the Demographic Transition', unpublished PhD thesis, Pennsylvania.

DIETRICH, (1902), 'Säuglingsernährung und Wöchnerinnen-Asyle', *Centralblatt für allgemeine Gesundheitspflege*, **21**, 46–53.

DIETRICH, E. (1908), 'Das Fürsorgewesen für Säuglinge', *Zeitschrift für Säuglingsfürsorge*, **2**, 1–61.

DODD, F. LAWSON (1905), *Municipal Milk and Public Health*, Fabian Tract No. 122, London.

DORNEDDEN, H. (1939), 'Der Einfluß der Seuchen auf die deutsche Bevölkerungsentwicklung', *Archiv für soziale Hygiene und Demographie*, **5**, 217–30.

DREYFUSS, I. (1899), 'Ueber die Sterblichkeitsabnahme in deutschen Grossstädten im Laufe der letzten drei Dezennien', *Vierteljahrsschrift für gerichtliche Medicin und öffentliches Sanitätswesen*, **17**, Supplement 1, 145–232.

DUBOS, R. (1988), *Pasteur and Modern Science*, Madison.

Düsseldorf im Jahre 1898. Festschrift den Theilnehmern an der 70. Versammlung deutscher Naturforscher und Ärzte dargereicht von der Stadt Düsseldorf (1898), Düsseldorf.

Düsseldorf und seine Bauten. (1904), Architekter und Ingenièur-verein zu Düsseldorf, Düsseldorf.

DWORK, D. (1987), *War is Good for Babies and Other Young Children. A History of the Infant and Child Welfare Movement in England 1898–1918*, London/New York.

DYHOUSE, C. (1978), 'Working-Class Mothers and Infant Mortality in England, 1895–1914', *Journal of Social History*, **12**, 248–67.

DYOS. H. J. and M. WOLFF (eds) (1973), *The Victorian City: Images and Realities*, 2 vols, London.

EBERSTADT, R. (1909; 3rd edn 1917; 4th edn 1920), *Handbuch des Wohnungswesens und der Wohnungsfrage*, Jena.

EMMERICH, R. and F. WOLTER (1906), *Die Entstehungsursachen der Gelsenkirchener Typhusepidemie von 1901*, Jubiläumsschrift zum 50jährigen Gedenken der Begründung der lokalistischen Lehre Max von Pettenkofer's, Munich.

ENGEL, S. and H. BEHRENDT (1927), 'Säuglingsfürsorge', in A. Gottstein, A. Schlossmannn and L. Teleky (eds), *Handbuch der Sozialen Hygiene und Gesundheitsfürsorge*, Vol. 4, Berlin, 28–194.

ENGELS, F. (1892), *The Condition of the Working-Class in England in 1844*, London.

Die Entwicklung Münchens unter dem Einflusse der Naturwissenschaften während der letzten Dezennien. Festschrift der 71. Versammlung deutscher Naturforscher und Ärzte (1899), Munich.

ESCHE, P. vor dem (1954a), 'Die Verbreitung der Ärzte im Deutschen Reich bzw. in der Bundesrepublik von 1876–1950', *Archiv für Hygiene und Bakteriologie*, **138**, 373–85.

ESCHE, P. vor dem (1954b), 'Die Versorgung der Bevölkerung mit Krankenhäusern in Deutschland von 1876 bis zur Gegenwart', *Archiv für Hygiene und Bakteriologie*, **138**, 386–98.

ESCHERICH, T. (1887), 'Die Ursachen und Folgen des Nichtstillens bei der Bevölkerung Münchens', *Münchener Medicinische Wochenschrift*, **34**, 233–35, 256–59.

EVANS, R. (1987), *Death in Hamburg. Society and Politics in the Cholera Years 1830–1910*, Oxford.

EVANS, R. J. and W. R. LEE (eds) (1986), *The German Peasantry. Conflict and Community in Rural Society from the Eighteenth to the Twentieth Centuries*, London.

EYLER, J. M. (1979), *Victorian Social Medicine. The Ideas and Methods of William Farr*, London.

FALKUS, M. (1977), 'The Development of Municipal Trading in the Nineteenth Century', *Business History*, **19**, 134–61.

FARR, W. (1974 reprint), *Mortality in Mid 19th Century Britain* (originally published in 1837 as 'Vital Statistics or the Statistics of Health, Sickness, Disease and Death', in J. R. McCulloch (ed.), *A Statistical Account of the British Empire*), Farnborough.

FEINSTEIN, C. (1990a), 'What Really Happened to Real Wages?: Trends in Wages, Prices and Productivity in the United Kingdom, 1880–1913', *Economic History Review*, 2nd ser. **63**, 329–55.

FEINSTEIN, C. (1990b), 'New Estimates of Average Earnings in the United Kingdom, 1880–1913', *Economic History Review*, 2nd series, **63**, 595–632.

Festschrift Nürnberg 1892, dargeboten den Mitgliedern und Teilnehmern der 65. Versammlung der Gesellschaft deutscher Naturforscher und Ärzte vom Stadtmagistrate Nürnberg. Herausgegeben im Auftrage desselben von W. Beck, F. Goldschmidt and E. Hecht (1892), Nuremberg.

FILDES, V. (1992), 'Breast-feeding in London', *Journal of Biosocial Science*, **24**, 53–70.

FINER, S. E. (1952), *The Life and Times of Sir Edwin Chadwick*, New York/London.

FINKELNBURG, R. (1882), 'Über den hygienischen Gegensatz von Stadt und Land, insbesondere in der Rheinprovinz', *Zentralblatt für allgemeine Gesundheitspflege*, **1**, 4–15, 43–54.

First Report of the Commissioners for Inquiring into the State of the Large Towns and Populous Districts, London (1844).

FISCHER, A. (1933), *Geschichte des deutschen Gesundheitswesens*, 2 vols, Berlin.

FISCHER, O. (1913), 'Die organisierte Typhusbekämpfung im Südwesten des Reichs mit Berücksichtigung ihrer militärischen Bedeutung und der Mitwirkung der Heeresverwaltung', *Deutsche militärärztliche Zeitschrift*, 151–66.

FLINN, M. W. (1974), 'The Stabilisation of Mortality in Pre-Industrial Western Europe', *Journal of European Economic History*, **3**, 285–318.

FLINN, M. W. (1981), *The European Demographic System 1500–1820*, Brighton.

FLORA, P. (1973), 'Die Bildungsentwicklung im Prozess der Staaten- und Nationenbildung. Eine vergleichende Analyse', in P. C. Ludz (ed.), *Soziologie und Sozialgeschichte. Aspekte und Probleme*, Opladen, 294–319.

FLORA, P. (1975), *Indikatoren der Modernisierung. Ein historisches Datenhandbuch*, Opladen.

FLOUD, R., K. WACHTER and A. GREGORY (1990), *Height, Health and History: Nutritional Status in the United Kingdom*, Cambridge.

FLÜGGE, C. (1894), 'Die Aufgaben und Leistungen der Milchsterilisierung gegenüber den Darmkrankheiten der Säuglinge', *Zeitschrift für Hygiene und Infectionskrankheiten*, **17**, 272–342.

FLÜGGE, C. (1916), *Großstadtwohnungen und Kleinhaussiedlungen in ihrer Einwirkung auf die Volksgesundheit*, Jena.

FOGEL, R. W. (1986), 'Nutrition and the Decline in Mortality since 1700: Some Preliminary Findings', in S. L. Engerman and R. E. Gallmann (eds), *Long-Term Factors in American Economic Growth*, Chicago, 439–555.

Forty-Second Annual Report of the Local Government Board, 1912–13. Supplement in Continuation of the Report of the Medical Officer of the Board for 1912–13, containing a Second Report on Infant and Child Mortality by the Medical Officer of the Board (1913), London.

FRÄNKEL, B. (1911), 'Tuberkulosesterblichkeit in Preußen in der Stadt- und Landbevölkerung', *Zeitschrift für Tuberkulose*, **17**, 534–35.

Frankfurt am Main in seinen hygienischen Verhältnissen und Einrichtungen. Festschrift zur Feier des 50-jährigen Doctorjubiläums des Herrn Geh. Sanitätsrath Dr. G. Varrentrapp, herausgegeben von Collegen, Freunden und Mitbürgern des Jubilars (1881), Frankfurt am Main.

FRANZOI, B. (1984), 'Domestic Industry. Work Options and Women's Choice', in J. C. Fout (ed.), *German Women in the Nineteenth Century. A Social History*, New York, 256–69.

'Die Frauenerwerbsarbeit im Deutschen Reich nach den Ergebnissen der Berufszählungen von 1882–1910', *Statistische Beilage des Correspondenz-Blatt*, **3** (27 April 1912), 68–77.

FRAZER, W. M. (1950), *A History of English Public Health, 1834–1939*, London.

FREVERT, U. (1984), 'The Civilizing Tendency of Hygiene. Working-Class Women under Medical Control in Imperial Germany', in J. C. Fout (ed.), *German Women in the Nineteenth Century. A Social History*, New York, 320–44.

FRÖHLICH, H. (1886), 'Die Stadt Leipzig in medicinischer und insbesondere in militär-sanitärer Beziehung', *Münchener medicinische Wochenschrift*, **41**, 726–28, 745–47, 763–66, 783–85.

FROSCH, P. (1907), 'Die Grundlagen und erste Erfahrungen in der modernen Typhusbekämpfung', *Klinisches Jahrbuch*, **17**, 115–44.

FUCHS, C. J. (1911), 'Wohnungsfrage', in *Handwörterbuch der Staatswissenschaften*, Vol. 8, Jena, 873–928.

GALE, A. H. (1959), *Epidemic Diseases*, London.

GÄRTNER, A. (1904), 'Zur Hygiene der Wasserversorgung', *Schillings Journal für Gasbeleuchtung und verwandte Beleuchtungsarten sowie für Wasserversorgung*, **XLVII**, 20 August, 757–62.

GAULDIE, E. (1974), *Cruel Habitations. A History of Working-Class Housing 1780–1918*, London.

GEISSLER, (1883), 'Rückblick auf die Fruchtbarkeits- und Sterblichkeits-Verhältnisse in den grösseren Städten während des Fünfjahrts 1877–1881', *Schmidts Jahrbücher*, **200**, 281–97.

Die Gesundheitsverhältnisse Hamburgs im neunzehnten Jahrhundert. Den ärztlichen Theilnehmern der 73. Versammlung Deutscher Naturforscher und Ärzte gewidmet von dem Medicinal-Collegium (1901), Hamburg.

GEUSEN, C. (1908), 'Die Kanalisationsanlagen Düsseldorfs', in T. Weyl (ed.), *Die Assanierung der Städte in Einzeldarstellungen, Vol. 2.2: Die Assanierung von Düsseldorf*, Leipzig, 31–71.

GLASS, D. V. (1964), 'Some Indicators of Differences between Urban and Rural Mortality in England and Wales and Scotland', *Population Studies*, **17**, 263–67.

GLASS, D. V. (1973), *Numbering the People. The Eighteenth-Century Population Controversy and the Development of Census and Vital Statistics in Britain*, Farnborough.

GÖMMEL, R. (1979), *Realeinkommen in Deutschland. Ein internationaler Vergleich*, Vorträge zur Wirtschaftsgeschichte, ed. H. Kellenbenz and J. Schneider, Vol. 4, Nuremberg.

GOTTSTEIN, A. (1901a), *Geschichte der Hygiene*, Berlin.

GOTTSTEIN, A. (1901b), 'Beiträge zur Epidemiologie der Diphtherie', *Therapeutische Monatshefte*, **15**, 605–11.

GOTTSTEIN, A. (1903), *Die Periodizität der Diphtherie und ihre Ursachen. Eine epidemiologische Untersuchung*, Berlin.

GOTTSTEIN, A. (1912), 'Diphtherie', in A. Grotjahn and J. Kaup (eds), *Handwörterbuch der Sozialen Hygiene*, Vol. 1, Leipzig, 209–15.

GOTTSTEIN, A. (1927), 'Epidemiologie und Soziologie der akuten Infektionskrankheiten', in A. Gottstein, A. Schlossmann and L. Teleky (eds), *Handbuch der sozialen Hygiene und Gesundheitsfürsorge*, Vol. 5, Berlin, 425–80.

GOTTSTEIN, A. (1929), *Die Lehre von den Epidemien*, Berlin.

GOTTSTEIN, A., A. SCHLOSSMANNN and L. TELEKY (eds) (1925, 1926 and 1927), *Handbuch der Sozialen Hygiene und Gesundheitsfürsorge*, 6 vols, Berlin.

GOUBERT, J.-P. (1975), 'Eaux publiques et démographie historique dans la France urbaine du XIXe siècle. Le cas de Rennes', *Annales de Démographie Historique*, 115–21.

GRAHN, E. (1883), *Die Art der Wasserversorgung der Städte des Deutschen Reiches mit mehr als 5000 Einwohnern*, Munich and Leipzig.

GRAHN, E. (1898–1902), *Die städtische Wasserversorgung im Deutschen Reiche sowie in einigen Nachbarländern*, 2 Vols, Vol. 1: *Königreich Preussen,* Munich and Leipzig, 1898; Vol. 2, Part 1: *Königreich Bayern*, Munich and Leipzig, 1899; Vol. 2, Part 2: *Die deutschen Staaten außer Preussen und Bayern*, Munich and Berlin, 1902.

GRAHN, E. (1904a), 'Die städtischen Wasserwerke', in R. Wuttke (ed.), *Die deutschen Städte*. Vol. 1, Leipzig, 301–44.

GRAHN, E. (1904b), 'Die Typhusepidemie in Gelsenkirchen, deren Entstehung, Verlauf und Ursache', *Schillings Journal für Gasbeleuchtung und verwandte Beleuchtungsarten sowie für Wasserversorgung*, **XLVII**, 23 January, 67–75.

GRAHN, E. (1904c), 'Zur Geschichte der hygienischen Beurteilung des Wassers bis Ende 1902', *Schillings Journal für Gasbeleuchtung und verwandte Beleuchtungsarten sowie für Wasserversorgung*, **XLVII**, 29 October, 973–82.

GRANSCHE, E. and F. ROTHENBACHER (1888), 'Wohnbedingungen in der zweiten Hälfte des 19. Jahrhunderts 1861–1910', *Geschichte und Gesellschaft*, **14**, 64–95.

GREENHOW, E. H. (1858), *Papers Relating to the Sanitary State of the People of England*, General Board of Health, HMSO, London.

GROTJAHN, A. (1915 2nd edn; 1923 3rd edn), *Soziale Pathologie. Versuch einer Lehre von den sozialen Beziehungen der menschlichen Krankheiten als Grundlage der sozialen Medizin und der sozialen Hygiene*, Berlin.

GROTJAHN, A. and J. KAUP (1912), *Handwörterbuch der Sozialen Hygiene*, 2 vols, Leipzig.

HAINES, M. R. (1991), 'Conditions of Work and Mortality Decline', in R. Schofield, D. Reher and A. Bideau (eds), *The Decline of Mortality in Europe*, Oxford, 177–95.

HAMLIN, C. (1988), 'Muddling in Bumbledom: On the Enormity of Large Sanitary Improvements in Four British Towns, 1855–1885', *Victorian Studies*, **32**, 55–83.

HAMLIN, C. (1991), *A Science of Impurity. Water Analysis in Nineteenth Century Britain*, Berkeley and Los Angeles.

HARDY, A. (1993), *The Epidemic Streets. Infectious Disease and the Rise of Preventive Medicine, 1856–1900*, Oxford.

HARRIS, B. (1994), 'Health, Height, and History: An Overview of Recent Developments in Anthropometric History', *Social History of Medicine*, **7**, 297–320.

HARTOG, R. (1962), *Stadterweiterungen im 19. Jahrhundert*, Stuttgart.

HASSAN, J. A. (1985), 'The Growth and Impact of the British Water Industry in the Nineteenth Century', *Economic History Review*, **38**, 531–47.

HAWES, R. A. (1991), 'The Paradise of Every Nuisance. The Development of Municipal Public Health Services in St Helens, 1868–1914', unpublished PhD thesis, Liverpool.

HEALTH DEPARTMENT (1901), *Report on the Health of the City of Liverpool during 1900*, Liverpool.

HEALTH DEPARTMENT (1911), *Report on the Health of the City of Liverpool during 1910*, Liverpool.

HECKER, R. (1923), 'Studien über Sterblichkeit, Todesursachen und Ernährung Münchener Säuglinge', *Archiv für Hygiene*, **93**, 280–94.

HEIMANN, G. (1906), 'Die Zuverlässigkeit der amtlichen Erhebungen über die Todesursachen, besonders in Berlin', *Medizinische Klinik*, 2, 20–24.

HENNOCK, E. P. (1973), *Fit and Proper Persons: Ideal and Reality in Nineteenth-century Urban Government*, London.

HENNOCK, E. P. (1987), *British Social Reform and German Precedents. The Case of Social Insurance 1880–1914*, Oxford.

HERBERT, U. (1986), *Geschichte der Ausländerbeschäftigung in Deutschland 1880 bis 1980. Saisonarbeiter, Zwangsarbeiter, Gastarbeiter*, Berlin.

HIETALA, M. (1987), *Services and Urbanization at the Turn of the Century. The Diffusion of Innovations*, Helsinki.

HIGGS, E. (1987), 'Women, Occupations and Work in the Nineteenth Century Censuses', *History Workshop*, **23**, 59–80.

HIGGS, E. (1993), 'Causes of Death Registration in England and Wales 1837–1920: Design, Accident or Cuckoo in the Nest', unpublished paper presented at a conference on the History of the Registration of Causes of Death, 11–14 November 1993 at Indiana University, Bloomington, Indiana, USA.

HIGGS, R. (1979), 'Cycles and Trends in Mortality in 18 Large American Cities, 1871–1900', *Explorations in Economic History*, **16**, 381–408.

HIGGS, R. and D. BOOTH (1979), 'Mortality Differentials within Large American Cities', *Human Ecology*, **7**, 353–70.

HIRSCH, A. (1886), *Handbuch der Historisch-Geographischen Pathologie*, 2nd edn, 3 vols, Stuttgart.

HIRT, L. (1873), *Die gewerbliche Thätigkeit der Frauen vom hygienischen Standpunkte aus. Mit speciellen Hinweisen auf die an eine Fabrikgesetzgebung zu stellenden Anforderungen*, Breslau and Leipzig.

HOBRECHT, J. (1868), *Ueber öffentliche Gesundheitspflege und die Bildung eines Central-Amts für öffentliche Gesundheitspflege im Staate*, Stettin.

HOFFMANN, W. G. (1965), *Das Wachstum der deutschen Wirtschaft seit der Mitte des 19. Jahrhunderts*, Berlin.

HOHLFELD, M. (1905), 'Ueber den Umfang der natürlichen Säuglingsernährung in Leipzig', *Deutsche Medizinische Wochenschrift*, **31**, 1391–94.

HOHORST G., J. KOCKA and G. A. RITTER (1975), *Sozialgeschichtliches Arbeitsbuch. Materialien zur Statistik des Kaiserreichs 1870–1914*, Munich.

HOWARD-JONES, N. (1973), 'Gelsenkirchen Typhoid Epidemic of 1901, Robert Koch, and the Dead Hand of Max von Pettenkofer', *British Medical Journal*, 103–05.

HUDSON, P. and W. R. LEE (1990), 'Women's Work and the Family Economy in Historical Perspective', in P. Hudson and W. R. Lee (eds), *Women's Work and the Family Economy in Historical Perspective*, Manchester, 2–47.

HUEPPE, F. (1887), 'Der Zusammenhang der Wasserversorgung mit der Entstehung und Ausbreitung von Infectionskrankheiten und hieraus in hygienischer Beziehung abzuleitende Folgerungen', *VI. Internationaler Congress für Hygiene und Demographie zu Wien 1887, Nr. 2, Arbeiten der Hygienischen Sectionen*, Vienna, 1–22.

HUERKAMP, C. (1980), 'Ärzte und Professionalisierung in Deutschland. Überlegungen zum Wandel des Arztberufs im 19. Jahrhundert', *Geschichte und Gesellschaft*, **6**, 349–82.

HUME, E. E. (1927), *Max von Pettenkofer. His Theory of the Etiology of Cholera, Typhoid Fever & other Intestinal Diseases. A Review of his Arguments and Evidence*, New York.

Hygiene und Soziale Fürsorge in München, ed. Statistishe Amt, Munich, 1907.

IMHOF A. E. (1979), 'Die Übersterblichkeit verheirateter Frauen im fruchtbaren Alter. Eine Illustration der "condition féminine" im 19. Jahrhundert', *Zeitschrift für Bevölkerungswissenschaft*, **5**, 487–510.

IMHOF, A. E. (1981a), *Die gewonnenen Jahre. Von der Zunahme unserer Lebensspanne seit dreihundert Jahren oder der Notwendigkeit einer neuen Einstellung zu Leben und Sterben. Ein historischer Essay*, Munich.

IMHOF, A. E. (1981b), 'Unterschiedliche Säuglingssterblichkeit in Deutschland, 18. bis 20. Jahrhundert—Warum?', *Zeitschrift für Bevölkerungswissenschaft*, **7**, 343–82.

IMHOF, A. E. (1981c), 'Women, Family and Death: Excess Mortality of Women of Child-Bearing Age in Four Communities in Nineteenth-Century Germany', in R. J. Evans and W. R. Lee (eds), *The German Family. Essays on the Social History of the Family in Nineteenth- and Twentieth-Century Germany*, London, 148–74.

IMHOF, A. E. (1985), 'From the Old Mortality Pattern to the New: Implications of a Radical Change from the Sixteenth to the Twentieth Century', *Bulletin of the History of Medicine*, **59**, 1–29.

IMHOF, A. E. (1990), *Lebenserwartungen in Deutschland vom 17. bis 19. Jahrhundert*, Weinheim.

IMHOFF, K. L. (1979), 'Die Entwicklung der Abwasserreinigung und des Gewässerschutzes seit 1868', *Das Gas- und Wasserfach, Ausgabe Wasser/Abwasser*, **120**, 563–75.

JOHANSSON, S. RYAN (1984), 'Deferred Infanticide: Excess Female Mortality During Childhood', in G. Hausfater and S. B. Hrdy (eds), *Infanticide. Comparative and Evolutionary Perspectives*, New York, 462–85.

JOHANSSON, S. RYAN (1991), 'Welfare, Mortality, and Gender. Continuity and Change in Explanations for Male/Female Mortality Differences over Three Centuries', *Continuity and Change*, **6**, 135–77.

JOHN, A. V. (ed.) (1986), *Unequal Opportunities. Women's Employment in England 1800–1918*, Oxford.

JONES, H. R. (1894), 'The Perils and Protection of Infant Life', *Journal of the Royal Statistical Society*, **57**, 1–103.

Das Kaiserliche Gesundheitsamt. Rückblick auf den Ursprung sowie auf die Entwickelung und Thätigkeit des Amtes in den ersten zehn Jahren seines Bestehens (1886), Berlin.

KASPARI, C. (1989), 'Alfred Grotjahn (1869–1931) Leben und Werk', unpublished PhD thesis, Bonn.

KASTEN, A. (1928), 'Die deutsche Reichs- und Landesgesundheitsstatistik', *Allgemeines statistisches Archiv*, **17**, 122–56.

KEARNS, G. (1988a), 'The Urban Penalty and the Population History of England', in A. Brändström and L.-G. Tedebrand (eds), *Society, Health and Population during the Demographic Transition*, Stockholm, 213–36.

KEARNS, G. (1988b), 'Private Property and Public Health Reform in England 1830–70', *Social Science Medicine*, **26**, 187–99.

KEARNS, G. (1989), 'Zivilis or Hygaeia: Urban Public Health and the Epidemiologic Transition', in R. Lawton (ed.), *The Rise and Fall of Great Cities*, London, 96–124.

KEARNS, G. (1991), 'Biology, Class and the Urban Penalty', in G. Kearns and C. J. Withers (eds), *Urbanising Britain: Essays on Class and Community in the Nineteenth Century*, Cambridge, 12–30.

KEARNS, G. (1993), 'Le handicap urbain et le déclin de la mortalité en Angleterre et au Pays de Galles 1851–1900', *Annales de Démographie Historique*, 75–105.

KEARNS, G., W. R. LEE and J. ROGERS (1989), 'The Interactions of Political and Economic Factors in the Management of Urban Public Health', in C. Nelson and J. Rogers (eds), *Urbanisation and the Epidemiologic Transition*, Uppsala, 9–81.

KINDLEBERGER, C. P. (1975), 'Germany's Overtaking of England 1806–1914', *Weltwirtschaftliches Archiv*, **111**, 253–81, 477–504.

KINTNER, H. J. (1982), 'The Determinants of Infant Mortality in Germany from 1871 to 1933', unpublished PhD thesis, Michigan.

KINTNER, H. J. (1985), 'Trends and Regional Differences in Breastfeeding in Germany from 1871 to 1937', *Journal of Family History*, 163–82.

KINTNER, H. J. (1986), 'Classifying Causes of Death during the Late Nineteenth and Early Twentieth Centuries: The Case of German Infant Mortality', *Historical Methods*, **19**, 45–54.

KINTNER, H. J. (1987), 'The Impact of Breastfeeding Patterns on Regional Differences in Infant Mortality in Germany, 1910', *European Journal of Population*, **3**, 233–61.

KINTNER, H. J. (1993), 'Recording the Epidemiologic Transition in Germany, 1816–1934', unpublished paper presented at a conference on the History of the Registration of Causes of Death, 11–14 November 1993 at Indiana University, Bloomington, Indiana, USA.

KIPLE, K. F. (1993), *The World History of Human Diseases*, Cambridge.

KISSKALT, K. (1921), 'Die Sterblichkeit im 18. Jahrhundert', *Zeitschrift für Hygiene und Infectionskrankheiten*, **93**, 439–511.

KISSKALT, K. (1922), 'Die Sterblichkeit in der ersten Hälfte des 19. Jahrhunderts in den deutschen Städten', *Zeitschrift für Hygiene und Infectionskrankheiten*, **98**, 1–21.

KISSKALT, K. (1948), *Max von Pettenkofer*, Stuttgart.

KLEßMANN, C. (1978), *Polnische Bergarbeiter im Ruhrgebiet 1870–1945. Soziale Integration und nationale Subkultur einer Minderheit in der deutschen Industriegesellschaft*, Göttingen.

KNODEL, J. (1974), *The Decline of Fertility in Germany, 1871–1939*, Princeton.

KNODEL, J. (1977), 'Town and Country in Nineteenth-Century Germany: A Review of Urban-Rural Differences in Demographic Behaviour', *Social Science History*, **1**, 356–82.

KNODEL, J. (1988), *Demographic Behavior in the Past. A Study of Fourteen German Village Populations in the Eighteenth and Nineteenth Centuries*, Cambridge.

KNODEL, J. and H. KINTNER (1977), 'The Impact of Breastfeeding Patterns on the Biometric Analysis of Infant Mortality', *Demography*, **14**, 391–409.

KNODEL, J. and E. VAN DE WALLE (1967), 'Breast Feeding, Fertility and Infant Mortality: An Analysis of some Early German Data', *Population Studies*, **21**, 109–31.

KNORR, M. (1958), 'Die Salubrität vor 100 Jahren und ihr Einfluß auf die Entwicklung der Wasserhygiene', *Das Gas- und Wasserfach, Ausgabe Wasser/Abwasser*, **99**, 681–87.

KOCH, E. (1911), *Die städtische Wasserleitung und Abwasserbeseitigung volkswirtschaftlich sowie finanzpolitisch beleuchtet*, Jena.

KOCH, G. (1886), 'Ueber die Wohnverhältnisse, insbesondere der unbemittelten Bevölkerungsklassen Hamburgs, sowie Versuche, welche zur Besserung dieser Verhältnisse unternommen worden sind', *Schriften des Vereins für Socialpolitik*, **30**, 41–55.

KOCH, R. (1888), *Die Bekämpfung der Infektionskrankheiten insbesondere der Kriegsseuchen. Rede gehalten zur Feier des Stiftungstages der militär-ärztlichen Bildungsanstalten am 2. August 1888*, Berlin

KOCH, R. (1902), 'Seuchenbekämpfung im Kriege', in *Vorträge über Aerztliche Kriegswissenschaft*, ed. Zentralkomitee für das ärztliche Fortbildungswesen in Preussen, Vol. 9, Jena.

KOCKA, J. (1983), *Lohnarbeit und Klassenbildung. Arbeiter und Arbeiterbewegung in Deutschland 1800–1875*, Berlin/Bonn.

KOHLER, W. F. (1991), 'Quellen zur Statistik des Gesundheitswesens in Deutschland', in W. Fischer and A. Kunz (eds), *Grundlagen der historischen Statistik von Deutschland*, Opladen, 275–98.

KÖLLMANN, W. (1974), *Bevölkerung in der industriellen Revolution*, Göttingen.

KRABBE, W. (1979), 'Munizipalsozialismus und Interventionsstaat. Die Ausbreitung der städtischen Leistungsverwaltung im Kaiserreich', *Geschichte in Wissenschaft und Unterricht*, **30**, 265–83.

KRABBE, W. R. (1983), 'Die Entfaltung der kommunalen Leistungsverwaltung in deutschen Städten während des späten 19. Jahrhunderts'; in H.-J. Teuteberg (ed.), *Urbanisierung im 19. und 20. Jahrhundert*, Cologne, 373–91.

KRABBE, W. R. (1985), *Kommunalpolitik und Industrialisierung*, Stuttgart.

KREI, T. (1995), *Gesundheit und Hygiene in der Lehrerbildung. Strukturen und Prozesse*, Cologne.

KRUSE, W. (1897), 'Die Verminderung der Sterblichkeit in den letzten Jahrzehnten und ihr jetziger Stand', *Zeitschrift für Hygiene und Infectionskrankheiten*, **25**, 113–67.

KRUSE, W. (1912), 'Was lehren uns die letzten Jahrzehnte und der heisse Sommer 1911 über die Säuglingssterblichkeit und ihre Bekämpfung', *Centralblatt für allgemeine Gesundheitspflege*, **31**, 175–201.

KUCZYNSKI, J. (1965), *Die Geschichte der Lage der Arbeiter unter dem Kapitalismus, Part 2, Vol. 24: Darstellung der Lage der Arbeiter in England von 1832 bis 1900*, Berlin.

KUCZYNSKI, J. (1967), *Die Geschichte der Lage der Arbeiter unter dem Kapitalismus, Part 1, Vol. 4: Darstellung der Lage der Arbeiter in Deutschland von 1900 bis 1917/18*, Berlin.

KUCZYNSKI, R. (1897), *Der Zug nach der Stadt. Statistische Studien über Vorgänge der Bevölkerungsbewegung im Deutschen Reiche*, Stuttgart.

KÜHNEMANN, O. (1911), 'Neuere Erfahrungen über Epidemiologie und Bekämpfung des Typhus', *Zeitschrift für Medizinalbeamte*, **24**, 81–89.

KUNITZ, S. J. (1983), 'Speculations on the European Mortality Decline', *Economic History Review*, 2nd Series, **36**, 349–64.

KUNITZ, S. J. and S. L. ENGERMAN (1992), 'The Ranks of Death: Secular Trends in Income and Mortality', *Health Transition Review, Supplement to Volume 2: Historical Epidemiology and the Health Transition*, ed. J. Landers, 29–46.

LABISCH, A. (1986), 'Gemeinde und Gesundheit. Zur historischen Soziologie des kommunalen Gesundheitswesens', in B. Blanke, A. Evers and H. Wollmann (eds), *Die Zweite Stadt. Neue Formen der Arbeits- und Sozialpolitik,* Leviathan. Zeitschrift für Sozialwissenschaft, Sonderheft 7/1986, Opladen, 275–305.

LABISCH, A. (1988), 'Kommunale Gesundheitssicherung im rheinisch-westfälischen Industriegebiet (1869–1934)—ein Beispiel zur Soziogenese öffentlicher Gesundheitsleistungen', in H. Schadewaldt and K.-H. Leven (eds), *XXX. Internationaler Kongreß für Geschichte der Medizin, Düsseldorf 31.8.–5.9.1986, Actes/Proceedings*, Düsseldorf, 1077–94.

LABISCH, A. (1992), *Homo Hygienicus. Gesundheit und Medizin in der Neuzeit*, Frankfurt and New York.

LABISCH, A. and F. TENNSTEDT (1985), *Der Weg zum 'Gesetz über die Vereinheitlichung des Gesundheitswesens' vom 3. Juli 1934. Entwicklungslinien und -momente des staatlichen und kommunalen Gesundheitswesens in Deutschland*, Düsseldorf.

LADD, B. (1990), *Urban Planning and Civic Order in Germany, 1860–1914*, Cambridge, Massachusetts.

LAMBERTSEN, G. (1989), *Liverpool Cowkeepers, Milk Supply and Public Health 1850–1914*, MA Dissertation, Liverpool.

LANCASTER, H. O. (1990), *Expectations of Life. A Study in the Demography, Statistics, and History of World Mortality*, New York.

LANDES, D. S. (1969), *The Unbound Prometheus*, Cambridge.

LANGEWIESCHE, D. (1977), 'Wanderungsbewegungen in der Hochindustrialisierungsperiode. Regionale, interstädtische und innerstädtische Mobilität in Deutschland, 1880–1914', *Vierteljahrschrift für Sozial- und Wirtschaftsgeschichte*, **64**, 1–40.

LANGEWIESCHE, D. (1979), 'Mobilität in deutschen Mittel- und Großstädten. Aspekte der Binnenwanderung im 19. und 20. Jahrhundert', in W. Conze and U. Engelhardt (eds), *Arbeiter im Industrialisierungsprozeß. Herkunft, Lage und Verhalten*, Stuttgart, 70–93.

LANGSTEIN, L. and F. ROTT (eds) (1918; reprint 1989), *Atlas der Hygiene des Säuglings und Kleinkindes*, Berlin (repr. Lübeck).

LAUX, H.-D. (1983), 'Demographische Folgen des Verstädterungsprozesses. Zur Bevölkerungsstruktur und natürlicher Bevölkerungsentwicklung deutscher Städtetypen 1871–1914', in H.-J. Teuteberg (ed.), *Urbanisierung im 19. und 20. Jahrhundert. Historische und geographische Aspekte*, Cologne, 65–93.

LAUX, H.-D. (1985), 'Mortalitätsunterschiede in preussischen Städten 1905: Ansätze zu einer Erklärung', in F.-J. Kemper, H.-D. Laux and G. Thieme (eds), *Geographie als Sozialwissenschaft. Beiträge zu ausgewählten Problemen kulturgeographischer Forschung. W. Kuls zum 65. Geburtstag*, Bonn, 50–82.

LAUX, H.-D. (1989), 'The Components of Population Growth in Prussian Cities, 1875–1905 and their Influence on Urban Population Structure', in R. Lawton and R. Lee (eds), *Urban Population Development from the Late-Eighteenth to the Early-Twentieth Century*, Liverpool, 120–48.

LAW, C. (1967), 'The Growth of the Urban Population of England and Wales, 1801–1911', *Transactions of the Institute of British Geographers*, **41**, 125–43.

LAWTON, R. (1978), 'Census Data for Urban Areas', in R. Lawton (ed.), *The Census and Social Structure. An Interpretative Guide to Nineteenth Century Censuses for England and Wales*, London, 82–145.

LAWTON, R. (1983), 'Urbanization and Population Change in Nineteenth-Century England', in J. Patten (ed.), *The Expanding City. Essays in Honour of Professor Jean Gottmann*, London, 179–224.

LAWTON, R. (1989), 'Population Mobility and Urbanization: Nineteenth-Century British Experience', in R. Lawton and R. Lee (eds), *Urban Population Development from the Late-Eighteenth to the Early-Twentieth Century*, Liverpool, 149–77.

LAWTON, R. and C. G. POOLEY (1976), 'The Social Geography of Merseyside in the Nineteenth Century, Final Report to the S.S.R.C.', unpublished typescript, Liverpool.

LAXTON, P. and N. WILLIAMS (1989), 'Urbanization and Infant Mortality in England: A Long Term Perspective and Review', in C. Nelson and J. Rogers (eds), *Urbanisation and the Epidemiologic Transition*, Uppsala, 109–35.

LEE, W. R. (1979), 'Germany', in W. R. Lee (ed.), *European Demography and Economic Growth*, London, 144–95.

LEE, W. R. (1980), 'The Mechanism of Mortality Change in Germany, 1750–1850', *Medizinhistorisches Journal*, **15**, 244–88.

LEE, W. R. (1984a), 'Mortality Levels and Agrarian Reform in Early 19th Century Prussia: Some Regional Evidence', in T. Bengtsson, G. Fridlizius and R. Ohlsson (eds), *Pre-Industrial Population Change. The Mortality Decline and Short-Term Population Movements*, Stockholm, 161–90.

LEE, W. R. (1984b), 'The Impact of Agrarian Change on Women's Work and Child Care in Early-Nineteenth-Century Prussia', in J. C. Fout (ed.), *German Women in the Nineteenth Century. A Social History*, New York, 234–55.

LEE, W. R. (1988), 'Economic Development and the Role of the State in Nineteenth-Century Germany', *Economic History Review*, **41**, 346–67.

LEE, W. R. (forthcoming), 'Forschungen und Hypothesen zur Bevölkerungsentwicklung europäischer Hafenstädte: Stralsund im Vergleich', in W. R. Lee and W. Urban (eds), *Stadt und Bevölkerung bis zum Ende des 19. Jahrhunderts. Pommern im Vergleich*, Stralsund.

LENGER, F. (1990), 'Bürgertum und Stadtverwaltung in rheinischen Großstädten des 19. Jahrhunderts', in L. Gall (ed.), *Stadt und Bürgertum im 19. Jahrhundert*, Historische Zeitschrift, Beihefte (Neue Folge), Vol. 12, 97–169.

LEUTHOLD (1886), 'Von welchen gesetzlichen Bestimmungen kann Minderung der Wohnungsnoth in unseren Großstädten erwartet werden?', *Schriften des Vereins für Socialpolitik*, **30**, 1–40.

LEWIS, J. (1984), *Women in England 1870–1950: Sexual Divisions and Social Change*, Brighton.

LEWIS, J. (1986), 'The Working-Class Wife and Mother and State Intervention, 1870–1918', in J. Lewis (ed.), *Labour and Love. Women's Experience of Home and Family, 1850–1940*, Oxford, 73–98.

LEWIS, R. E. (1952), *Edwin Chadwick and the Public Health Movement, 1832–1914*, London; repr. New York, 1970.

LINDEMANN, H. (1901), 'Wohnungsstatistik', *Schriften des Vereins für Socialpolitik, **94**: Neuere Untersuchungen über die Wohnungsfrage, Vol. 1: Deutschland und Österreich*, Leipzig, 261–384.

LINDEMANN, U. (1986), 'Die Geschichte der Krankheitsbezeichnung "Typhus" und der Wandel der Typhuslehre im 19. Jahrhundert in Deutschland', unpublished PhD thesis, Berlin.

LOEFFLER, (1908), 'Inwieweit hat sich die Morbidität und Mortalität bei Diphtherie in Deutschland während der ersten 10 Jahre der Serumbehandlung, 1895–1905, verändert?', *Bericht über den XIV. Internationalen Kongress für Hygiene und Demographie, Berlin, 23.–29. September 1907*, Vol. IV, Berlin, 123–30.

LUCKIN, B. (1984), 'Evaluating the Sanitary Revolution: Typhus and Typhoid in London, 1851–1900', in R. Woods and J. Woodward (eds), *Urban Disease and Mortality in Nineteenth-Century England*, London, 102–19.

LUCKIN, B. (1986), *Pollution and Control. A Social History of the Thames in the Nineteenth Century*, Bristol.

MAIER, K. (1871), 'Die Sterblichkeit der Kinder im ersten Lebensjahr in Bayern', *Journal für Kinderkrankheiten*, **57**, 153–98.

Manchester Corporation, Council Proceedings 1884–85.

MARSCHALCK, P. (1984), *Bevölkerungsgeschichte Deutschlands im 19. und 20. Jahrhundert*, Frankfurt am Main.

MARSCHALCK, P. (1987), 'The Age of Demographic Transition: Mortality and Fertility', in K. J. Bade (ed.), *Population, Labour and Migration in 19th- and 20th-Century Germany*, Leamington Spa, Hamburg and New York, 15–33.

MATZERATH, H. (1980 2nd edn), 'Städtewachstum und Eingemeindungen im 19. Jahrhundert', in J. Reulecke (ed.), *Die deutsche Stadt im Industriezeitalter*, 2nd edn Wuppertal, 67–89.

MATZERATH, H. (1984), 'Regionale Unterschiede im Verstädterungsprozeß: Der Osten und Westen Preußens im 19. Jahrhundert', in H. Matzerath (ed.), *Städtewachstum und innerstädtische Strukturveränderungen. Probleme des Urbanisierungsprozesses im 19. und 20. Jahrhundert*, Stuttgart, 65–95.

MATZERATH, H. (1985), *Urbanisierung in Preußen 1815-1914*, Stuttgart.

MAYR, G. (1870), 'Die Sterblichkeit der Kinder während des ersten Lebensjahres in Süddeutschland, insbesondere in Bayern', *Zeitschrift des königlich bayerischen statistischen Bureau*, **2**, 201–47.

McCLEARY, G. F. (1904), *Infantile Mortality and Infant Milk Depots*, London.

McFARLANE, N. (1989), 'Hospitals, Housing and Tuberculosis in Glasgow, 1911–51', *Social History of Medicine*, **2**, 59–86.

McKEOWN, T. (1976), *The Modern Rise of Population*, London.

McKEOWN, T., R. G. BROWN and R. G. RECORD (1972), 'An Interpretation of the Modern Rise of Population', *Population Studies*, **26**, 345–82.

McKEOWN, T. and R. G. RECORD (1962), 'Reasons for the Decline of Mortality in England and Wales during the Nineteenth Century', *Population Studies*, **16**, 94–122.

Medizinalstatistische Mitteilungen aus dem Reichsgesundheitsamte, **1** (1893) onwards.

MEEKER, E. (1972), 'The Improving Health of the United States, 1850–1915', *Explorations in Economic History*, **9**, 353–73.

MERCER, A. (1990), *Disease, Mortality and Population in Transition. Epidemiological-Demographic Change in England Since the Eighteenth Century as Part of a Global Phenomenon*, Leicester, London and New York.

MEYER, F. A. (1894), *Das Wasserwerk der freien und Hansestadt Hamburg unter besonderer Berücksichtigung der in den Jahren 1891–1893 ausgeführten Filteranlage*, Hamburg.

MIDWINTER, E. C. (1969), *Social Administration in Lancashire 1830–1860*, Manchester.

MITCHELL, B. R. (1988), *British Historical Statistics*, Cambridge.

Mittheilungen des Statistischen Amtes der Stadt Leipzig (1887), 18 Heft, Leipzig.

Mittheilungen des Statistischen Amtes der Stadt München, Band XVII, Munich (1900–1902); Band XXII, Munich (1910–1913); Band XXIII, Munich (1910–1911).

Mittheilungen des Statistischen Bureaus der Stadt Dresden, (1877) Heft 4a und Heft V, Dresden .

Mittheilungen des Statistischen Bureaus der Stadt Leipzig, **10** (1876) and **11** (1877).

Mittheilungen des Statistischen Bureaus der Stadt München, Band II, Munich (1880); Band VIII, Munich (1887); Band IX, Munich (1886–1888).

MOMBERT, P. (1908), 'Die Gemeindebetriebe in Deutschland. Allgemeine Darstellung', *Schriften des Vereins für Socialpolitik*, **128**, 1–77.

MOMMSEN, W. J. (ed. in collaboration with W. Mock) (1981), *The Emergence of the Welfare State in Britain and Germany 1850–1950*, London.

MOMMSEN, W. J. (1986), *Britain and Germany 1800 to 1914. Two Developmental Paths Towards Industrial Society. The 1985 Annual Lecture of the German Historical Institute London*, London.

MORGAN, C. J. (1980), 'Demographic Change, 1771–1911', in D. Fraser (ed.), *A History of Modern Leeds*, Manchester, 46–71.

MORGENROTH, W. (1913), 'Die Sommersterblichkeit der Säuglinge in den deutschen Großstädten', *Zeitschrift für die gesamte Staatswissenschaft*, **99**, Vol. 2, 312–23.

MULHALL, M. G. (1886), *Dictionary of Statistics*, 2nd edn, London.

MULHALL, M.G. (1903), *Dictionary of Statistics*, 4th edn, London.

München unter dem Einflusse der öffentlichen Wohlfahrtspflege. Festschrift der 27. Versammlung des Deutschen Vereins für öffentliche Gesundheitspflege gewidmet von der Stadt München (1902), Munich.

NEEFE, M. (1886), 'Hauptergebnisse der Wohnungsstatistik deutscher Großstädte', *Schriften des Vereins für Socialpolitik*, **30**, 161–91.

NEUMANN, H. (1902), 'Über die Häufigkeit des Stillens', *Deutsche Medicinische Wochenschrift*, **28**, 795.

NEUMANN, H. (1906), 'Die Krämpfe in der Mortalitätsstatistik der Säuglinge', *Die medicinische Reform*, **14**, 2–5.

NEWSHOLME, A. (1898), *Epidemic Diphtheria*, London.

NEWSHOLME, A. (1935), *Fifty Years in Public Health. A Personal Narrative with Comments*, London.

NIEDNER, O. (1903), *Die Kriegsepidemien des 19. Jahrhunderts*, Berlin.

NIETHAMMER, L. with the collaboration of F. Brüggemeier (1976), 'Wie wohnten Arbeiter im Kaiserreich?', *Archiv für Sozialgeschichte*, **16**, 61–134.

NIETHAMMER, L. (1979), 'Ein langer Marsch durch die Institutionen. Zur Vorgeschichte des preußischen Wohnungsgesetzes von 1918', in L. Niethammer (ed.), *Wohnen im Wandel. Beiträge zur Geschichte des Alltags in der bürgerlichen Gesellschaft*, Wuppertal, 363–84.

O'DAY, R. and D. ENGLANDER (1993), *Mr Charles Booth's Inquiry: Life and Labour of the People in London Reconsidered*, London.

ODDY, D. J. (1982), 'The Health of the People', in T. Barker and M. Drake (eds), *Population and Society in Britain, 1850–1980*, London, 120–41.

ODDY, D. J. and D. S. MILLER (eds) (1976), *The Making of the Modern British Diet*, London.

OESTERLEN, F. R. (1874), *Handbuch der medicinischen Statistik*, 2nd edn, Tübingen.

OLDENDORFF, A. (1904), 'Die Sterblichkeitsverhältnisse Berlins mit besonderer Berücksichtigung der Verhandlungen der Berl. med. Gesellschaft über den Einfluss hygienischer Maassnahmen auf die Gesundheit Berlins', *Centralblatt für allgemeine Gesundheitspflege*, **23**, 327–52.

OMRAN, A. R. (1971), 'The Epidemiologic Transition. A Theory of the Epidemiology of Population Change', *Milbank Memorial Fund Quarterly*, **49**, 509–38.

OMRAN, A. R. (1977), 'Epidemiologic Transition in the United States. The Health Factor in Population Change', *Population Bulletin*, **32**, 1–42.

ORSAGH, T. J. (1969), 'Löhne in Deutschland 1871–1913. Neue Literatur und weitere Ergebnisse', *Zeitschrift für die gesamte Staatswissenschaft*, **125**, 476–83.

OTTO, R., R. SPREE and J. VÖGELE (1990), 'Seuchen und Seuchenbekämpfung in deutschen Städten während des 19. und frühen 20. Jahrhunderts. Stand und Desiderate der Forschung', *Medizinhistorisches Journal*, **25**, 286–304.

PELLING, M. (1978), *Cholera, Fever and English Medicine, 1825–1865*, Oxford.

PFAFFENHOLZ (1902a), 'Wichtige Aufgaben der öffentlichen und privaten Wohlfahrtspflege auf dem Gebiet der künstlichen Ernährung der Säuglinge', *Centralblatt für allgemeine Gesundheitspflege*, **21**, 393–416. See also the contributions to the discussion by Dietrich and Cramer at the end.

PFAFFENHOLZ (1902b), 'Säuglings-Sterblichkeit und Kindermilch', *Centralblatt für allgemeine Gesundheitspflege*, **21**, 183–200.

POLLARD, S. (1987), ' "Made in Germany"—die Angst vor der deutschen Konkurrenz im spätviktorianischen England', *Technikgeschichte*, **53**, 183–95.

POOLEY, C. G. (1992), 'England and Wales', in C. G. Pooley (ed.), *Housing Strategies in Europe, 1880–1930*, Leicester, 73–104.

POOLEY, M. E. and C. G. POOLEY (1984), 'Health, Society and Environment in Nineteenth-Century Manchester', in R. Woods and J. Woodward (eds), *Urban Disease and Mortality in Nineteenth-Century England*, London, 148–75.

PRAUSNITZ, W. (1923), *Grundzüge der Hygiene*, 12th edn, Munich.

PRESTON, S. H. (1975), 'The Changing Relation between Mortality and Level of Economic Development', *Population Studies*, **29**, 231–48.

PRESTON, S. H. (1976), *Mortality Patterns in National Populations. With Special Reference to Recorded Causes of Death*, New York.

PRESTON, S. H. and M. R. HAINES (1991), *Fatal Years. Child Mortality in Late Nineteenth-Century America*, Princeton.

PRESTON, S. H. and E. VAN DE WALLE (1978), 'Urban French Mortality in the Nineteenth Century', *Population Studies*, **32**, 275–97.

Preußische Statistik, **16** (1869), **39** (1877), **48**, **2** (1879), **50** (1879), **200** (1906), **214** (1908) and **234** (1913).

PRINZING, F. (1899), 'Die Entwicklung der Kindersterblichkeit in den europäischen Staaten', *Jahrbücher für Nationalökonomie und Statistik*, 3rd series, **17**, 577–635.

PRINZING, F. (1900), 'Die Kindersterblichkeit in Stadt und Land', *Jahrbücher für Nationalökonomie und Statistik*, 3rd series, **20**, 593–644.

PRINZING, F. (1903), 'Die Sterbefälle an akuten Infectionskrankheiten in den europäischen Staaten 1891–1900', *Centralblatt für allgemeine Gesundheitspflege*, **22**, 441–72.

PRINZING, F. (1906), *Handbuch der medizinischen Statistik*, Jena.

PRINZING, F. (1912), 'Stadt und Land', in A. Grotjahn and J. Kaup (eds), *Handwörterbuch der sozialen Hygiene*, Vol. 1, Leipzig, 494–512.

PRINZING, F. (1913), 'Die Gesundheitsstatistik', in R. Abel (ed.), *Handbuch der praktischen Hygiene*, Vol. 1, Jena, 13–42.

PRINZING, F. (1914), 'Die Ursachen der Totgeburt', *Allgemeines Statistisches Archiv*, **7**, 21–49.

PRINZING, F. (1916), *Epidemics Resulting from Wars*, ed. H. Westergaard, Oxford.

PRINZING, F. (1930/31), *Handbuch der medizinischen Statistik*, 2nd edn, Jena.

Published Volumes of the Census of England and Wales (1851, 1871, 1891, 1911).

Quellen zur Bevölkerungs-, Sozial- und Wirtschaftsstatistik Deutschlands 1815–1875 (1980), Vol. 1, ed. W. Köllmann, Boppard.

de RANCE, C. E. (1882), *The Water Supply of England and Wales: Its Geology, Underground Circulation, Surface Distribution, and Statistics*, London.

RATH, G. (1969), 'Die Hygiene der Stadt im 19. Jahrhundert', in W. Artelt et al. (eds), *Städte-, Wohnungs- und Kleidungshygiene des 19. Jahrhunderts in Deutschland*, Stuttgart, 70–84.

REICH, E. (1912), *Der Wohnungsmarkt in Berlin von 1840–1910*, Staats- und sozialwissenschaftliche Studien, 164, Munich and Leipzig.

2. Sonderheft zum Reichsarbeitsblatte: Erhebung von Wirtschaftsrechnungen minderbemittelter Familien im Deutschen Reiche (1909), Bearbeitet im Kaiserlichen Statistischen Amte, Abteilung für Arbeiterstatistik, Berlin.

Das Reichsgesundheitsamt 1876–1926. Festschrift hrsg. vom Reichsgesundheitsamt aus Anlaß seines fünfzigjährigen Bestehens (1926), Berlin.

REINCKE, J. J. (1890), *Der Typhus in Hamburg mit besonderer Berücksichtigung der Epidemien von 1885 bis 1888*, Hamburg.

REINCKE, J. J. (1896), 'Zur Epidemiologie des Typhus in Hamburg und Altona', *Deutsche Vierteljahrsschrift für öffentliche Gesundheitspflege*, **28**, 409–30.

REINCKE, J. J. (1899), 'Das Verhalten von Cholera und Typhus an der Hamburg-Altonaer Grenze', *Münchener medicinische Wochenschrift*, **28**, 926–27.

REINSCH, A. (1894), 'Die Bakteriologie im Dienste der Sandfiltrationstechnik', *Centralblatt für Bakteriologie und Parasitenkunde*, **16**, 881–96.

Report of the Royal Sanitary Commission, Vol III: Tabular Abstract of Answers in Writing received to Circular Questions issued by the Commissioners (1987), London.

'Report of The Lancet Special Commission on the Relative Strength of Diphtheria Antitoxic Serums' (1896), *The Lancet*, **74**, 182–95.

REULECKE, J. (1985), *Geschichte der Urbanisierung in Deutschland*, Frankfurt am Main.

RICHTER, K. (1974), 'Seuchenbekämpfung und Expansionspolitik des preußisch-deutschen Militarismus zu Ausgang des 19. Jahrhunderts', *Wissenschaftliche Zeitschrift, Martin-Luther-Universität Halle-Wittenberg, Mathematisch-naturwissenschaftliche Reihe*, **23**, 50–55.

RILEY, J. C. (1989), *Sickness, Recovery and Death: A History and Forecast of Ill Health*, Iowa City.

RITTER, G. A. (1986), Social Welfare in Germany and Britain. Origins and Development, Leamington Spa and New York. (Translation of German original, Sozialversicherung in Deutschland und England. Entstehung und Grundzüfge im Vergleich, Munich, 1983.).

RITTER, G. A. (1989), *Der Sozialstaat: Entstehung und Entwicklung im internationalen Vergleich*, Munich.

ROBERTS, E. (1988), *Women's Work 1840–1940*, Houndmills.

RODGER, R. (1989), *Housing in Urban Britain 1789–1914: Class, Capitalism and Construction*, Houndmills.

ROSEN, G. (1958), *A History of Public Health*, New York.

ROSEN, G. (1973), 'Disease, Debility, and Death', in H. J. Dyos and M. Wolff (eds) *The Victorian City: Images and Realities*, 2 vols, London, Vol. 2, 625–67.

ROTHENBACHER, F. (1982), 'Zur Entwicklung der Gesundheitsverhältnisse in Deutschland seit der Industrialisierung', in E. Wiegand and W. Zapf (eds), *Wandel der Lebensbedingungen in Deutschland. Wohlfahrtsentwicklung seit der Industrialisierung*, Frankfurt am Main, 335–424.

ROWNTREE, B. S. (1971), *Poverty: A Study of Town Life*, New York (reprint of the 1922 edition).

ROYAL COMMISSION ON WATER SUPPLY (1869), *Report of the Commissioners*, London.

RUPRECHT (1884), *Die Wohnungen der arbeitenden Klasse in England*, Göttingen.

RÜRUP, R. (1984), *Deutschland im 19. Jahrhundert 1815–1871*, Göttingen.

von SALDERN, A. (1979), 'Kommunalpolitik und Arbeiterwohnungen im Deutschen Kaiserreich', in L.

Niethammer (ed.), *Wohnen im Wandel. Beiträge zur Geschichte des Alltags in der bürgerlichen Gesellschaft*, Wuppertal, 344–62.

SALOMON, H. (1907 and 1911), *Die städtische Abwasserbeseitigung in Deutschland. Wörterbuchartig angeordnete Nachrichten und Beschreibungen städtischer Kanalisations- und Kläranlagen in deutschen Wohnplätzen. (Abwässer-Lexikon).* Vol. 2, *Erster Ergänzungsband*, Jena.

SALOMON, W. (1923), 'Säuglingskrankheiten', in A. Grothjahn (ed.), *Soziale Pathologie*, Berlin, 211–35.

SAUL, W. J. (1980), *Industrialisation and De-Industrialisation? The Interaction of the German and British Economies before the First War. The 1979 Annual Lecture of the German Historical Institute London*, London.

SCHLOSSMANN, A. (1897), 'Studien über Säuglingssterblichkeit', *Zeitschrift für Hygiene und Infektionskrankheiten*, **24**, 93–188.

SCHNECK, P. (1975), 'Die gesundheitlichen Verhältnisse der Fabrikarbeiterinnen', *Jahrbuch für Wirtschaftsgeschichte*, **16**, 53–72.

SCHOFIELD, R., D. REHER and A. BIDEAU (eds) (1991), *The Decline of Mortality in Europe*, Oxford.

SCHÖLLER, P. (1985), 'Die Großstadt des 19. Jahrhunderts—ein Umbruch der Stadtgeschichte', in H. Stoob (ed.), *Die Stadt. Gestalt und Wandel bis zum industriellen Zeitalter*, Cologne, 275–314.

SCHOMERUS, H. (1979), 'Lebenszyklus und Lebenshaltung in Arbeiterhaushalten des 19. Jahrhunderts', in W. Conze and U. Engelhardt (eds), *Arbeiter im Industrialisierungsprozeß. Herkunft, Lage und Verhalten*, Stuttgart, 195–200.

SCHOTT, S. (1912), *Die großstädtischen Agglomerationen des Deutschen Reichs, 1871–1910*, Breslau.

SCHRAKAMP, F. (1908), 'Gesundheitswesen', in T. Weyl (ed.), *Die Assanierung der Städte in Einzeldarstellungen*, Vol. 2.2: *Die Assanierung von Düsseldorf*, Leipzig, 83–119.

SEIDLMAYER, H. (1937), *Geburtenzahl, Säuglingssterblichkeit und Stillung in München in den letzten 50 Jahren*, Munich.

SELTER, (1902), 'Die Nothwendigkeit der Mutterbrust für die Ernährung der Säuglinge', *Centralblatt für allgemeine Gesundheitspflege*, **21**, 377–92.

SHEARD, S. (1993), 'Nineteenth Century Public Health. A Study of Liverpool, Belfast and Glasgow', unpublished PhD thesis, Liverpool.

SILBERGLEIT, H. (1896), 'Kindersterblichkeit in europäischen Grossstädten', *Huitième Congrès International d'Hygiène et de Démographie*, Tome VII, Budapest, 443–56.

SILVERTHORNE, A. (1884), *London and Provincial Water Supplies with the Latest Statistics of Metropolitan and Provincial Waterworks*, London.

SIMMONDS, M. (1886), 'Die Typhusepidemie in Hamburg im Jahre 1885', *Deutsche Vierteljahrsschrift für öffentliche Gesundheitspflege*, **18**, 537–44.

SINGER, K. (1895), *Die Abminderung der Sterblichkeitsziffer Münchens. Ein Beitrag zur Frage hygienischer und sozialpolitischer Maassnahmen auf die Gesundheit der Städte*, Munich.

SMITH, F. B. (1979), *The People's Health, 1830–1910*, London.

SMITH, N. (1978), *Mensch und Wasser*, Munich.

SNOW, J. (1855), *On the Mode of Communication of Cholera*, London.

SOMBART, W. (1903), *Die deutsche Volkswirtschaft im 19. Jahrhundert*, Berlin.

SOXHLET, F. (1886), 'Ueber Kindermilch und Säuglings-Ernährung', *Münchener Medicinische Wochenschrift*, **33**, 253–56, 276–78.

SPIEGEL, L. (1908), 'Kommunale Milchversorgung', *Schriften des Vereins für Socialpolitik*, **128**, 219–43.

SPREE, R. (1980), 'Die Entwicklung der differentiellen Säuglingssterblichkeit in Deutschland seit der Mitte des 19. Jahrhunderts (Ein Versuch zur Mentalitätsgeschichte)', in A. E. Imhof (ed.), *Mensch und Gesundheit in der Geschichte*, Husum, 251–78.

SPREE, R. (1981a), *Soziale Ungleichheit vor Krankheit und Tod. Zur Sozialgeschichte des Gesundheitsbereichs im Deutschen Kaiserreich*, Göttingen. (English translation: *Health and Social Class in Imperial Germany. A Social History of Mortality, Morbidity and Inequality*, Oxford and Hamburg 1988.)

SPREE, R. (1981b), 'Zu den Veränderungen der "Volksgesundheit" zwischen 1870 und 1913 und ihren Determinanten (vor allem in Preussen)', in W. Conze and U. Engelhardt (eds), *Arbeiterexistenz im 19. Jahrhundert. Lebensstandard und Lebensgestaltung deutscher Arbeiter und Handwerker*, Stuttgart, 235–92.

SPREE, R. (1986), 'Veränderungen des Todesursachen-Panoramas und sozio-ökonomischer Wandel—Eine Fallstudie zum "Epidemiologischen Übergang"', in G. Gäfgen (ed.), *Ökonomie des Gesundheitswesens*, Berlin, 73-100.

SPREE, R. (1988), ' "Volksgesundheit" und Lebensbedingungen in Deutschland während des frühen 19. Jahrhunderts', *Jahrbuch des Instituts für Geschichte der Medizin der Robert Bosch Stiftung*, **7**, 75–113.

SPREE, R. (1995), *On Infant Mortality Change in Germany since the Early 19th Century*, Münchener Wirtschaftswissenschaftliche Beiträge, Nr. 95–03, Munich.

STANBRIDGE, H. H. (1976), *History of Sewage Treatment in Britain*, 6 vols, Maidstone, Kent.

Statistik des Deutschen Reichs, NF **44** (1892); NF **207**, 1 (1909); NF **207**, 2 (1910).

Statistik des Hamburgischen Staates, **8** (1876); **14** (1887); **14**, 2. Abteilung (1887); **15**, 2. Abteilung (1894); **17** (1895); **22** (1904); **27** (1918).

Statistische Monatsberichte der Stadt (1891) Düsseldorf (1907 and 1910), Beilagen.

Statistisches Bundesamt (ed.) (1972), *Bevölkerung und Wirtschaft 1872–1972*, Stuttgart and Mainz.

Statistisches Handbuch für den Hamburgischen Staat (1891), ed. Statistisches Bureau der Steuer-Deputation, 4th edn, Hamburg

Statistisches Handbuch für den Hamburgischen Staat (1921), ed. Statistisches Landesamt, 5th edn, Hamburg.

Statistisches Jahrbuch der Landeshauptstadt Düsseldorf (1979/80).

Statistisches Jahrbuch der Stadt Berlin, **32** (1913).

Statistisches Jahrbuch der Stadt Leipzig, **2** (1912).

Statistisches Jahrbuch Deutscher Städte, **1** (1890) onwards.

Statistisches Jahrbuch für das Deutsche Reich (1881; 1896).

Statistisches Jahrbuch für die Stadt Dresden 1900, (1901) Dresden .

Statistisches Jahrbuch für die Stadt Dresden 1901, (1902) Dresden.

Statistisches Jahrbuch der Stadt Dresden, **12** (1910), Dresden 1912, and **14** (1912), Dresden 1913.

STEDMAN JONES, G. (1971), *Outcast London: A Study in the Relationship between Classes in Victorian Society*, Oxford.

STEFANSKI, V.-M. (1984), *Zum Prozeß der Emanzipation und Integration von Außenseitern: Polnische Arbeitsmigranten im Ruhrgebiet*, Dortmund.

STERN, W. M. (1954), 'Water Supply in Britain: The Development of a Public Service', *Royal Sanitary Institute Journal*, **74**, 998–1004.

STEUER, P. (1912), *Die Wasserversorgung der Städte und Ortschaften. Ihre wirtschaftliche Entwicklung und Analyse*, Berlin.

STÖCKEL, S. (1986), 'Säuglingssterblichkeit in Berlin von 1870 bis zum Vorabend des ersten Weltkriegs—Eine Kurve mit hohem Maximum und starkem Gefälle', *Berlin-Forschungen*, **1**, Berlin, 219–64.

STRANG, J. (1859), 'On Water Supply to Great Towns', *Journal of the Statistical Society of London*, **12**, 232–49.

STUMPF, (1886), contribution to the discussion of F. Soxhlet's 'Ueber Kindermilch und Säuglings-Ernährung', *Münchener Medicinische Wochenschrift*, **33**, 438.

SUTCLIFFE, A. (1974), 'Introduction', in A. Sutcliffe (ed.), *Multi-Storey Living. The British Working-Class Experience*, London, 1–18.

SUTCLIFFE, A. (1981), *Towards the Planned City: Germany, Britain, the United States and France*, Oxford.

SYDENSTRICKER, E. (1933), *Health and Environment*, New York and London.

SYRUP-GLEIWITZ, F. (1914), 'Der Altersaufbau der industriellen Arbeiterschaft', *Archiv für exacte Wirtschaftsforschung (Thünen-Archiv)*, **6**, 14–115.

SZRETER, S. (1988), 'The Importance of Social Intervention in Britain's Mortality Decline 1850–1914, A Reinterpretation of the Role of Public Health', *Social History of Medicine*, **1**, 1–37.

SZRETER, S. (1991), 'The General Record Office and the Public Health Movement in Britain, 1837–1914', *Social History of Medicine*, **4**, 435–63.

SZRETER, S. (1994), 'Mortality in England in the Eighteenth and Nineteenth Centuries: A Reply to Sumit Guha', *Social History of Medicine*, **7**, 269–82.

TAYLOR, I. C. (1974), 'The Insanitary Housing Question and Tenement Dwellings in Nineteenth-Century Liverpool', in A. Sutcliffe (ed.), *Multi-Storey Living. The British Working-Class Experience*, London, 41–87.

TAYLOR, I. C. (1976), ' "Black Spot on the Mersey". A Study of Environment and Society in Eighteenth and Nineteenth Century Liverpool', unpublished PhD thesis, Liverpool.

TELEKY, L. (1914), *Vorlesungen über Soziale Medizin*, Jena.

TELEKY, L. (1950), *Die Entwicklung der Gesundheitsfürsorge, Deutschland, England, USA*, Berlin.

TENNSTEDT, F. (1976), 'Sozialgeschichte der Krankenversicherung', in M. Blohmke et al. (eds), *Sozialmedizin in der Praxis*, Vol. 3, Stuttgart, 385–492.

TENNSTEDT, F. (1981), *Sozialgeschichte der Sozialpolitik in Deutschland. Vom 18. Jahrhundert bis zum Ersten Weltkrieg*, Göttingen.

TENNSTEDT, F. (1983), *Vom Proleten zum Industriearbeiter. Arbeiterbewegung und Sozialpolitik in Deutschland 1800 bis 1914*, Cologne.

TEUTEBERG, H. J. (1972), 'Studien zur Volksernährung unter sozial- und wirtschaftsgeschichtlichen Aspekten', in H. J. Teuteberg and G. Wiegelmann (eds), *Der Wandel der Nahrungsgewohnheiten unter dem Einfluß der Industrialisierung*, Göttingen, 21–221.

TEUTEBERG, H. J. (1979), 'Der Verzehr von Nahrungsmitteln in Deutschland pro Kopf und Jahr seit Beginn der Industrialisierung (1850–1975). Versuch einer quantitativen Langzeitanalyse', *Archiv für Sozialgeschichte*, **19**, 331–88.

TEUTEBERG, H. J. (ed.) (1985), *Homo Habitans. Zur Sozialgeschichte des ländlichen und städtischen Wohnens in der Neuzeit*, Münster.

TEUTEBERG, H. J. (ed.) (1992), *European Food History. A Research Review*, Leicester.

TEUTEBERG, H. J. and G. WIEGELMANN (1986), *Unsere tägliche Kost. Geschichte und regionale Prägung*, Münster.

TEUTEBERG, H. J. and G. WIEGELMANN (1992), 'Germany', in C. G. Pooley (ed.), *Housing Strategies in Europe, 1880–1930*, Leicester, 240–67.

THOMPSON, B. (1984), 'Infant Mortality in Nineteenth-Century Bradford', in R. Woods and J. Woodward (eds), *Urban Disease and Mortality in Nineteenth-Century England*, London, 120–47.

TILLY, L. A. and J. W. SCOTT (1978), *Women, Work, and Family*, New York.

TILLY, R. and T. WELLENREUTHER (1985), 'Bevölkerungswanderung und Wohnungsbauzyklen in deutschen Großstädten im 19. Jahrhundert', in H. J. Teuteberg (ed.) *Homo Habitans. Zur Sozialgeschichte des ländlichen und städtischen Wohnens in der Neuzeit*, Münster, 273–300.

TITMUSS, R. (1943), *Birth, Poverty and Wealth*, London.

TREBLE, J. H. (1979), *Urban Poverty in Britain 1830–1914*, London.

TREUE, W. (1969), 'Haus und Wohnung im 19. Jahrhundert', in W. Artelt et al. (eds), *Städte-, Wohnungs- und Kleiderhygiene des 19. Jahrhunderts in Deutschland*, Stuttgart, 34–51.

TRUMPP, J. (1908), 'Die Milchküchen und Beratungsstellen im Dienste der Säuglingsfürsorge', *Zeitschrift für Säuglingsfürsorge*, **2**, 119–37.

TUGENDREICH, G. (1908), 'Bericht über die Säuglingsfürsorgestellen der Schmidt-Gallischstiftung in Berlin', *Zeitschrift für Säuglingsfürsorge*, **2**, 62–86.

TUTZKE, D. (1969), 'Die Entwicklung der Geburts- und Sterbestatistik einschließlich der Todesursachenstatistik', *NTM—Schriftenreihe für Geschichte der Naturwissenschaften, Technik und Medizin*, **6**, 33–110.

TYSZKA, C. von (1914), 'Löhne und Lebenskosten in Großbritannien im 19. Jahrhundert', *Schriften des Vereins für Sozialpolitik*, **145**, Part 3: Löhne und Lebenskosten in Westeuropa im 19. Jahrhundert (Frankreich, England, Spanien, Belgien), 69–224.

UFFELMANN, J. (1874), *Darstellung des auf dem Gebiete der öffentlichen Gesundheitspflege in ausserdeutschen Ländern bis jetzt Geleisteten*, Berlin.

VARRENTRAPP, G. (1868), *Über Entwässerung der Städte, über Werth oder Unwerth der Wasserclosette, über deren angebliche Folgen: Verlust werthvollen Düngers, Verunreinigung der Flüsse, Benachteiligung der Gesundheit, mit besonderer Rücksicht auf Frankfurt am Main*, Berlin.

VARRENTRAPP, G. (1880), 'Offener Brief an Herrn Dr. Erhardt, ersten rechtskundigen Bürgermeister von München', *Deutsche Vierteljahrsschrift für öffentliche Gesundheitspflege*, **12**, 545–66.

Veröffentlichungen des Kaiserlichen Gesundheitsamtes (Beilagen), **2** (1878) onwards.

Verwaltungsbericht des Rathes der Stadt Leipzig für das Jahr 1886 (1888), Leipzig.

VÖGELE, J. (1989), *Getreidemärkte am Bodensee im 19. Jahrhundert. Strukturen und Entwicklungen*, St Katharinen.

VÖGELE, J. (1991), 'Die Entwicklung der (groß)städtischen Gesundheitsverhältnisse in der Epoche des Demographischen und Epidemiologischen Übergangs', in J. Reulecke and A. Castell (eds), *Stadt und Gesundheit. Zum Wandel von 'Volksgesundheit' und kommunaler Gesundheitspolitik im 19. und frühen 20. Jahrhundert*, Stuttgart, 21–36.

VÖGELE, J. (1992), 'Sanitäre Reformen in deutschen und englischen Städten—Ansätze eines Vergleichs', *Informationen zur modernen Stadtgeschichte*, 11–14.

VÖGELE, J. (1994), 'Urban Infant Mortality in Imperial Germany', *Social History of Medicine*, **7**, 401–25.

VÖGELE, J. (forthcoming a), 'The Urban Mortality Decline in Germany, 1870–1913: Some Preliminary Results', in G. Kearns, W. R. Lee, M. C. Nelson and J. Rogers (eds): *Improving the Public Health: Essays in Medical History*, Liverpool.

VÖGELE, J. (forthcoming b), 'Typhus und Typhusbekämpfung in historischer Perspektive', in W. R. Lee and W. Urban (eds), *Stadt und Bevölkerung bis zum Ende des 19. Jahrhunderts. Pommern im Vergleich*, Stralsund.

von VOIT, C. (1902), *Max von Pettenkofer zum Gedächtniss*, Munich.

VONDE, D. (1989), *Revier der großen Dörfer. Industrialisierung und Stadtentwicklung im Ruhrgebiet*, Essen.

WALLICHS (1891), 'Eine Typhusepidemie in Altona, Anfang des Jahres 1891', *Deutsche medicinische Wochenschrift*, **17**, 811–13.

WARD, W. P. (1993), *Birth Weight and Economic Growth: Women's Living Standards in the Industrializing West*, Chicago.

WARDLE, T. (1893), *Sewage Treatment and Disposal*, London.

WATTERSON, P. A. (1988), 'Infant Mortality by Father's Occupation from the 1911 Census of England and Wales', *Demography*, **25**, 289–306.

WEBER, A. (1912), 'Das Berufsschicksal der Industriearbeiter', *Archiv für Sozialwissenschaft und Sozialpolitik*, **34**, 377–405.

WEBER, A. F. (1899), *The Growth of the Cities in the Nineteenth Century. A Study in Statistics*, New York.

WEHLER, H.-U. (1987), *Deutsche Gesellschaftsgeschichte*, Vol. 2, Munich.

WEIGEL, P. (1909), 'Die Gemeindebetriebe der Stadt Leipzig', *Schriften des Vereins für Socialpolitik*, **129**, Part 7, Vol. 2, Leipzig.

WEINDLING, P. (1989), *Health, Race and German Politics between National Unification and Nazism, 1870–1945*, Cambridge.

WEINDLING, P. (1992a), 'From Isolation to Therapy. Children's Hospitals and Diphtheria in fin de siècle Paris, London and Berlin', in R. Cooter (ed.), *In the Name of the Child. Health and Welfare, 1880–1940*, London and New York, 124–45.

WEINDLING, P. (1992b), 'From Medical Research to Clinical Practice: Serum Therapy for Diphtheria in the 1890s', in J. Pickstone (ed.), *Medical Innovations in Historical Perspective*, Basingstoke, 72–83.

WEISSENFELD, J. (1900), 'Die Veränderungen der Sterblichkeit an Diphtherie und Scharlach', *Centralblatt für allgemeine Gesundheitspflege*, **19**, 319–34.

WELTON, T. A. (1911), *England's Recent Progress. An Investigation of the Statistics of Migrations, Mortality, &c. in the Twenty Years from 1881 to 1901 as Indicating Tendencies Towards the Growth or Decay of Particular Communities*, London.

WEYER, M. (1989), 'Die Gelsenkirchener Typhusepidemie von 1901 und ihr gerichtliches Nachspiel', unpublished dissertation, Essen.

WEYL, T. (1904), 'Assanierung', in T. Weyl (ed.), *Soziale Hygiene. Handbuch der Hygiene. 4. Supplement-Band*, Jena, 1–27.

WILBERT, P. (1891), *Ueber den Einfluss der Ernährungsweise auf die Kindersterblichkeit*, Bonn.

WILCKENS, M. (1898), 'Eine durch Milchinfection hervorgerufene Typhus-Epidemie, beobachtet zu Hamburg im August-September 1897', *Zeitschrift für Hygiene und Infectionskrankheiten*, **27**, 244–71.

WILLIAMS, N. (1989), 'Infant and Child Mortality in Urban Areas of Nineteenth-century England and Wales. A Record-linkage-study', unpublished PhD thesis, Liverpool.

WILLIAMS, N. (1992), 'Death in its Season: Class, Environment and the Mortality of Infants in Nineteenth-Century Sheffield', *Social History of Medicine*, **5**, 71–95.

WILLIAMS, N. and G. MOONEY (1994), 'Infant Mortality in an "Age of Great Cities": London and the English Provincial Cities Compared, c. 1840–1910', *Continuity and Change*, **9**, 185–212.

WILLIAMSON, J. G. (1987), *Underinvestment in Britain's Cities during the Industrial Revolution*, Harvard Institute for Economic Research, Discussion Paper No. 1344, Cambridge, Massachusetts.

WILLIAMSON, J. G. (1990), *Coping with City Growth During the British Industrial Revolution*, Cambridge, Massachusetts

WILSON, A. (1990), 'Technology and Municipal Decision Making. Sanitary Systems in Manchester 1868–1900', unpublished PhD thesis, Manchester.

WINSLOW, C.-E. A. (1943), *The Conquest of Epidemic Disease. A Chapter in the History of Ideas*, Princeton (reprint Wisconsin 1980).

WINTER, J. M. (1982), 'The Decline of Mortality in Britain 1870–1950', in T. Barker and M. Drake (eds), *Population and Society in Britain, 1850–1980*, London, 100–20.

WISCHERMANN, C. (1983), *Wohnen in Hamburg vor dem Ersten Weltkrieg*, Münster.

WOHL, A. S. (1971), 'The Housing of the Working Classes in London, 1815–1914', in S.D. Chapmann, *The History of Working-Class Housing. A Symposium*, Totowa, 13–54.

WOHL, A. S. (1977), *The Eternal Slum. Housing and Social Policy in Victorian London*, London.

WOHL, A. S. (1983), *Endangered Lives. Public Health in Victorian Britain*, London.

WOODS, R. (1984a), 'Mortality and Sanitary Conditions in Late Nineteenth-Century Birmingham', in R. Woods and J. Woodward (eds), *Urban Disease and Mortality in Nineteenth-Century England*, London, 176–202.

WOODS, R. (1984b) 'Mortality Patterns in the Nineteenth Century', in R. Woods and J. Woodward (eds), *Urban Disease and Mortality in Nineteenth-Century England*, London, 37–64.

WOODS, R. (1985), 'The Effect of Population Redistribution on the Level of Mortality in Nineteenth Century England and Wales', *Journal of Economic History*, **45**, 645–51.

WOODS, R. and P. R. A. HINDE (1987), 'Mortality in Victorian England: Models and Patterns', *Journal of Interdisciplinary History*, **18**, 27–54.

WOODS, R., P. A. WATTERSON and J. H. WOODWARD (1988/89), 'The Causes of Rapid Infant Mortality Decline in England and Wales', *Population Studies*, **42**, 343–66; **43**, 113–32.

WOODS, R., N. WILLIAMS and C. GALLEY (1993), 'Infant Mortality in England, 1550–1950. Problems in the Identification of Long-Term Trends and Geographical and Social Variations', in C. A. Corsini and P. P. Viazzo (eds), *The Decline of Infant Mortality in Europe, 1800–1950. Four National Case Studies*, Florence, 35–50.

WOODS, R. and J. WOODWARD (eds) (1984), *Urban Disease and Mortality in Nineteenth-Century England*, London.

WOODWARD, J. (1984), 'Medicine and the City: the Nineteenth Century Experience', in R. Woods and J. Woodward (eds), *Urban Disease and Mortality in Nineteenth-Century England*, London, 65–78.

WRAY, J. D. (1978), 'Maternal Nutrition, Breast-feeding and Infant Survival', in W. H. Mosley (ed.), *Human Nutrition and Reproduction*, New York, 197–230.

WRIGHT, L. (1963), *Clean and Decent. The Fascinating History of the Bathroom and the Water Closet*, 4th edn, London.

WRIGLEY, E. A. and R. S. SCHOFIELD (1981), *The Population History of England 1541–1871. A Reconstruction*, London.

WÜRZBURG, A. (1887/88), 'Die Säuglingssterblichkeit im Deutschen Reiche während der Jahre 1875 bis 1877', *Arbeiten aus dem Kaiserlichen Gesundheitsamte*, **2**, 208–22, 343–446; **4**, 28–108.

WÜRZBURGER, E. (1909–1914), *Die Bearbeitung der Statistik der Bevölkerungsbewegung durch die*

Statistischen Ämter im Deutschen Reiche (Allgemeines statistisches Archiv, Bd. 7, Ergänzungsheft), Göttingen.

WÜRZBURGER, E. (1930), 'Die Häufigkeit der ärztlichen Beglaubigung von Todesursachen in Sachsen', *Bulletin de l'Institut International de Statistique*, **24**, 189–203.

ZADEK, I. (1909), *Hygiene der Städte, I: Die Trinkwasser-Versorgung*, Berlin.

ZAMAGNI, V. (1989), 'An International Comparison of Real Industrial Wages, 1890–1913: Methodological Issues and Results', in P. Scholliers (ed.), *Real Wages in 19th and 20th Century Europe. Historical and Comparative Perspectives*, New York, 107–244.

ZAPF, W. (1983), 'Die Wohlfahrtsentwicklung in Deutschland seit der Mitte des 19. Jahrhunderts', in W. Conze and M. R. Lepsius (eds), *Sozialgeschichte der Bundesrepublik Deutschland. Beiträge zum Kontinuitätsproblem*, Stuttgart, 47–65.

ZIMMERMANN, C. (1991), *Von der Wohnungsfrage zur Wohnungspolitik. Die Reformbewegung in Deutschland 1845–1914*, Göttingen.

INDEX